Treatment of Elbow Lesions

New Aspects in Diagnosis and Surgical Techniques

Andrea Celli
Luigi Celli
Bernard F. Morrey

ANDREA CELLI • LUIGI CELLI • BERNARD F. MORREY

Treatment of Elbow Lesions

New Aspects in Diagnosis and Surgical Techniques

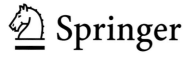 Springer

ANDREA CELLI
Department of Orthopaedic and
Traumatology Surgery
University of Modena
Modena, Italy

LUIGI CELLI
Department of Orthopaedic and
Traumatology Surgery
University of Modena
Modena, Italy

BERNARD F. MORREY
Department of Orthopedics
Mayo Medical School
Rochester, MN, USA

Cover illustration: Leonardo da Vinci, Codice Windsor Vol. A foglio 2 verso (detail).
The Royal Collection © 2007 Her Majesty Queen Elizabeth II

Library of Congress Control Number: 2007929133

ISBN 978-88-470-0317-0 Springer Milan Berlin Heidelberg New York
e-ISBN 978-88-470-0591-4

Springer is a part of Springer Science+Business Media
springer.com
© Springer-Verlag Italia 2008

Cover design: Simona Colombo, Milan, Italy
Typesetting: C & G di Cerri e Galassi, Cremona, Italy
Printer: Printer Trento Srl, Trento, Italy
Printed in Italy

Springer-Verlag Italia S.r.l.,Via Decembrio 28, I-20137 Milan, Italy

PREFACE

Because of the relatively low incidence of involvement efforts to enhance the diagnosis and management of elbow pathology are not common. Nonetheless, because of a rapidly expanding knowledge base, both with regard to a more refined understanding of elbow pathology, coupled with exciting and emerging approaches and options for management, it is appropriate and timely to address this deficiency in the orthopedic literature. This volume, therefore, was produced in order to provide current and relevant information with content that is drawn from a very well received symposium of the same name as this book and convened in Modena, Italy recently. As with the symposium, the specific goals of this text are to provide the most updated concepts in the management of a full spectrum of elbow pathology. The content, therefore, is comprehensive in nature, but with a focus on emerging options in the management of traumatic conditions as well as reconstructive options for the sequelae of trauma. These topics are covered in detail in the 31 chapters which comprise this text. The focus of each chapter was specifically designed to address the topic in the most timely fashion and with less of an emphasis on the historical context and more focus on current thinking. The references documenting content are intended to be efficient and focused. In addition, the popular and appropriate expectation of the orthopedic community of enhanced explanation of technique are featured in the appropriate chapters. Probably the most important aspect of the text to allow the attainment of this goal is the involvement of surgeons from the Mayo Clinic as well as the participation of world renowned international surgeons. This group was assembled to serve both as a faculty for the symposium and also to document their experience as contributors to this text.

The organization of this volume is designed to be logical and user friendly. The early chapters include basic information on an array of diagnostic topics and techniques. In this context a very important, but basic, discussion of surgical exposures is provided. A full 8 chapters deal with traumatic conditions of the elbow and 7 assess the rapidly emerging field of radial head deficiency and its management with fixation or prosthetic replacement. The consequences of elbow trauma are addressed in detail with an emphasis on the open and arthroscopic management of the stiff elbow.

Current concepts in elbow joint replacement are discussed with a focus on several design concepts as well as outcomes based on presenting diagnosis. Finally, the postoperative management including the use of continuous motion machine, braces and examination under anesthesia is discussed. Overall, therefore, the editors feel as though the goals of the symposium and the documentation of the proceedings have been well realized with the publication of this volume. It is our expectation that this textbook will provide a useful tool to the busy orthopedic surgeon to enhance the diagnosis and effective management for this difficult spectrum of elbow pathology.

In closing, it should be noted that this documentation of our current thinking on these topics has become a reality due to the drive and vision of Professor Luigi Celli and the organizational skills of his son, Andrea Celli, of the University of Modena, Italy. Their vision and leadership, coupled with the international contributions and a spectrum of thought processes, provides a useful and unique perspective to this joint that has heretofore deserved the dubious reputation for the challenges it poses to the orthopedic community. Hopefully, this text will, therefore, in some measure, provide insight and a successful management for this "problem joint".

September 2007   *B.F. Morrey, M.D.*

TABLE OF CONTENTS

LIST OF CONTRIBUTORS

JULIE E. ADAMS
Department of Orthopedic Surgery
Mayo Clinic
Rochester, MN, USA

ROBERTO ADANI
Department of Orthopaedic Surgery
University of Modena and Reggio Emilia
Modena, Italy

YVES ALLIEU
Hand Institute
Clémentville Clinic
Montpellier, France

LUCA BALDINI
Department of Diagnostic Imaging
AUSL Modena
NOCSE Nuovo Ospedale Civile
S. Agostino and Estense
Baggiovara (MO), Italy

ELISABETTA BERTELLINI
Anesthesia Unit Chief
Department of Critical Care
AUSL Modena
Carpi Hospital
Carpi (MO), Italy

GIANLUCA BONANNO
Department of Orthopaedic and
Traumatology Surgery
University of Modena
Modena, Italy

ANDREA CELLI
Department of Orthopaedic and
Traumatology Surgery
University of Modena
Modena, Italy

LUIGI CELLI
Department of Orthopaedic and
Traumatology Surgery
University of Modena
Modena, Italy

MAURIZIO FONTANA
Orthopaedic and Traumatology Unit
Faenza Hospital
AUSL Ravenna, Italy

FABIO GAZZOTTI
Anesthesia Unit
Department of Surgery
University Hospital Policlinico di Modena
Modena, Italy

MATTHIAS HANSEN
Klinik für Unfallchirurgie
Klinikum Worms
Worms, Germany

MICHAEL W. HARTMAN
Department of Orthopedic surgery
Mayo Clinic
Rochester, MN, USA

ANDREAS HINSCHE
Queen Elizabeth Hospital
Gateshead, United Kingdom

LUCIO V. INDRIZZI
Anesthesia Unit
Department of Surgery
University Hospital Policlinico di Modena
Modena, Italy

STEEN L. JENSEN
Shoulder and Elbow Clinic
Aalborg University Hospital
Aalborg, Denmark

GRAHAM J.W. KING
Hand and Upper Limb Centre
Division of Orthopaedic Surgery
University of Western Ontario
London, Ontario, Canada

GIOVANNI LEO
Department of Orthopaedic and
Traumatology Surgery
University of Modena
Modena, Italy

GIUSEPPE MAGNI
Anesthesia Unit
Department of Surgery
University Hospital Policlinico di Modena
Modena, Italy

ALESSANDRO MARINELLI
Rizzoli Orthopaedic Institute
Bologna, Italy

MARIA C. MARONGIU
Department of Orthopaedic and
Traumatology Surgery
University of Modena
Modena, Italy

BRUNO MARTINELLI
Department of Orthopaedic Surgery
University of Trieste
Hospital of Cattinara
Trieste, Italy

CLAUDIO MINERVINI
Department of Orthopaedic and
Traumatology Surgery
University of Modena
Modena, Italy

BERNARD F. MORREY
Department of Orthopedics
Mayo Medical School
Rochester, MN, USA

LARS P. MÜLLER
Johannes Gutenberg Universität Mainz
Klinik für Unfall - Wiederherstellungs -
und Handchirurgie
Mainz, Germany

PHILIPPE DE MOURGUES
Department of Orthopedics
St. Joseph Clinic
Chambéry, France

SHAWN W. O'DRISCOLL
Department of Orthopedics
Mayo Clinic
Rochester, MN, USA

JEAN-PIERRE PEQUIGNOT
Nice, France

KARL J. PROMMERSBERGER
Orthopädische Klinik Markgröningen
Stuttgart, Germany

POL M. ROMMENS
Orthopädische Klinik Markgröningen
Stuttgart, Germany

ROBERTO ROTINI
Rizzoli Orthopaedic Institute
Bologna, Italy

CLAUDIO ROVESTA
Department of Orthopaedic and
Traumatology Surgery
University of Modena
Modena, Italy

ALBERTO G. SCHNEEBERGER
Shoulder & Elbow Surgery
University of Zurich
Zurich, Switzerland

VINCENZO SPINA
Department of Diagnostic Imaging
AUSL MO
Civil Hospital B. Ramazzini
Carpi (MO), Italy

DAVID STANLEY
Shoulder and Elbow Unit
Northern General Hospital
Sheffield, United Kingdom

SCOTT P. STEINMANN
Department of Orthopedic Surgery
Mayo Clinic
Rochester, MN, USA

LUIGI TARALLO
Department of Orthopaedic and
Traumatology Surgery
University of Modena
Modena, Italy

ALBERTO TASSI
Anesthesia Unit Chief
Department of Surgery
University Hospital Policlinico di Modena
Modena, Italy

MATTHIAS WINTER
Department of Orthopedics
and Traumatology
St. Roch Hospital
Nice, France

KEN YAMAGUCHI
Shoulder and Elbow Service
Washington University Orthopedics
Barnes-Jewish Hospital
Saint Louis, MO, USA

CHAPTER 1

Anatomy and Biomechanics of the Elbow

A. Celli

Introduction

The elbow is a complex structure that provides an important function as the mechanical link in the upper extremity between the hand, the wrist, and the shoulder. Its primary functions are to position the hand in the space; loss of this ability can cause significant disability for the activities of daily living. The elbow and the wrist joints associated with the ulna and radius bones linked with the interosseous membrane constitute the anatomical and functional unit of the forearm. This unit provides the rotational movements of the forearm and allows the forces transmission from the hand to the elbow when the elbow joint is the stable fulcrum needed for powerful grasping and fine motions. The elbow joint consists of three separate articulations: the ulnohumeral, radio-capitellar, and proximal radio-ulnar joints, together inside a small capsule with a volume of 15-20 cc. The soft tissue are divided into passive stabilizers (the lateral collateral ligament, the medial collateral ligament, and the capsula) and into active stabilizers as the muscle that provides joint compressive forces and functions. This chapter begins with an overview of the anatomical features, including some anatomical tables of the nonarticular structures, and examines the passive structures of the elbow that are related to joint function and motion. The second section discusses the elbow biomechanics including kinematics, and force transmission through the elbow.

Anatomy of the Elbow

Bone Anatomy

The distal humerus comprises two condyles that form the articular surface of the capitellum laterally and the trochlea medially (Fig. 1). The more prominent medial epicondyle is the region (Fig. 2) where the ulnar collateral ligament and the flexor-pronator muscles are attached. The less prominent lateral epicondyle (Fig. 3) is the attached point for the lateral collateral ligament and the extensor supinator muscles. The articular surface is angled approximately 30° anterior to the axis of the humerus shaft. The medial ridge of the trochlea is larger than the lateral ridge; this gives to the articular surface a slight valgus position, approximately 6° from the epicondylar axis (Figs. 4, 5). During the flexion extension the olecranon moves on the articular surface of the trochlea like a screw tapping on it and it allows the normal valgus angle in extension and the varus in flexion (carrying angle) [1-7]. The coronoid fossa and the olecranon fossa proximally to the articular surface accommodates the olecranon process during the extension and the coronoid tip during the flexion movements, increasing the osseous stability of the joint in these positions [1, 4, 8]. Laterally a small radial fossa accepts the contour of the radial head with the elbow in full flexion.

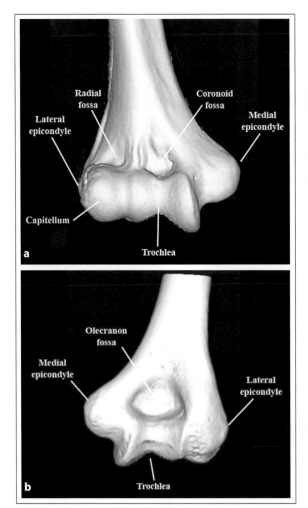

Fig. 1 a, b. The anterior and posterior aspects of the distal humerus with the bone landmarks (TC 3D reconstruction)

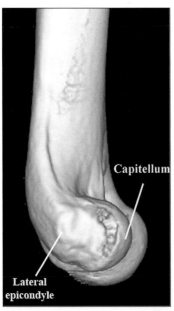

Fig. 3. The lateral aspect of the distal humerus (TC 3D reconstruction)

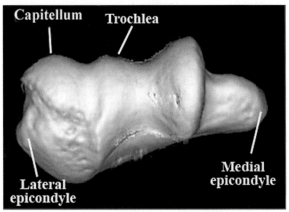

Fig. 4. The distal humerus articular surface: TC 3D reconstruction with bone landmarks

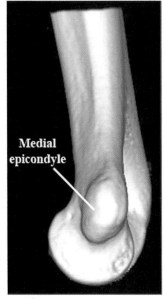

Fig. 2. The medial aspect of the distal humerus (TC 3D reconstruction)

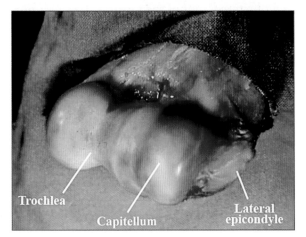

Fig. 5. The distal humerus articular surface anatomical picture with bone landmarks

The proximal ulna provides the elbow articulation; it is divided into the greater sigmoid notch from the coronoid process anteriorly to the tip of the olecranon posteriorly. The contour of the articular surface is not a semicircle but rather is ellipsoid, the articular cartilage is usually discontinuous centrally (nonarticular portion); the forces are distributed on to the articulation into the two functional facets anteriorly and posteriorly [3, 9] (Fig. 6). The greater sigmoid notch is oriented approximately 30° of posterior angulation to match with the anterior angulation of distal humerus. On the frontal plane the shaft is angulated 1°-6° laterally and this contributes in part to the formation of the carrying angle [10]. The coronoid process is constituted laterally by the lesser sigmoid notch, a depression with an arc of 70° that allows the articulation with the radial head [3]. Distally to the lesser sigmoid notch there is an anatomical point called crista supinatoris; it is the insertion of the lateral ulnar collateral ligament (Fig. 7). The medial side of the coronoid provides the insertion of the anterior band of the medial collateral ligament.

The proximal radius includes the cylindrical shape of the radial head with concave disc which articulates with the capitellum and with the lesser sigmoid notch (Fig. 8). The radial margin, which articulates with the ulna, is approximately 240°, the antero-lateral third (120°) of the radial head is void of cartilage. The transverse cross section of

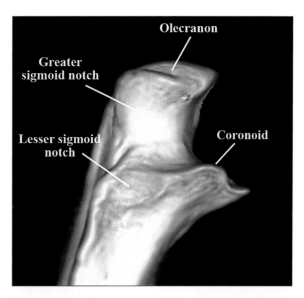

Fig. 7. The olecranon aspect with the bone landmarks (TC 3D reconstruction)

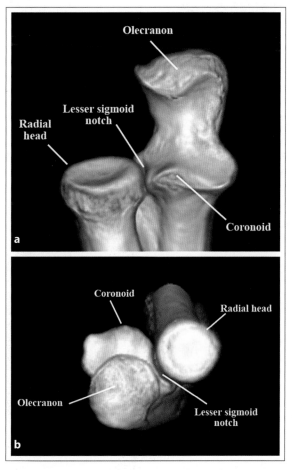

Fig. 8 a, b. The proximal ulna and radius aspects with the bone landmarks (TC 3D reconstruction)

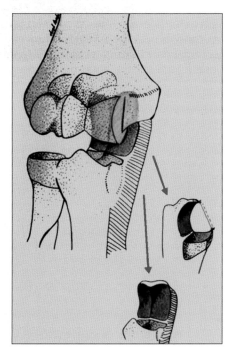

Fig. 6. The articular surface of the olecranon is usually discontinuous centrally (nonarticular portion)

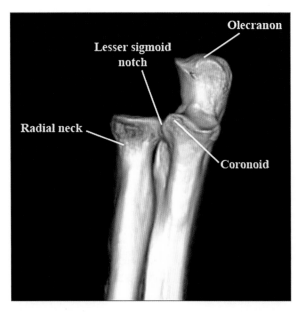

Fig. 9. The proximal radius forms an angle of approximately 15° from the neck and the head

the radial head is not circular but elliptical in shape; the head and the neck form an angle of approximately 15° with the long axis of the proximal radius opposite to the radial tuberosity [3] (Fig. 9). Distal to the neck is the radial bicipital tuberosity which is extra-articular.

Soft Tissue Anatomy

The stability of the elbow is the result of the combination of articulate congruence of the ulno-humer- al and radio-capitellum joints and its capsulo-liga- mentous structures [11].

The medial collateral complex originates from the distal portion of the medial epicondyle and in particular from the anteroinferior surface of the epicondyle and not from the condilar part of the trochlea [8, 12-16]. The ligament structure consists of three parts; anterior bundle, posterior bundle, and transverse segment [8, 12, 15, 17] (Fig. 10). The anterior bundle is more prominent than the poste- rior bundle and it is subdivided into anterior, cen- tral, and posterior bands [3]. The posterior bundle is thin and inserted into the postero-medial margin of the greater sigmoid notch [8, 12, 15]. The trans- verse ligament is variable in its definition and ap- pears to have no significant role in stabilizing the elbow. The anterior bundle is stronger than the posterior part and its insertion is in the anterome- dial margin of the coronoid, its fibers are sequen- tially tightened moving the elbow from 20° of ex- tension to 120° of flexion [15, 16, 18]. Morrey and An valuated an average increase of 18% in length of the anterior bundle from full extension to 120° of flex- ion [9, 17]. The posterior bundle is more posterior to the rotation axis; the change in length was greater than the anterior bundle, with an average of 39% of the resting length [19]. The posterior bundle provides also a minimal stability to valgus stress and provides constraint to hyperflexion.

The lateral collateral complex consists of three parts: the annular ligament, the radial collateral, and the ulnar collateral ligaments [8, 18, 20-22] (Fig. 11). The origin of the lateral collateral complex is on the lateral epicondyle near the axis of rotation of the el- bow. The radial part terminates along the course of the annular ligaments; the ulnar part is inserted on

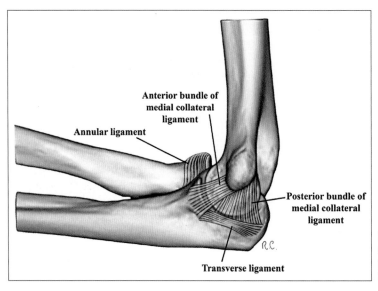

Fig. 10. The medial collateral ligament complex. The ligament consists of three parts: anterior and posterior bundles and transverse segment

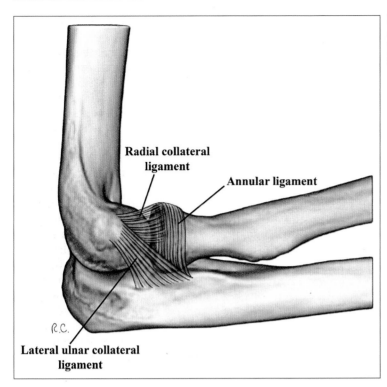

Fig. 11. The lateral collateral ligament complex. The ligament consists of three parts: the annular ligament and the ulnar and radial collateral ligaments

the crista supinatoris of the ulna and has been considered to be an important stabilizer of the elbow. The lateral collateral ligament is almost uniformly taut during the flexion-extension range of motion with little change in distance between the origin and the insertion during the motion (isometric position) [23]. The annular ligament is inserted on the anterior and posterior margins of the less sigmoid notch and it maintains the radial head in contact with the ulna [15] (Fig. 12). The anterior insertion becomes taut during the supination and the posterior insertion during the pronation [16, 22]; this is because the radial head is not a pure circular dish. The annular ligament with the radial part of the lateral collateral ligament are important stabilizers of the radial head avoiding the postero-lateral subluxation. The capsule of the elbow is attached to the articular margins of the joint and its fibers are connected to the annular ligament [24]. Anteriorly it includes the coronoid and the radial fossa, posteriorly the olecranon fossa. Its maximum distension is with the elbow at 70°-80° of flexion. The contribution of the capsule as a passive stabilizer is a controversial point; some studies have suggested no change in the joint laxity after complete capsulotomy and on the other side Morrey reported that this structure has an important function as stabilizer to varus-valgus and distraction loading in extension but not in flexion [17]. The anterior capsule has a transverse and oblique bands that seem to provide

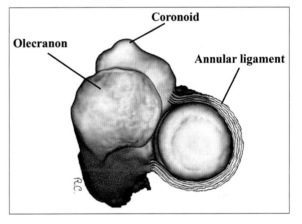

Fig. 12. The annular ligament, which is inserted on the anterior and posterior margin of the less sigmoid notch and it maintains the radial head in contact with the ulna

a significant stability in extension [19]; on the other side the posterior capsule becomes taut in flexion and may have a role as a static stabilizer.

The Muscles and Neuro-Vascular Structures

The muscle and the neuro-vascular structures across the elbow can be divided into four main groups. Posteriorly, the triceps tendon crosses the elbow joint with the ulnar nerve; laterally, the extensor and supinator muscles (brachio-radialis, extensor carpi radialis longus, extensor radialis brevis, the finger extensors, the extensor carpi ulnaris, and the anconeus) with the radial nerve; anteriorly, the elbow flexors cross the joint with the median nerve; and medially, the flexor-pronator group (pronator teres, flexor carpi radialis, palmaris longus, flexor carpi ulnaris, and the flexor digitorum). The majority of the muscles crossing the elbow work to rotate the forearm and flex and extend the wrist and the fingers. Only a few muscles have an action on moving the elbow joint. The primary elbow flexors are the brachialis, biceps brachii, and brachio-radialis; secondary elbow flexors include the pronator teres, extensor carpi radialis longus, and the flexor carpi radialis. The triceps and the anconeus are the mean extensor muscles of the elbow. Pronation is provided by the pronator teres and pronator quadratus. Supination is performed mainly by the biceps, with assistance from the supinator muscle. Muscle loading results in a compressive force generated across the articulation of the elbow; muscle activities may also produce a dynamic stabilization (compressing the articular surfaces together) and protect the static ligaments constraints [1, 2, 23, 25, 26].

The ulnar nerve derives from the medial cord of the brachial plexus and it descends in the arm posterior to the pectoralis major muscle and medially to the brachial artery. At the inferior border of the pectoralis major the nerve moves medially from the brachial artery and pierces the medial intermuscular septum about 8 cm above the medial epicondyle. A thick fascial band, the arcade of Struthers, is present in 20%-70% of the upper limbs and extends from the medial head of the triceps to the intermuscular septum and it can be a potential point of compression. The ulnar nerve along with the ulnar artery, a branch of the brachial artery, descend distally and medially on the anterior surface of the medial head of the triceps muscle. The artery runs with the nerve as it enters the interval between the medial epicondyle of the humerus and the olecranon. The nerve passes into the ulnar groove on the dorsal aspect of the medial epicondyle, then it passes into a fibrosus arcade (Osborne's arcade), which attaches to the medial epicondyle and the olecranon and connects the ulnar and humeral heads of origin of the flexor carpi ulnaris muscle (Fig. 13). In the first part of the cubital tunnel the nerve provides a small articula branch. In the second portion of the tunnel, it supplies two branches to the flexor carpi ulnaris muscle; the main branch leaves the main trunk horizontally and supplies the humeral head of the flexor carpi ulnaris. The second branch courses distally for several centimeters before entering in the muscle (Figs. 13, 14). As the nerve leaves the cubital tunnel it

runs between the flexor carpi ulnaris and the flexor digitorum profundus muscles. The nerve maintains this relationship through the proximal and medial forearm and then it end with sensitive and motor terminal branches in the hand. While the ulnar nerve does not innervate any muscle in the arm, distally at the elbow it supplies the flexor carpi ulnaris (above 0.5-1 cm the medial epicondyle) and the ulnar half of the flexor digitorum profundus muscles.

The radial nerve derives from the posterior cord of the brachial plexus behind the third portion of the axillary artery. In the proximal third of the arm, the nerve descends behind the brachial artery, anterior to the subscapularis muscle, the teres major and the latissimus dorsi tendons, and the long head of the triceps. The nerve crosses the posterior aspect of the humerus next to the bone without interposition of muscle fibers and it sends branches only to the lateral triceps head, and no branch is sent to the medial head. At the humerus lateral aspect the nerve branches off the common branch of the medial head and anconeus and the lower lateral brachial cutaneous nerve while the radial nerve pierces the inter-

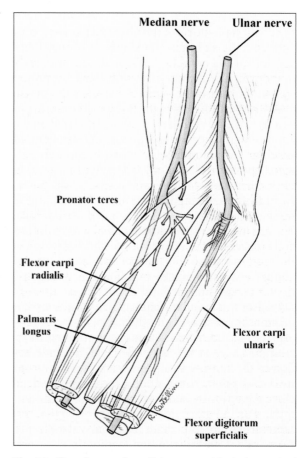

Fig. 13. The ulnar and medial nerves with their terminal branches on the medial side of the elbow

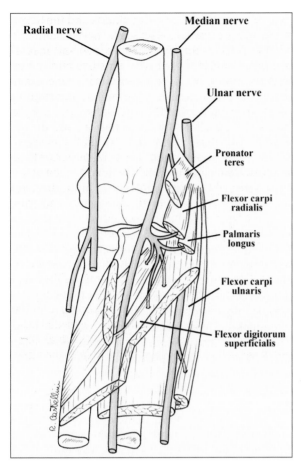

Fig. 14. The ulnar, radial, and medial nerves and their terminal branches on the anterior side of the elbow

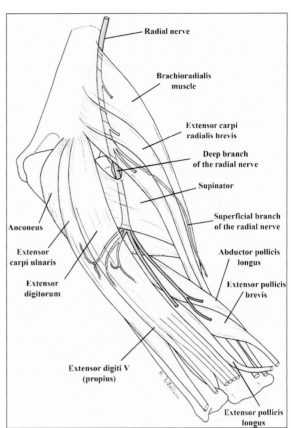

Fig. 15. The radial nerve and its terminal branches at the elbow

muscular septum (at 10-12 cm on average from the lateral epicondyle) (Fig. 15). At the lateral border of the medial head of the triceps muscle, the nerve leaves the extensor compartment and enters in the flexor compartment of the arm, and it runs distally between the brachialis and the brachioradialis muscles. Proximal to the elbow, the radial nerve supplies the brachioradialis and the extensor carpi radialis longus and occasionally medially the brachialis. Then it divides into terminal branches, one superficial sensory and the other deep motor. Those terminal branches passes 1 cm distally to the biceps tendon (Fig. 16). The superficial radial nerve (superficial to the supinator muscle) continues distally on the deep surface of the brachio-radialis muscle and pierces the fascia on the ulnar side of this tendon, about 7 cm above the wrist. Descending in the dorsoradial side of the wrist, it terminates at the hand. The posterior interosseous nerve courses obliquely through the supinator muscle and crossing the proximal radius, to enter into the extensor compartment of the forearm. The motor branches to the extensor carpi radi-

alis brevis arises for the posterior interosseous nerve prior to entering the supinator. The posterior interosseous nerve is separated by the radius from the deep head of the supinator muscle (Fig. 16). As the posterior interosseous nerve exits from the supinator muscle, the variability of its branches becomes so great that only generalizations can be made. The proximal branch heading and supply the extensor carpi ulnaris by one or more little branches. The distal division of the posterior interosseus nerve consists of at least two branches, one to the abductor pollicis longus and sometimes to the extensor pollicis brevis. The most distally innervated muscle is usually the extensor indicis proprius. The terminal portion of the nerve passes deep to the extensor pollicis longus on the interosseous membrane to provide sensory innervation to the wrist. From a surgical point of view, it is important to remember the terminal branches in the arm. From the nerve in the arm arrises cutaneous nerves and several muscular branches and articular fibers supplying the elbow joint. The posterior cutaneous nerve is the first branch arising from the main trunk of the nerve in the axilla, the second branch arising about 7 cm be-

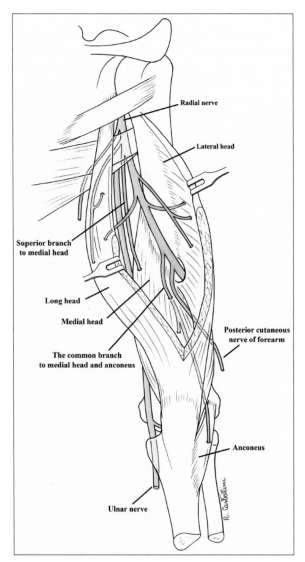

Fig. 16. The radial nerve and its terminal branches at the arm

two its major brances: the posterior interosseus nerve and the superficial sensitive radial nerve.

The median nerve originates from the medial and lateral cords of the brachial plexus then it runs with the artery. The nerve descends in the arm posteriorly to the pectoralis major muscle and laterally to the artery. It runs in the anteromedial side of the brachialis muscle and posteromedial to the biceps muscle. It crosses the medial side of the elbow, where it lies superficial to the brachialis, just deep to the bicipital aponeurosis (Figs. 13, 14). Distally it runs between the two heads of the pronator teres into the forearm between the two flexor digitorum muscles (superficial and profondus). The median nerve does not provide innervation to muscles of the arm. It innervates in the forearm; the pronator teres, flexor carpi radialis, flexor digitorum superficialis, and in most cases the flexor digitorum profondus. Distally in the end, it supplies the index and middle finger lombricalis, abductor pollicis brevis, opponens pollicis, and the flexor pollicis brevis. The anterior interosseous nerve branches supplies the flexor digitorum profundus-2, flexor pollicis longus and the pronator quadratus.

At the elbow the brachial artery enters the cubital fossa on the anterior surface of the brachialis laterally to the median nerve, then both pass under the aponeurosis. In the cubital fossa the artery divides into the radial and ulnar arteries. The radial runs medial to the biceps tendon and then distally superficial to the supinator and to the pronator teres. The ulnar artery passes deep to the head of the pronator teres and runs distally beneath the flexor carpi ulnaris and the flexor digitorum superficialis on the surface of the flexor digitorum profundus.

Kinematics of the Elbow

The elbow has been generally likened to a trochoginglymoid joint in that it has 2° of freedom: flexion-extension (0°-140°) and prono-supination (75°-85°). According to the Morrey's study, the arc of motion necessary to perform most of the activities of daily living is 30°-130° of flexion-extension and 50°-50° of prono-supination [3, 23]. The axis of rotation of the elbow passes through the capitellum in line with the bottom of the trochlea solcus. During the flexion-extension arc of motion, this axis has approximately 3°-5° of internal rotation with respect to the plane of the medial and lateral epicondyles and 4°-8° of valgus with respect to the long axis of the humerus [3, 15, 23, 27, 28]. This is possible because the center of rotation of the el-

low the tip of the acromion supplies the long head of the triceps. The branch to the medial portion of the medial head arises just distally to the branch for the long head. As the nerve passes deep to the long head it provides additional branches to this muscle. The posterior muscular branches arise from the main trunk as it lies between the lateral and medial heads near to the spiral groove of the humerus. This is the largest muscular branch of the radial nerve in the arm and it innervates the medial and lateral heads of the triceps. The nerve to the anconeus descends distally within the substance of the medial heads of the triceps muscle, giving several branches to this muscle. Above the elbow it innervates the brachio radialis and the extensor carpi radialis longus and at level of the radio-capitellum joint the radial nerve divides in

bow in flexion extension is not a fixed single point but rather moves within an area. The olecranon moves on the trochlea (as a screw) during the flexion extension and this justifies the movement of the elbow from the valgus in extension to the varus in flexion (Fig. 17). This movement produces the carry angle, defined as the angle between the long axis of the humerus and the long axis of the ulna measured in the frontal plane [10, 29] (Fig. 18). This angle is generally higher in women than in men,

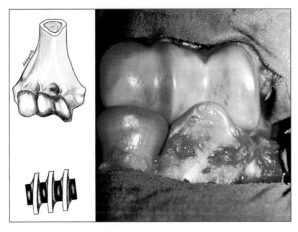

Fig. 17. The olecranon moves on the articular surface of the trochlea like a screw tapping on it

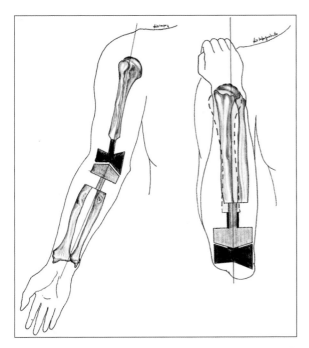

Fig. 18. During the flexion-extension movements the elbow moves from valgus to the varus, producing an angle defined as carry angle

the average has been reported to vary between 7°-12° in men and 2° or 3° greater in women [19]. During the flexion extension the primary constraints of the ulno-humeral joint are as follows: in extension, the posterior part of the olecranon impacts the olecranon fossa associated with the anterior capsula and the ligaments restrained. In flexion, the constraint is the impact of the radial head and of the coronoid process in the corresponding fossa. The forearm motion is clearly influenced by the morphology of the radial head; the axis of rotation of the forearm passes through the center of the radial head proximally and the fovea of the ulna at the base of the ulnar styloid distally [8]. During the forearm rotation, the edge of the radial head maintains contact with the lesser sigmoid notch, and the radial shaft moves away and toward the ulna, in the transverse plane.

Articular and Capsulo-Ligamentous Stabilizers

The structures that stabilize the elbow during motion can be also divided into two main groups: passive and active stabilizers, which have different actions during the range of motion of the elbow [30-35].

The radial head is a secondary stabilizer to the valgus stress. Morrey et al. have shown that selective radial head resection does not influence the valgus instability as long as the medial ulnar collateral ligament is intact [9, 36]. When the ulnar collateral ligament is released the radial head becomes the primary constraint to the valgus instability [3, 9, 36, 37]. The radial head is the main longitudinal stabilized when the interosseous membrane is injured [38]. Biomechanical tests suggest that the radial head contributes about 30% of the valgus stability in both flexion and extension [19, 23, 38]. The complete release of the ulnar collateral ligament produces an average increase of 18° of valgus laxity and this increases to 36° after radial head excision [19]. The axis loading produces a stress distribution of 40% across the ulna and 60% across the radius; the transmission across the radial head increases when the elbow is 0°-35° of flexion and it also increases when it is placed in supination [19, 23].

The role of the olecranon has been analyzed in different biomechanical studies. An et al., showed that 75%-85% of valgus stress was resisted by the proximal half of the olecranon, and 60%-67% of varus stress was resisted by the coronoid [23]. The olecranon engages the olecranon fossa of the humerus at 20°; at this point the elbow becomes more stable against varus-valgus laxity. The coronoid process plays an important role in preventing the posterior dislocation of the elbow. O'Driscoll et al. reported that when the collateral ligaments are injured and the radial head is compromised, the resection of 30% of the coronoid produces instability [39, 40]. The fracture of the coronoid, even small fragments, can decrease the stability of the elbow in particular when it is associated with ligament injuries. The coronoid is also essential to varus stability when the collateral ligaments are intact [27]. The elbow becomes more unstable as successive portions of the coronoid are damaged; the radial head resection produces an increase in instability correlated to the type of the coronoid fracture [11].

The passive soft tissue stabilizers include the medial and lateral collateral ligaments complexes [30]. Their activities during the elbow motion were analyzed by Morrey and An [9, 23]. At 90° of flexion, the anterior band of the medial collateral ligament is the primary stabilizer to the valgus stress, whereas in extension the medial collateral ligament, the anterior capsula and bony fit are equally resistant to the valgus stress. Its posterior component is more important in higher degrees of flexion. During the elbow motion the midportion and the anterior band of the medial collateral ligament maintain tension; the posterior bundle is taut at 65° to full flexion [8, 27]. The section of this posterior portion to recover the full flexion does not significantly increase the valgus instability [27, 41, 42]. Morrey et al. show that the primary restraint to the valgus stress is the medial collateral ligaments and the secondary stabilizer is the radial head; the radial head becomes the primary restraint to the valgus in case of a medial ligaments complex insufficiency [3, 23].

The lateral collateral ligament was analyzed in different studies. The lateral collateral ligament remains taut throughout elbow range of motion; this is because its origin lies close to the axis of rotation of the elbow. The anterior portion of the annular ligament is taut during the supination; instead the posterior portion is taut in pronation. The function of the lateral collateral ligament was analyzed by O'Driscoll et al.; they described it as the primary ligamentous stabilizer to varus and postero-lateral rotatory instability [39].

The active stabilizers are the muscles crossing the elbow joint; they can be divided into four compartments as previously described [31, 33]. The line of pull and contraction of these muscles create compressive forces around the humerus, ulna, and radius. These forces function as dynamic stabilizers of the joint. The largest force was seen axially at the distal humerus near full extension and decreases when the elbow moves in flexion [23, 25, 26, 43].

Acknowledgements

The Author thanks Dr. Stefano Colopi for his contribution in creating the support to this paper with TC 3D reconstructions.

References

1. Bernstein AD, Jazrawi LM, Rokito AS, Zuckerman JD (2000) Elbow joint biomechanics: basic science and clinical applications. Orthopedics 23:1293-1301
2. Werner FW, An KN (1994) Biomechanics of the elbow and forearm. Hand Clin 10:357-373
3. Morrey BF (ed) (2000) Anatomy of the elbow joint. The elbow and its disorders, 3rd edn. W.B Saunders, Philadelphia, pp 13-42
4. Zimmerman NB (2002) Clinical application of advances in elbow and forearm anatomy and biomechanics. Hand Clin 18:547
5. Werner SI, Fleisig GS, Dillman CJ (2003) Biomechanics of the elbow during baseball pitching. Orthop Sports Phys Ther 17:274-278
6. Duck TR, Dunnig CE, King GJ (2003) Variability and repeatability of the flexion axis at the ulnohumeral joint. J Orthop Res 21:399-404
7. Morrey BF, Tanaka S, An KN (1991) Valgus stability of the elbow. A definition of primary and secondary constraints. Clin Orthop Relat Res 265:187-195
8. Pomianowski S, O'Driscoll SW, Neale PG et al (2001) The effect of forearm rotation on laxity and stability of the elbow. Clin Biomech 16:401-407
9. Morrey BF, An KN (1983) Articular and ligamentous contributions to the stability of the elbow joint. Am J Sports Med 5:315-319
10. Paraskevas G, Papadopoulos A, Papaziogas B et al (2004) Study of the carrying angle of the human elbow joint in full extension: a morphometric analysis. Surg Radiol Anat 26:19-23
11. Fornalski S, Gupta R, Lee T (2003) Anatomy and biomechanics of the elbow joint. Tech Hand Up Extrem Surg 7:168-178
12. Floris S, Olsen BS, Dalstra M et al (1998) The medial collateral ligament of the elbow joint: anatomy and kinematics. J Shoulder Elbow Surg 4:345-351
13. Hannouche D, Begue T (1999) Functional anatomy of the lateral collateral ligament complex of the elbow. Surg Radiol Anat 21:187-191
14. Rongieres M, Akhavan H, Mansat P et al (2001) Functional anatomy of the medial ligamentous complex of the elbow. Its role in anterior posterior instability. Surg Radiol Anat 23:301-305
15. Regan WD, Korinek SL, Morrey BF, An KN (1991) Biomechanical study of ligaments around the elbow joint. Clin Orthop Relat Res 271:170-179
16. Eygendaal D, Olsen BS, Jensen SL et al (1999) Kinematics of partial and total ruptures of the medial collateral ligament of the elbow. J Shoulder Elbow Surg 8:612-616
17. Morrey BF, An KN (1985) Functional anatomy of the ligaments of the elbow. Clin Orthop Relat Res 201:84-90

18. Dunning CE, Zarzour ZD, Patterson SD et al (2001) Ligamentous stabilizers against posterolateral rotatory instability of the elbow. J Bone Joint Surg Am 83:1823-1828

19. King GJ, An KN (1997) Biomechanics and fuctional anatomy of the elbow. In: Norris T (ed) Shoulder and Elbow (Orthopaedic Knowledge Update) ASES published by AAOS

20. Olsen BS, Sojbjerg JO, Dalstra M, Sneppen O (1996) Kinematics of the lateral ligamentous constraints of the elbow joint. J Shoulder Elbow Surg 5:333-341

21. Nielsen KK, Olsen BS (1999) No stabilizing effect of the elbow joint capsule. A kinematic study. Acta Orthop Scand 70:6-8

22. Olsen BS, Vaesel MT, Sojbjerg JO et al (1996) Lateral collateral ligament of the elbow joint: anatomy and kinematics. J Shoulder Elbow Surg 5:103-112

23. An K, Morrey BF (2000) Biomechanics of the elbow. In: Morrey BF (ed) The elbow and its disorders, 3rd edn. W.B. Saunders, Philadelphia, pp 43-60

24. O'Driscoll SW, Morrey BF, An KN (1990) Intraarticular pressure and capacity of the elbow. Arthroscopy 6:100-103

25. An KN, Hui FC, Morrey BF et al (1981) Muscles across the elbow joint: A biomechanical analysis. J Biomech 14:659-669

26. Funk DA, An KN, Morrey BF, Daube JR (1987) Electromyographic analysis of muscles across the elbow joint. J Orthop Res 5:529-538

27. Alcid JG, Ahmad CS, Lee TQ (2004) Elbow anatomy and structural biomechanics. Clin Sports Med 23:503-517

28. Stroyan M, Wilk KE (1993) The functional anatomy of the elbow complex. J Orthop Sports Phys Ther 17:279-288

29. An KN, Morrey BF, Chao EY (1984) Carrying angle of the human elbow joint. J Orthop Res 1:369-378

30. Safran MR, Baillargeon D (2005) Soft-tissue stabilizers of the elbow. J Shoulder Elbow Surg 14[1 Suppl S]:179S-185S

31. Davidson PA, Pink M, Perry J, Jobe FW (1995) Functional anatomy of the flexor pronator muscle group in relation to the medial collateral ligament of the elbow. Am J Sports Med 2:245-250

32. Dunning CE, Zarzour ZD, Patterson SD et al (2001) Muscle forces and pronation stabilize the lateral ligament deficient elbow. Clin Orthop Relat Res 388:118-124

33. Park MC, Ahmad CS (2004) Dynamic contributions of the flexor-pronator mass to elbow valgus stability. J Bone Joint Surg Am 86:2268-2274

34. Hotchkiss RN, Weiland AJ (1987) Valgus stability of the elbow. J Orthop Res 5:372-377

35. Stein J, Murthi AM (2005) Current concepts in elbow kinematics and biomechanics. Curr Opin Orthop 16:276-279

36. Morrey BF, An KN (2005) Stability of the elbow: Osseous constraints. J Shoulder Elbow Surg 14[1 Suppl S]:174S-178S

37. Cohen MS, Bruno RJ (2001) The collateral ligaments of the elbow: anatomy and clinical correlation. Clin Orthop Relat Res 383:123-130

38. Morrey BF, An KN, Stormont TJ (1988) Force transmission through the radial head. J Bone Joint Surg Am 70:250-256

39. O'Driscoll SW, Bell DF, Morrey BF (1991) Postero lateral rotatory instability of the elbow. J Bone Joint Surg Am 73:440-446

40. O'Driscoll SW, Jaloszynski R, Morrey BF, An KN (1992) Origin of the medial ulnar collateral ligament. J Hand Surg Am 17:164-168

41. Callaway GH, Field LD, Deng XH et al (1997) Biomechanical evaluation of the medial collateral ligament of the elbow. J Bone Joint Surg Am 79:1223-1231

42. Sojbjerg JO, Ovesen J, Nielsen S (1987) Experimental elbow instability after transection of the medial collateral ligament. Clin Orthop Relat Res 218:186-190

43. Askew LJ, An KN, Morrey BF, Chao EY (1987) Isometric elbow strength in normal individuals. Clin Orthop Relat Res 222:261-266

CHAPTER 2

The Clinical Examination of the Elbow

A. HINSCHE, D. STANLEY

Introduction

In order to perform a satisfactory examination of the elbow it is essential for the clinician to have a sound knowledge of the anatomy of the elbow joint. This should include an understanding of the bony anatomy of the distal humerus and proximal radius and ulna. In addition, the attachment of the capsule and the medial and lateral collateral ligaments should be known, together with the arrangement of the muscles and tendons that encircle the joint. Finally, the relationship of the neurovascular structures to the joint must be appreciated. By applying this anatomical knowledge it is usually possible for the clinician who takes a careful history and performs a meticulous examination to reach a firm provisional diagnosis prior to understanding confirmatory diagnostic tests [1].

History

When taking the history it is important to know the patient's age, sex, hand dominance, and occupation since these factors are of special value in the initial assessment and will often give the first indication as to the possible cause of the patient's symptoms.

Age is the first discriminator. A child presenting with intermittent locking and swelling of the elbow is most likely to have a loose body within the joint secondary to osteochondritis dissecans, whereas the same symptoms in an adult over the age of 40 years would be consistent with degenerative arthritis. Progressive pain and swelling of the elbow in a female patient may suggest an early presentation of rheumatoid arthritis, which in turn would require specific investigations for that condition.

Symptoms affecting the dominant elbow may prevent the patient working, participating in sports, and at times undertaking activities of daily living. In this situation it is appropriate to enquire whether the patient believes their work or sporting activities are responsible for, or aggravate, the symptoms they experience.

In elbow disorders the symptoms most frequently noted by patients are pain often associated with local tenderness, reduced elbow movement, and intermittent swelling and locking. Less commonly the patient may complain of symptoms of elbow instability. At times combinations of symptoms will be present.

Past Medical History

A review of the patient's past medical history should also be performed and may identify previous elbow trauma, chronic inflammatory joint disease, psoriasis, haemophilia, or other local or generalised disease processes which may be of relevance to the patient's current complaints.

Presenting Symptoms

Pain

In the assessment of elbow pain it is always essential to specifically enquire about neck symptoms, since at times the elbow pain may be referred from a primary cervical spine pathology. Providing this is not the case the site of the elbow pain should be identified together with its duration, nature, and frequency. It is also important to note whether the pain is associated with elbow movement suggesting an articular pathology, or whether the pain is experienced at the end of movement, which would be consistent with impingement. Pain at rest suggests an inflammatory component or infection. Acute intermittent pain associated with locking is often caused by loose bodies within the joint or less commonly by intra-articular plicae.

Frequently patients will present with lateral or medial elbow pain suggesting lateral or medial epicondylitis. However, it should be remembered that these diagnoses are most uncommon below the age of 40 years and a differential diagnosis should be thought of, e.g. PIN syndrome [2]. In addition, pain on the medial aspect of the elbow may relate to ulnar nerve neuropathy, and for this reason specific note should be made as to whether the patient's pain radiates into the hand and whether there are symptoms of paraesthesia and intrinsic muscle weakness within the ulna nerve distribution [3].

Stiffness

Reduced elbow movement occurs most frequently as a result of elbow trauma [4]. This may be associated with an *intrinsic* joint abnormality due to malunion of a fracture or an *extrinsic* problem resulting from fibrosis and scarring of the soft tissues. The second cause for reduced elbow motion is of degenerative nature, causing loose bodies within the joint and particularly in the olecranon fossa as well as osteophyte formation at the tip of the olecranon and coronoid process [5].

Instability

Recurrent instability of the elbow is an uncommon problem which is often associated with a dislocation of the elbow joint occurring below the age of 15 years. The patient presents with recurrent clicking and giving way of the elbow. When asked the patient will state that the elbow cannot be locked fully in extension when pushing out of a chair or when attempting a "press-up". In these situations the patient is apprehensive that the elbow will dislocate.

Clinical Examination

Since the elbow is a subcutaneous joint, a careful examination will often indicate the likely cause of the patient's symptoms. In order, however, that no areas of the examination are missed it is essential that the clinician develops a methodical examination technique. The process we have found most useful is inspection, palpation, and movement, following Apley's classical principle of "Look, Feel and Move". The examination is completed by specific provocation tests concentrating on that part of the elbow, which is thought to be responsible for the patient's symptoms.

Inspection – "Look"

On initial inspection the posture of the symptomatic elbow should be noted. A painful elbow will often be protected by the contralateral arm and held closely to the side of the body. In contrast, an elbow lacking extension may be supported by placing the ipsilateral hand in the trouser pocket. Skin changes including scars from previous injury or surgical procedures together with olecranon bursae, rheumatoid nodules, and psoritic plaques must also be recorded.

Assessment of the carrying angle should be made with the elbow in full extension. Although some variation is common, the average valgus angulation is 15° in females and 10° in males. Varus deformity is always abnormal and is usually the result of a supracondylar fracture in childhood. Previous bony injury of the lateral humeral condyle may result in an increased valgus angulation, which can cause ulna neuropathy (cubitus tarda).

It is important to remember that with the elbow fully extended the forearm is in valgus relative to the upper arm, whilst in full flexion the forearm is in varus, facilitating the movement of the hand towards the face.

Palpation – "Feel"

Palpation should be performed systematically working progressively around the elbow. Our preferred starting point is lateral, moving anteriorly to the medial side and ending posteriorly.

Lateral

On the lateral side the palpation begins on the lateral supracondylar ridge and progresses distally (Fig. 1). The extensor carpi radialis longus and brevis are identified and palpated for tenderness. The typical trigger point for lateral epicondylitis is just distal and anterior to the lateral epicondylar ridge over the origin of extensor carpi radialis brevis [6]. If tenderness is detected it is reasonable at this stage to perform the appropriate provocation test to confirm the diagnosis. However, a posterior interosseous nerve syndrome should be excluded by palpating the extensor mass deep and medial to the radial neck.

Tenderness over the capitellum in a child may indicate osteochondritis dissecans, which can be associated with an effusion detectable in the infracondylar recess between the capitellum and radial head. At times this recess may have a boggy feel consistent with inflammatory process within the joint.

The radial head should then be palpated with respect to its position and orientation with the capitellum and with regards to tenderness and crepitus on movement. In all positions of the arm the radial head aligns with the capitellum, and if it is subluxed or dislocated as the result of injury or a congenital abnormality this should be identifiable at this stage. Crepitus at the radiocapitellar joint, best appreciated by getting the patient to grip the examiner's fingers and undertake pronation and supination movement, may indicate a recent injury to either the radial head or capitellum. Alternatively, if there is no history of recent trauma, crepitus is consistent with degenerative or inflammatory arthritis.

Anterior

Palpation from lateral to medial across the anterior aspect of the elbow allows identification of the brachioradialis muscle, biceps tendon and aponeurosis, brachial artery, and median nerve (Fig. 2). Of these structures avulsion of the biceps insertion is the one most likely to present pathologically. The patient usually has a history of recent injury with significant bruising around the anterior aspect of the elbow and proximal prominence of the biceps muscle [7]. Loss of flexion and supination strength will be found on specific muscle testing. Occasionally if the patient has suffered a previous dislocation of the elbow, palpation of the anterior aspect of the elbow will reveal bony hardness consistent with myositis ossificans.

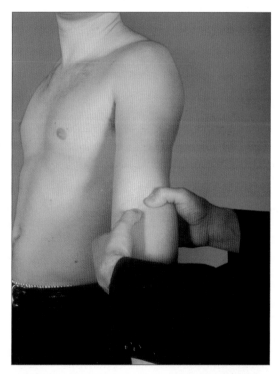

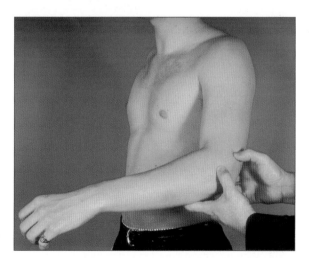

Fig. 1. Examination of the lateral aspect of the elbow. The lateral supracondylar ridge, extensor carpi radialis longus and brevis, capitellum and radial head can be palpated

Fig. 2. Examination of the anterior aspect of the elbow allows indentification of brachioradialis, the biceps tendon and aponeurosis, brachial artery and median nerve

Medial

The two structures that are easily palpated on the medial aspect of the elbow are the common flexor origin and the ulnar nerve (Fig. 3). Tenderness anteriorly over the common flexor origin is consistent with medial epicondylitis, and, as with epicondylitis on the lateral side of the joint, it is appropriate on eliciting tenderness to perform the confirmatory provocation tests [8].

The ulnar nerve lies more posteriorly behind the medial epicondyle, although in up to 10% of patients it may subluxate anteriorly during flexion of the elbow. A subluxing ulnar nerve is a cause of medial elbow pain. More commonly, however, ulnar nerve symptoms arise because of entrapment of the nerve, usually between the two heads of flexor carpi ulnaris. Associated with this the patient may complain of pins and needles or numbness affecting the ipsilateral little and ring fingers. Specific testing may reveal sensory disturbance in these fingers together with small-muscle wasting in the hand. A comparison with the unaffected hand should always be performed [9].

Posterior

The bony anatomy of the elbow can be easily palpated posteriorly (Fig. 4). In the uninjured extended elbow the lateral epicondyle, tip of the olecranon, and medial epicondyle form a straight line. When the elbow is flexed at 90° these bony structures form an isosceles triangle. If, however, there has been a previous fracture this arrangement of the bony architecture may be disrupted.

Palpation of the triceps insertion may reveal local tenderness suggesting a partial tear, whilst an inability to extend the elbow against gravity indicates a complete avulsion. In this situation a defect between the distal triceps and olecranon is usually palpable [10].

Finally palpation of the posterior aspect of the elbow will, if present, reveal an olecranon bursa or rheumatoid nodules.

Movement – "Move"

In order to avoid missing subtle abnormalities the range of movement of the symptomatic elbow

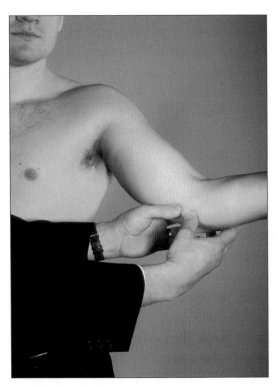

Fig. 3. On the medial aspect of the elbow the common flexor origin and ulnar nerve can be palpated

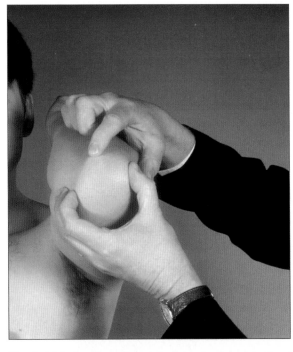

Fig. 4. With the elbow flexed the lateral epicondyle, tip of the olecranon and medial epicondyle form an isosceles triangle. When the elbow is fully extended these structures form a horizontal straight line

should be compared with the asymptomatic joint. The normal range of flexion and extension at the elbow is 140°. This is measured from 0° when the forearm is supinated and fully extended to 140° when fully flexed. Ten degrees of hyperextension is not uncommon, but a greater amount suggests hypermobility or previous bony injury. Hyperextension is recorded as a negative integer [11].

Loss of extension is an early sign of an intra-articular abnormality. Although loss of extension may not be appreciated by the patient, loss of flexion is usually noted. The functional range of movement at the elbow is 100°, and once patients have less than this their ability to work and perform activities of daily living becomes compromised.

Assessment of pronation and supination should be undertaken with compensatory shoulder movement excluded. This is achieved by stabilising the elbow joint against the side of the body with the elbow flexed at 90°. Average supination is 85° whilst pronation is usually a few degrees less. For functional rotation the patient requires approximately half the normal supination and pronation movement. Loss of supination has traditionally been regarded as the more serious functional loss, although in today's world as keyboards are used extremely commonly, loss of pronation may also now be a significant handicap.

Instability

Valgus Instability

Valgus instability results from damage to the ulnar collateral ligament of the elbow. It is most commonly seen in throwing athletes who may sustain either an acute or chronic injury. It can be demonstrated by fully externally rotating the arm to stabilise the shoulder, flexing the elbow approximately 30° to unlock the olecranon from the fossa, and applying a valgus force whilst palpating the ulnar collateral ligament. Opening of the elbow, together with local pain and tenderness, are compatible with damage to the ligament.

Partial tears of the ligament can be assessed using O'Brien's test. This involves holding the patient's thumb with the elbow fully flexed. Pain over the medial ligament suggests a partial tear of the ligament.

Varus Instability

Assessment of the integrity of the lateral collateral ligament is achieved by fully internally rotating the shoulder, flexing the elbow to approximately 30° to

unlock the olecranon from its fossa, and applying a varus stress to the elbow. If the lateral collateral ligament is deficient, the gap between the capitellum and radial head will increase.

Rotatory Instability

Posterolateral rotatory instability results from insufficiency of the lateral ulnar collateral ligament. It is best assessed by performing the lateral pivot shift test. This is undertaken with the patient in the supine position and with the shoulder and elbow flexed to 90°. The patient's forearm is fully supinated, and with the examiner holding the patient's wrist and forearm a valgus and axial compression force is applied to the elbow whilst the elbow is slowly extended. This will often reproduce the patient's symptoms and produce apprehension such that the patient prevents further movement. The radius and ulna sublux from the humerus producing a prominence posterolaterally and a dimple between the radial head and capitellum. At approximately 40° of flexion the ulna suddenly reduces with a palpable and visible clunk [12].

Instability testing is best appreciated if performed under general anaesthesia using image intensification. This provides a permanent record of the ligament injury and is of assistance when reconstruction is being planned (Fig. 5).

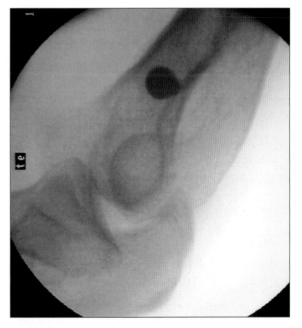

Fig. 5. Rotatory instability is demonstrated by the lateral pivot shift test and confirmed under general anaesthesia using image intensification

Specific Tests

The clinical examination is completed by performing specific tests based on the clinical findings so far.

Provocation Tests

Lateral Epicondylitis

Several provocation tests can be performed for lateral epicondylitis:
1. Resisted wrist extension with the wrist in neutral results in localised pain over the extensor origin at the elbow epicondyle (Fig. 6).
2. Resisted extension of the middle finger with the wrist in extension and radial deviation produces pain over the origin of extensor carpi radialis brevis.
3. Passive volar flexion of the wrist with the forearm pronated and the elbow extended also produces pain at the lateral epicondyle.

If any of these tests are positive the diagnosis can be confirmed by injecting a small amount of local anaesthetic. The injection should be at the common extensor origin and should obliterate the patient's symptoms.

Medial Epicondylitis

Provocation tests for medial epicondylitis include:
1. Resisted wrist flexion which should produce pain at the medial epicondyle (Fig. 7).
2. Passive extension of the wrist and elbow results in medial epicondylar pain.

Local anaesthetic injected at the common flexor origin should obliterate the symptoms to confirm the diagnosis. Care, however, should be taken when the injection is performed in order to be certain that local anaesthetic does not affect the ulnar nerve, which can also be a cause of medial elbow pain.

Impingement Tests

Impingement of the elbow may involve both the posterior or anterior elbow compartments. Normally it results from osteophytes on the tip of the olecranon impinging in the olecranon fossa or osteophytes on the coronoid process impinging into the coronoid fossa. Posterior impingement is more common and occurs due to repetitive hyperextension movements of the elbow. Classically it is stated to occur in "boxers", although we have seen it more commonly in those undertaking racquet sports. It can be demonstrated by applying a hyperextension force to the elbow. This manoeuvre which normally

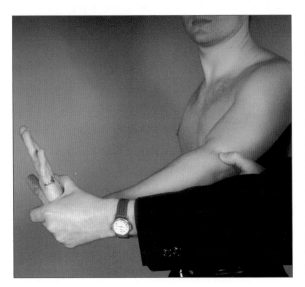

Fig. 6. Provocation test for lateral epicondylitis. Resisted wrist extension results in localised pain over the extensor origin at the lateral epicondyle

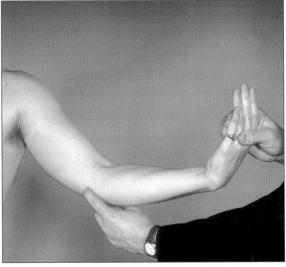

Fig. 7. Provocation test for medial epicondylitis. Resisted wrist flexion results in localised pain over the flexor origin at the medial epicondyle

is pain-free results in posterior elbow pain in patients with posterior elbow impingement. Hyperflexion will similarly demonstrate anterior elbow impingement by causing anterior elbow pain.

Clinical Examination Checklist

Look

– Swelling, deformity, scarring, wasting
– Skin changes, e.g. RA nodules, eczema, erythema
– Carrying angle
– Resting position

Feel

– Bony surface landmarks
– Extensor origin
– Radial head
– PIN
– Biceps tendon
– Flexor-pronator origin
– Ulna nerve
– Olecranon tip and fossa

Move

– Extension
– Flexion
– Supination
– Pronation
– Valgus/varus stress testing
– Pivot shift test
– Provocation tests
– Impingement test
Always examine and compare both elbows.

Common Pathologies ("The Big 10")

• Lateral/medial epicondylitis
• Cubital tunnel syndrome
• RA, OA
• Dislocated radial head (congenital/acquired)
• Altered carrying angle (previous supracondylar fracture)
• Bony lump (myositis ossificans, nonunion)
• Bicipital avulsion/tendonitis
• Radio-ulna synostosis
• Post-traumatic stiffness
• Instability

Presenting Problem and Differential Diagnosis

• Pain lateral side
  – Lateral epicondylitis
  – Lateral compartment OA
  – PIN syndrome
  – Nonunion
  – Acute avulsion fracture lateral (epi-) condyle
  – Radial head fracture
  – Osteochondritis dissecans
  – Varus instability
  – Posterolateral instability
• Pain medial side
  – Medial epicondylitis
  – Cubital tunnel syndrome
  – Nonunion
  – Acute avulsion fracture medial (epi-) condyle
  – Valgus instability
• Anterior elbow pain
  – Biceps tendonitis
  – Biceps avulsion
  – Anterior impingement
• Posterior elbow pain
  – Posterior impingement
  – Triceps tendon injury
  – Olecranon spur
  – Olecranon bursitis
• Elbow stiffness
  – Intrinsic
    – Post-traumatic
    – Degenerative
    – Inflammatory
    – Infective
  – Extrinsic
    – Post-traumatic
  – Neurological
• Elbow instability
  – Medial
  – Lateral
  – Rotatory
  – Complex
Don't forget systemic disease; e.g. Ehlers-Danlos and Marfan Syndrome.

References

1. Doyle JR (2003) Elbow in doyle and botte. Surgical anatomy of the hand and upper extremity. Lippincott, Williams and Wilkins, Philadelphia
2. Andrews JR, Whiteside JA (1993) Common elbow problems in the athlete. J Orthop Sports Phys Ther 17:289-295
3. Major HP (1883) Lawn tennis elbow. BMJ 2:557
4. Thompson H, Garcia A (1967) Myositis ossificans: Aftermath of elbow injuries. Clin Orthop 50:129-134

5. Stanley D (1994) Prevalence and aetiology of symptomatic elbow osteoarthritis. J Shoulder Elbow Surg 3:386-389

6. Nirschl RP (1992) Elbow tendinosis/tennis elbow. Clin Sports Med 4:851-870

7. Baker BE, Bierwagen D (1985) Rupture of the distal tendon of biceps brachii. Operative versus non-operative treatment. J Bone Joint Surg 67:414-417

8. Gabel GT, Nirschl RP (2002) Medial Epicondylitis. In: Morrey BF (ed) Masters techniques: The elbow. Lippincott, Williams and Wilkins, Philadelphia

9. Spinner M, Kaplan EP (1976) The relationship of the ulnar nerve to the medial intermuscular septum in the arm and it's clinical significance. Hand 8:239-242

10. Holleb PD, Bach BR (1990) Triceps brachii injuries. Sports Med 10:273-276

11. Morrey BF, Chow EY (1976) Passive motion of the elbow joint. J Bone Joint Surg Am 58:501-508

12. O'Driscoll SW, Bell DF, Morrey BF (1991) Postero-lateral rotatory instability of the elbow. J Bone Joint Surg Am 73:440-446

CHAPTER 3
Imaging of the Elbow

V. Spina, L. Baldini

Introduction

The technological innovations of recent decades have greatly improved the diagnostic information offered by imaging modalities in the study of skeletal and joint diseases. This is due to the addition of multiplanar modalities with high contrast and spatial resolution, such as computed tomography (CT), magnetic resonance (MR), and ultrasonography (US) to traditional modalities like plain radiography (X-ray) and nuclear medicine (NM) [1-3]. Being that the elbow has traditionally been a challenging joint not only for the orthopedic surgeon but also for the radiologist, imaging has been limited for a long time by the complexity of the elbow's anatomy as well as technical difficulties. For example, elbow stiffness, a typical result of traumatic lesions, is the factor that more than others in the past made it difficult to obtain good diagnostic imaging. Nowadays, the existing variety of imaging modalities permit a detailed analysis of several joint diseases of the elbow by providing images of high quality [4-6]. The use of contrast agents in the intra-articular space (arthrography) combined with the tomographic view offered by CT (arthro-CT) and MR (arthro-MR) examinations makes the diagnostic information more accurate in the evaluation of joint lesions [7-10].

Plain Radiography

Radiographic examination makes use of standard and additional projections [11]. Standard projections consist of two orthogonal views: an anteroposterior view (AP) and a lateral view (LL).

In the anteroposterior (AP) projection, the forearm is in a supine position with the elbow completely extended and the fingers slightly flexed. The central X-ray beam is directed perpendicular to the elbow joint. The distal humerus, especially the profiles of the medial and lateral epicondyles, the radial head, and the proximal ulna are highly visible in this view. The criteria for a correct projection are a slight superimposition of the radial head, neck and biceps tuberosity over the proximal ulna, and the visualization of the humeroradial joint space (Fig. 1).

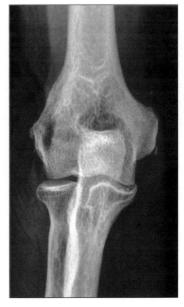

Fig. 1. Anteroposterior view of the elbow. This projection shows the medial and lateral epicondyles, the capitellum and the radial head, the olecranon fossa. The coronoid process is seen frontally and the olecranon is superimposed on the trochlea. Note a traction spur of the coronoid process and small calcification of collateral ligament. Calcific tendinitis of the common extensor tendon

In the laterolateral (LL) projection, the forearm is placed on the ulnar side with the elbow flexed 90° and the fingers slightly flexed. The central X-ray beam is directed perpendicular to the humeral epicondyle, highly visible in this position. It is important in this view to pay attention to the position of the shoulder, which must be positioned at the same level of the elbow. If this is not possible it would be necessary to use some devices to elevate the bearing surface so that shoulder, elbow, and forearm are at the same level. In the lateral view correctly obtained, the posterior part of the radial head is superimposed over the coronoid process and the trochlea is superimposed over the capitellum. The distal humerus, the olecranon process, and the anterior part of the radial head are highly visible in the lateral view (Fig. 2a).

This projection is also important to evaluate the periarticular fat pads anatomically present in the elbow. Such fat pads are intracapsular yet extrasinovial in location, being enveloped by the fibers of the joint capsule which separate them from the sinovial lining. They are located respectively anteriorly in the coronoid fossa and posteriorly in the olecranon fossa.

On a lateral radiograph of the elbow with 90° flexion the anterior fat pad is only normally seen as a radiolucent faint line parallel to the anterior profile of the distal humerus. The posterior fat pad is not normally seen because it is pressed into the deep olecranon fossa by the anconeus muscle and triceps tendon.

All pathological conditions that cause a distention of the joint capsule (effusion, synovitis, masses) produce a superior displacement of both fat pads with a consequent deformation of the normal morphology of the anterior fat pad, which assumes a convex shape (ship's sail configuration) while the posterior fat pad is visualized in a similar way posterior to the humeral condyles (Fig. 2b) [12].

The fat pad sign has proved crucial to predict an intra-articular disease process in the absence of any radiographically visible bone abnormalities. This sign is very useful particularly in the occult traumatic lesion because it shows the joint effusion, so that the fracture can be searched [13].

A false-negative fat pad sign can occur in some situations, including incorrect patient positioning, capsular rupture and extracapsular abnormalities (e.g., a massive soft-tissue swelling around the joint).

A false-positive fat pad sign can occur if the elbow is examined in extension. In this situation the triceps are relaxed, the posterior capsule is lax and the olecranon process displaces the posterior fat pad from the olecranon fossa. Normal displacement of the posterior fat pad with the elbow extended should not be mistaken for a sign of joint disease.

Radiographs, obtained with either conventional or digital techniques, represent in most cases the basic examination, which is able to show directly the morphology, structure, and articular relationships of bones and the presence of intra-articular or periarticular calcification (e.g., loose bodies) (Figs. 3, 4).

The additional projections are views which permit a better visualization of those elbow regions that are not well seen in standard projections. Additional projections include the lateral oblique view, the medial oblique view, the axial view, the radial head-capitellum view, and the cubital tunnel view.

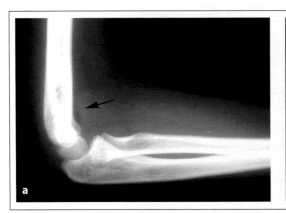 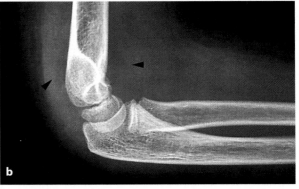

Fig. 2. (**a**) Lateral view of the elbow in a child shows the normal hockeystick appearance of the distal humerus. This projection demonstrates well the olecranon process and the anterior aspect of the radial head. The articular surface and the posterior aspect of the radial head are not well seen in this view due to overlap by the coronoid process. The capitellum is also obscured by the overlapping trochlea. The anterior fat pad appears as a radiolucent faint line parallel to the anterior profile of the distal humerus (*arrow*) while the posterior fat pad is not visualized. (**b**) On the lateral view of the elbow there is a positive posterior fat-pad sign, and the anterior fat-pad is clearly elevated (*arrowheads*)

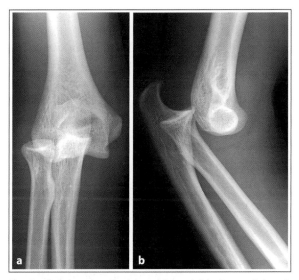

Fig. 3. Anteroposterior (**a**) and lateral (**b**) views of the elbow easily demonstrate the posterolateral displacement of the radius and the ulna without associated bone fracture

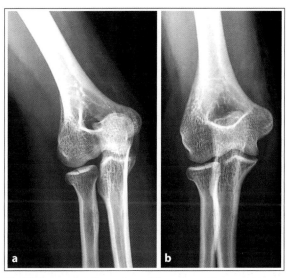

Fig. 5. External oblique view of the elbow (**a**) demonstrates a linear fracture of the radial head. On the anteroposterior view (**b**) the nearly invisible fracture line can be easily overlooked

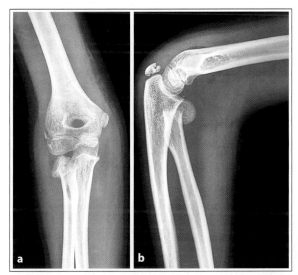

Fig. 4. Anteroposterior (**a**) and lateral (**b**) views of the elbow show a displaced fracture of radial epiphysis tilted more than 50°. On the lateral projection, posterior fat-pad becomes visible and the anterior fat-pad appears displaced indicating hemorrhagic effusion

The medial oblique view is performed with the elbow extended and the hand in prone position so that the anterior part of the forearm is at an angle of 40°-45° to the X-ray cassette [11]. The central X-ray beam is directed perpendicular to the midpoint of the joint. Even though there is a superimposition of the radial head and neck over the ulna, the profile of the coronoid process is easily seen in this projection (Fig. 6).

The radial head-capitellum view is extremely useful in traumatic diseases, especially when

In the lateral oblique view the elbow is extended and the hand is laterally rotated so that the forearm is at an angle of 40° to the X-ray cassette [11]. The central X-ray beam is centered perpendicular to the midpoint of the joint. This view permits elimination of the superimposition between radius and ulna, providing a better visualization of the radial head, neck, and biceps tuberosity (Fig. 5).

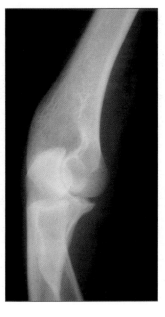

Fig. 6. Medial oblique view allows a better visualization of the trochlea, olecranon, and coronoid process. The radial head is obscured by the ulna

there is a strong clinical suspect of fracture, to detect occult radial heads fractures, which are not always evident in standard views [14]. The radial head-capitellum projection is performed, like lateral projection, with the elbow flexed at an angle of 90° and the hand placed on the ulnar side, with the exception that the central X-ray beam is not directed perpendicular but is angled 45° to the forearm and directed to the radial head, which is passed dorsoventrally in an oblique direction. As a result, the radial head is projected anteriorly to the coronoid process, and both the radial head and the coronoid process appear separately and as such can be easily evaluated (Fig. 7). The humeroradial joint space is also easily seen in this view.

In the axial view, the patient lays his arm with the extensor face upwards on the X-ray cassette and the elbow completely flexed [11]. The central X-ray beam is directed slightly oblique to the olecranon process. The axial view provides an axial representation of the olecranon process and of the cortical profile of medial and lateral epicondyles (Fig. 8). The sulcus between the olecranon process and the capitellum, a potential space for small loose bodies, is also shown.

The cubital projection is a technical variation of the axial projection in which the elbow, other than completely flexed, is also 15° externally rotated. The central X-ray beam is directed perpendicular to the cubital tunnel which is visualized in profile. This projection provides a good representation of the skeletal floor of the tunnel. The pro-

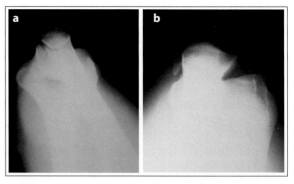

Fig. 8. Axial view of the elbow (**a**) provides an excellent visualization of the olecranon, trochlea, and epicondyles. This projection is helpful in detecting calcification or bone density lateral to the olecranon (**b**)

file of medial epicondyle and the olecranon process are easily visible.

Computed Tomography

Computed tomography (CT) has progressively replaced the conventional tomographic examination, providing an anatomic view of images also on an axial plane, with a high contrast and spatial resolution which allow simultaneous evaluation of bone and extraskeletal structures [15].

The advent and subsequent development of multislice CT, compared with conventional CT,

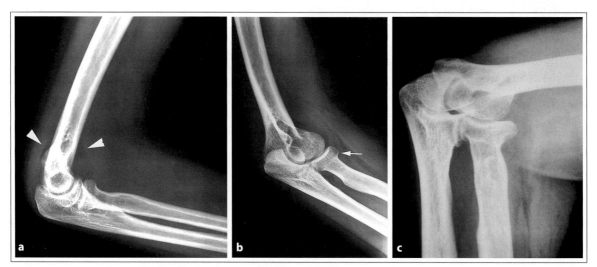

Fig. 7. On the lateral view of the elbow (**a**) there is a positive posterior fat-pad sign, and the anterior fat-pad is also clearly elevated (*arrowheads*); no evidence of abnormality. (**b**) On the radial head capitellum view the radial head is seen without overlap by the coronoid process and an subtle fracture of the radial neck is apparent (*arrow*). (**c**) The radial head-capitellum view shows in a different patient what appears to be easily visible degenerative changes involving the radioulnar joint

has brought further advantages in the study of bones and joints, giving increasing importance to this more recent technique [16]. In fact, multi-slice CT allows rather rapid examination of extended anatomic regions with very thin slices (thinner than 1 mm). In a single acquisition with very thin slices, a data set with isotropic properties can be obtained. This data set can be processed with software programs in independent and powerful workstations so that multiplanar (MPR) and three-dimensional (3D) images of high quality can be obtained [17]. MPR and 3D images have become an integral part of CT examination (Fig. 9).

MPR imaging permits representations in different planes of study (coronal, sagittal, oblique) and is very useful to reach a diagnosis. On the other hand, 3D imaging is able to represent quickly and in an easy manner complex spatial relationships of anatomic structures, and also the orthopedic surgeon is willing to approach 3D imaging, because it does not require mentally integrating multiple axial images.

There are different rendering techniques to create 3D images: volume rendering (VR), shaded surface display (SSD), and maximum intensity projection (MIP).

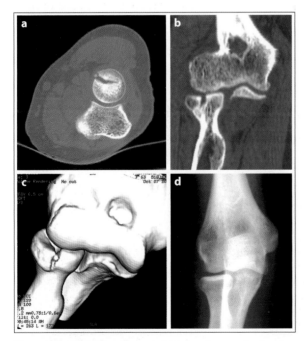

Fig. 9. CT scan of the elbow. Axial (**a**) and coronal reformatted CT images (**b**) demonstrate the linear fracture of articular surface of the radial head with a small fragment. (**c**) 3D reconstruction of the elbow. On AP view (**d**) the fracture is not clearly visualized

The major differences in the way these techniques process CT data sets are the reason for the different 3D images obtained.

With the SSD technique there is a detailed visualization of bones' contours, and fractures which interrupt the profile of the cortex are easily seen, while fractures which do not interrupt the cortex profile or that are parallel to the plane of scan are not easily seen.

VR technique provides an excellent representation of the anatomic model and is indicated to evaluate the spatial interrelationship of fracture fragments in case of complex skeletal trauma.

MIP images are most useful in the study of bone components when metal is present because of the low number of artifacts associated with this rendering technique compared to the others.

A correct technical execution of CT is crucial to obtain an examination of high quality and especially useful for diagnosis and treatment planning.

In the study of the elbow the patient is placed in a prone position with the involved arm above the head and the elbow slightly flexed, palm upwards. As this position might be uncomfortable and the patient has often pain, a careful immobilization of the joint with straps and blankets is required to avoid motion artifacts. Most studies require the use of thin slices and low pitch factors, which lead to a lower number of step artifacts.

To obtain MPR and 3D representations of high quality it is necessary, other than the use of thin slices, to reconstruct images with an increment of 50%-60% of the reconstructed section width; it is also important to use either a high resolution algorithm, excellent for axial and MPR images, or a standard or soft algorithm, particularly indicated for SSD and VR images. To obtain an optimal spatial resolution a small field of view should be preferred.

In the study of the elbow, CT is generally a second-choice modality, performed when radiographic examination is doubtful or when radiographic information is not sufficient for proper diagnostic and therapeutic management. CT is especially indicated in traumatic skeletal diseases to view subtle fractures not visible on radiographs (Fig. 10) and in case of complex fractures to have a detailed evaluation of the spatial inter-relationship of fracture fragments. It is also used for the complications in fracture healing, to search loose bodies (Fig. 11) and calcific plates in case of elbow stiffness (Figs. 12, 13), for bone tumors, in degenerative and infectious diseases, and to guide interventional procedures.

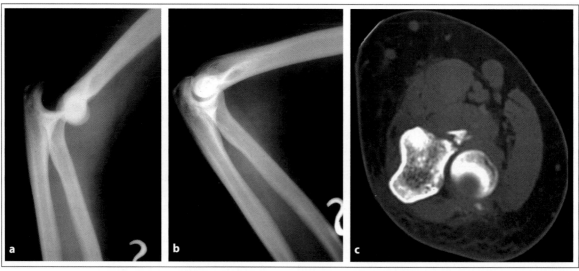

Fig. 10. (**a**) Lateral view demonstrates posterior dislocation of radius and ulna. (**b**) Lateral view postreduction. (**c**) Axial CT scan demonstrates a fracture through the base of the coronoid process

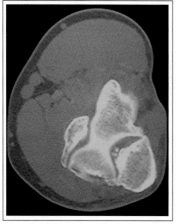

Fig. 11. Axial CT scan shows multiple loose bodies within the olecranon fossa adjacent to the olecranon tip

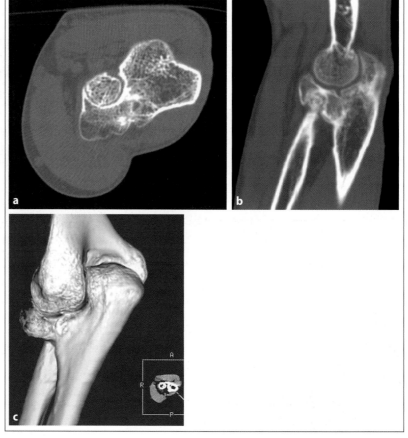

Fig. 12. CT scan demonstrates a synostosis between the radial and ulna as a result of original fracture of the radial metaphisas. Axial (**a**) and sagittal reformatted (**b**) CT images show a complete bony fusion between the radius and ulna; note the characteristic deformity of the radial shaft fracture resulting in a "pencil-in-cup". (**c**) Oblique coronal reconstructions of a 3D image

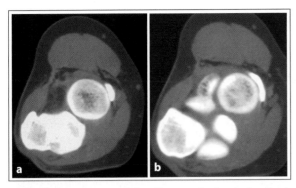

Fig. 13. Axial CT scan of the elbow at the level of radioulnar joint shows the ossification of annular ligament. Note that image (**a**) is more distal than image (**b**)

Ultrasonography

Ultrasonography (US) is a modality employing ultrasounds, particularly useful to evaluate the majority of periarticular anatomic structures. US is particularly indicated in the study of the elbow because of the superficial nature of the muscles and tendons of this region [18]. As technical advances continue to improve image quality, US will gain increasing importance in the study of musculoskeletal diseases. This modality can now rely on high-frequency probes (up to 16 Mhz) which are able to show the laminar structure of tendons and ligaments and the reticular structure of nerves [19] (Fig. 14); on the availability of Power and Color Doppler, which are very sensitive in vascular and sinovial pathologies; and eventually on the most recent use of dedicated contrast agents. Moreover, a characteristic feature of US is the possibility to perform dynamic examinations which often enable formulation of diagnoses that other methods can't always reach due to the impossibility

of offering a dynamic study of articular structures [20].

US study of the elbow makes use of a real-time technique, provided with linear high-frequency probes (7.5-10.13 MHz). The examination must be performed bilaterally, comparing the studied joint with the contralateral one that is considered "normal." Usually, an acknowledged series of acquisitions is performed, which enable evaluation of all the anatomic structures that can be seen with US. In most cases, US of the elbow should be preceded by standard radiographic examination. Note, for example, that a congenital abnormality of the bone structures alone would alter the US result.

US examination of the elbow enables detection of capsular distensions, bursal inflammations,

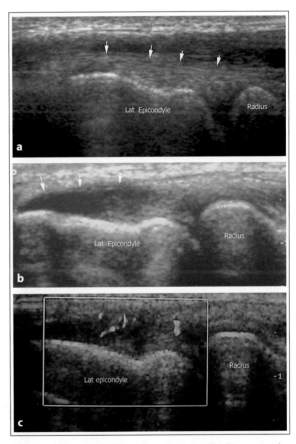

Fig. 15. Ultrasound of the elbow. Longitudinal image at the level of the lateral epicondyle (**a**) demonstrates the normal sonographic appearance of the common extensor tendon (*arrows*). (**b**) Lateral epicondylitis ("tennis elbow") The tendon is markedly thickened, heterogeneous, and has hypoechoic foci consistent with intrasubstance tears (*arrow*). (**c**) Corresponding Color Doppler image shows the vascularity of inflammatory tissue (courtesy of Enzo Silvestri, University of Genova, Italy)

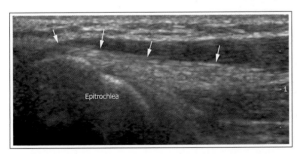

Fig. 14. Ultrasound of the elbow. Longitudinal image at the level of the epithroclea reveals the normal sonographic appearance of the common origin flexor and pronator tendon (*arrows*) (courtesy of Enzo Silvestri, University of Genova, Italy)

tendon pathologies (distal insertions of the tricipital and bicipital and insertion of the common tendons of the extensors and flexors) [21, 22] (Fig. 15), ligamental lesions, as well as nervous pathologies, in particular of the ulnar nerve in the cubital tunnel. Moreover, US is able to detect the presence of soft tissue masses (e.g., lipoma, angioma, lymph nodes) and in some cases to represent their content (either solid or fluid), as in the case of cystic ganglion (Fig. 16). This methodology can also be applied as a guide for surgical procedures, such as the drainage of fluid articular collections. For the study of bone structures, on the other hand, the use of US is highly limited because this technique only shows the bone profile and cartilage width.

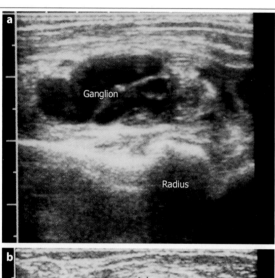

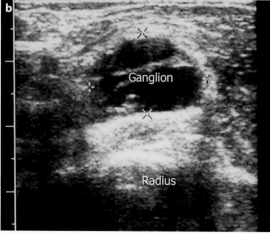

Fig. 16. Ganglion. Longitudinal (**a**) and transverse (**b**) ultrasound images of the radiocapitellar joint demonstrate a large loculated anechoic mass with posterior acoustic enhancement adjacent to the radial head

Magnetic Resonance

Magnetic Resonance (MR) is the most important technological innovation of recent years, representing a revolution for the study of joints, also being effectively employed in the study of the elbow [4-6, 23], as it permits an accurate analysis of several pathologies where other modalities (X-ray, CT, US, arthrography) have proved incomplete or inadequate.

MR is based on the principle that hydrogen protons, once placed in a strong, static magnetic field, resonate if subject to a radio frequency field [24]. In other words, the electromagnetic waves give up energy to the nuclei, thus leading to an increased width of their precession motion and to the passage from a stable to an unstable status. Furthermore, nucleis precession is timed, that is, follows a synchronous pattern. As a consequence, the overall magnetization of the tissue sample is modified and can be measured from outside, and relaxation phenomena arise, with the energy previously received given up towards the outside as electromagnetic waves. Such waves are measured by MR appliances and determine the characteristics of the images obtained with this technique.

The physical phenomenon previously described produces a signal whose intensity is influenced by various elements: first the density of the resonant nuclei, second the motion of hydrogen protons, which is strictly related to the function of the blood flow; finally, two chemical parameters defined as relaxation times T_1 and T_2, that are peculiar and variable yet not tissue-specific.

When a tissue is altered by a pathologic process, its relaxation values T_1 and T_2 change, thus differentiating the abnormal tissue from the normal one. The MR image consists of pixels generated by a computer according to the same process of image formation found in CT. The difference between the two image types lies in the fact that in MR the value of each pixel corresponds to the intensity of MR signal coming from the volume of tissue examined, while in CT it reflects the values of desitometric attenuation of the X-rays.

MR appliances differ depending upon the type of magnet determining the formation of the magnetic field: high field (3.0-1.5 Tesla), medium (1.0-Tesla) and low field (0.5-0.2 Tesla). The choice of the magnetic field highly influences the performance, price, and appearance of the appliances.

For the study of joints, radio-frequency coils are employed (Fig. 17), some of which, with dedicated geometry, enable improvement of the signal/noise ratio and consequently image quality.

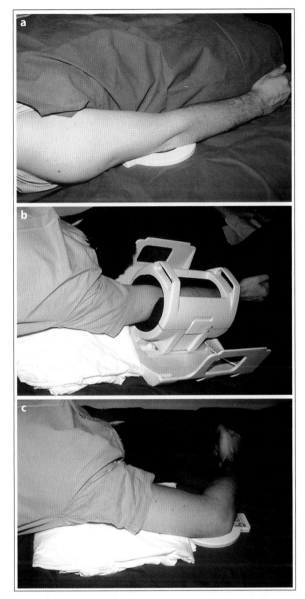

Fig. 17. MR technique: surface coils and patient positioning. (**a**) Patient may be scanned in a supine position with the elbow in extension and wrist in a neutral position. The circular surface coil is placed under the elbow. (**b**) The patient may be examined in a prone position with the arm extended overhead. The cylindrical extremity coil produces excellent elbow images but requires rapid scanning to avoid motion artifact. (**c**) The prone position with circular surface coil may be useful for patients unable to fully extend the elbow (elbow's stiffness)

In the study of joints, MR provides images of excellent quality thanks to the high spatial resolution and to the high resolution of the natural contrast between the various tissues [25]. Images are obtained freely in any spatial orientation (coronal, sagittal, axial, and oblique) with a wide variety of

impulse sequences. The most frequently used are the conventional Spin-echo (SE). T1-weighted images and STIR (short time inversion recovery) sequences are usually obtained in the coronal plane and are useful to demonstrate alterations of the bone marrow and to represent periarticular tendons and ligaments. Although the STIR sequence has relatively poor signal-noise ratio because of the suppression of signal from fat, pathology is often more evident because of the effects of additive T1 and T2 contrast.

Proton-density and T2-weighted images are typically obtained in the sagittal and axial planes to detect the presence of pathologic processes. Fast spin-echo sequences (FSE) may be substituted with the conventional T2-weighted spin-echo sequences if available; these more recent sequences permit a shorter examination and may be used to obtained higher-resolution T2-weighted images in the same time as the conventional spin-echo sequences or may simply be used to increase the speed of the examination (claustrophobic patients or uncomfortable position).

Additional sequences of study are those employing the Fat Suppression technique (SE Fat Sat), which is particularly sensitive to the visualization of tissue pathologies or hyaline articular cartilage. T1-weighted images with fat-suppression are useful whenever Gadolinium contrast is administered, either intravenously or directly into the elbow joint. Intravenous gadolinium may provide additional information in the evaluation of neoplastic or inflammatory processes about the elbow. Articular injection of saline or dilute gadolinium (arthro MRI) may be useful in patients without a joint effusion to detect loose bodies, to determine if the capsule is disrupted, or to determine if an osteochondral fracture fragment is stable.

Gradient-echo volume sequences (GE) allow acquisition of multiple very thin axial images, which may subsequently be reformatted in any plane using a computer workstation. These sequences make it possible to emphasize the natural contrast of the articular cartilage and fibrocartilage.

The anatomic structures of the elbow are depicted reliably with MR imaging [26, 27].

The coronal plane (Fig. 18) makes it possible to represent in an excellent way the humeroradial and humeroulnar joints, the articular cartilage of the humeral capitellum and trochlea, the tendon insertions of the flexor-pronator muscles and of the extensors of the hand, the collateral ligaments, both medial and lateral. The medial collateral ligament complex (MCL) is the most important stabilizer of the elbow, extending from the medial humeral epicondyle to the coronoid process of the ulna. It con-

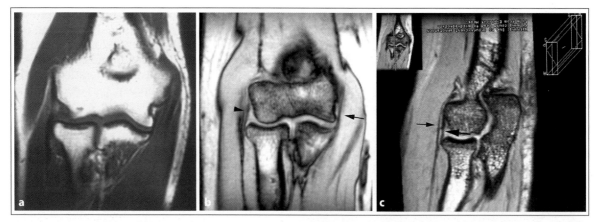

Fig. 18. MR anatomy of the elbow: coronal plane. (**a**) A T1-weighted SE sequence provides good evaluation of the medial and lateral epicondyles and the radiocapitellar articular surfaces. Assessment of the trochlear articular surface and of at least a portion of olecranon fossa is possible. (**b**) High resolution T2-weighted GE sequence (MPGR) shows the normal ulnar collateral ligament (*arrow*) extending from the medial humeral epicondyle to the proximal ulna and normal radial collateral ligament (*arrowhead*). (**c**) Oblique coronal image (3D GE) shows the radial collateral ligament (*large arrow*) as a linear band of signal void just deep to the extensor tendon group (*small arrow*)

sists of three aspects: anterior and posterior bundles as well as an oblique band also known as the transverse ligament. The largest and functionally most important is the anterior bundle, which is useful to provide the primary restraint to the valgus stress [28-30]. The lateral collateral ligament complex (LCL) is a more variable and less robust structure that extends from the lateral epicondyle to the annular ligament. A more posterior bundle, known as the lateral ulnar collateral ligament (LUCL), arises from the lateral epicondyle and extends along the posterior aspect of the radius to insert on the supinator crest of the ulna [31, 32]. This ligament provides the primary ligamentous restraint to varus stress and the disruption results in a posterolateral rotatory instability of the elbow [33, 34].

The sagittal plane (Fig. 19) is helpful to evaluate the trocheo-ulnar and radial-capitellum joints. Muscles are well visible in their whole major axes. This is particularly the case for the bicipital and the brachial muscles with the respective tendons at the distal insertions and the posterior part of the triceps with its tendon at the olecranon. The fat pads of the coronoid and olechranic fossae are also easily visible.

The axial plane (Fig. 20) is useful to evaluate the radio-ulnar and olecrano-humeral joints. It is possible to evaluate the radial head within the radial notch of the ulna and view the annular ligament. Disruption of the annular ligament results in proximal radioulnar joint instability. This plane is very important for the study of the muscular compartments and for the visualization of nerves. The ulnar nerve is positioned superficially at the elbow; it

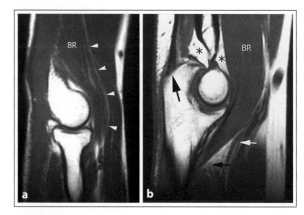

Fig. 19. MR anatomy of the elbow: sagittal plane. (**a**) A T1-weighted SE sequence permits a good visualization of the radial head and capitellum humeral. The radial nerve (*arrowshead*) courses distally, anterior to the brachialis muscle (BR). (**b**) A T1-weighted SE sequence obtained at the level of ulnotrochlear articulation depicts well the olecranon and coronoid tip, the trochlea humeral, the anterior and posterior fat pads (*asterisks*). The triceps tendon is attached to the proximal olecranon (*large black arrow*) and the brachialis muscle inserts on the ulna (*small black arrow*). A portion of the median nerve is visible anterior to the brachialis muscle (*long white arrow*)

runs in the cubital tunnel, along the posterior recurrent ulnar artery and vein and is covered by a thin arcuate ligament. The median nerve runs between the pronator teres and the brachial muscles. The radial nerve is situated in a fat plane between the brachial muscle and the long radial extensor muscle of the wrist, subsequently dividing under

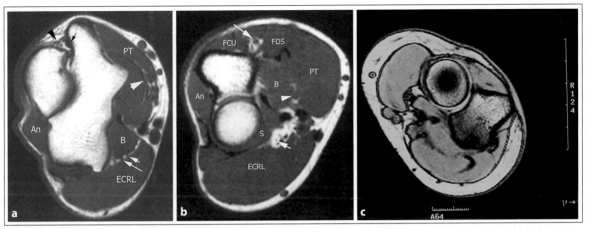

Fig. 20. MR anatomy of the elbow: axial plane. (**a**) A T1-weighted SE sequence obtained at the level of olecranon-humeral articulation shows the anatomy muscles and the cubital tunnel. The ulnar nerve (*black arrow*) is clearly delineated posterior to the medial epicondyle as well as the arcuate ligament (*black arrow-shead*). The superficial (*short white arrow*) and deep (*long white arrow*) radial nerve branches are clearly delineated between the brachialis (**b**) and extensor carpi radialis longus (ECRL) muscles. The median nerve is barely seen (*white arrowhead*) between the pronator teres (PT) and brachialis muscles. A T1-weighted SE sequence at the level of radio-ulnar proximal joint illustrates the ulnar nerve medially (*long white arrow*) between the flexor digitorum superficialis (FDS) and the flexor carp ulnaris (FCU) muscles. The median nerve (*white arrowhead*) is located posterior to the pronator teres muscle. The deep branch of the radial nerve (*short white arrow*) is anterior to the supinator (S) muscle and deep to the extensor carpi radialis longus (ECRL) muscle. (**c**) Axial MPGR sequence shows the annular ligament as a linear band of signal void around the radial head. Note the hyaline cartilage of articular surfaces

the elbow joint into the superficial and posterior interosseous branches.

MR imaging can provide important diagnostic information in the evaluation of the elbow pathology. MRI may help to establish the cause of elbow pain by accurately depicting the presence and extent of bone and soft tissue pathology, with superior detail relative to the conventional imaging techniques.

The extent of MCL injury secondary to a repetitive valgus stress or to elbow dislocations is well delineated with MR imaging [35, 36]. This injury is of-

ten associated with impaction injury on the radiocapitellar compartment. Athletes who throw present frequently with this constellation of abnormalities [37-39]. The ligament may be inflamed, stretched, partially [40] or complete torn, or avulsed from its humeral insertion (Fig. 21). Acute ruptures of the MCL are easily seen with standard MR imaging and appear as areas of high signal intensity on T2-weighted MR images. Partial ruptures are more difficult to diagnose with standard MR imaging and the detection is improved with intra-articular con-

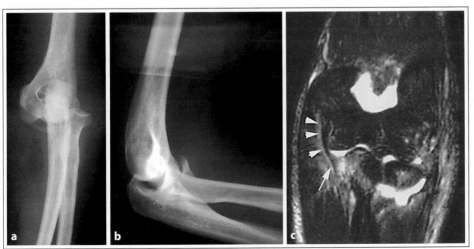

Fig. 21. Posterolateral dislocation of the elbow on anteroposterior view (**a**). The lateral view postreduction (**b**) shows residual posterolateral rotatory instability and fracture of coronoid process. Coronal STIR MR image (**c**) shows avulsion fracture of sublime tubercle with the intact medial collateral ligament (*arrowheads*) still attached to the surface of fracture fragment (*arrow*)

trast [41, 42]. Midsubstance MCL ruptures can be differentiated from proximal avulsions or distal avulsions [43]. The disrupted ligament cannot be seen at its usual location (Fig. 22) or may be seen coursing in an abnormal direction without continuity between the medial epicondyle and ulna.

High resolution coronal gradient-echo MR images are optimal for demonstrating disruption of the MCL. Chronic degeneration of MCL is characterized by thickening of the ligament secondary to scarring often accompanied by foci of calcification [44].

Injury to the RCL is less common and is usually caused by varus stress. The disrupted ligament cannot be seen at its usual location on MR images (Fig. 23) [45].

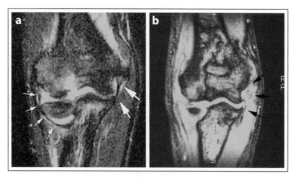

Fig. 22. A T2-weighted with fat saturation coronal image (**a**) reveals increased signal intensity throughout the medial collateral ligament (*arrows*) compatible with a ligament strain injury. The normal lateral ulnar collateral ligament is well seen on this image (*small arrows*). T2-weighted coronal image (**b**) shows poor definition and increased signal of a medial collateral ligament compatible with rupture (*black arrows*)

Lateral and medial epicondylitis, also known as "tennis elbow" and "golfer's elbow," are usually diagnosed clinically [46] but MR imaging can be useful to confirm a diagnosis or excluding complications [47-49]. Overall, 4%-10% of cases of lateral epicondylitis are resistant to conservative therapy [50]. The spectrum of damage to the muscle-tendon unit that may be characterized by MR imaging includes muscle strain injury, tendon degeneration (tendinosis), and tendon disruption. Coronal and axial T2-weighted or STIR MR images best depict injury to the flexor and extensor tendon origins. Degenerative tendinosis is manifested by normal to increased tendon thickness with increased signal intensity on T1-weighted images that is not as bright as fluid on properly windowed T2-weighted images. Partial tears are characterized by thinning of the tendon that is outlined by adjacent fluid on the T2-weighted images. Complete tears may be diagnosed on MR imaging by identifying a fluid-filled gap separating the tendon from its adjacent bony attachment site (Fig. 24). In addition to determining the degree of tendon damage, MR imaging also provides a more global assessment of the elbow (Fig. 25) and therefore is able to detect additional pathologic conditions that may explain the lack of a therapeutic response [51, 52].

MR is a useful imaging method to evaluate nerve disease in the elbow [53]. MRI can depict both normal anatomy and unsuspected space-occupying masses, as well as severe intrinsic nerve disease. Various nerve entrapment syndromes exist in the elbow [54]. The most common is the cubital tunnel syndrome as a result of the location ulnar nerve within the fibro-osseous tunnel posterior to the medial

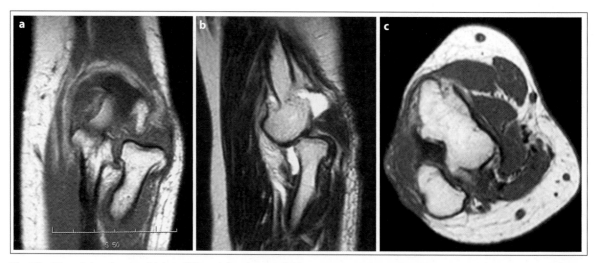

Fig. 23. T1-weighted coronal (**a**) and T2-weighted sagittal (**b**) images reveal posterior dislocation of the radius relative to the capitellum. The lateral collateral ligament is not visualized compatible with rupture. Note the effusion. The T1-weighted axial image (**c**) demonstrates dislocation of olecranon process due to posterolateral rotatory subluxation of the elbow

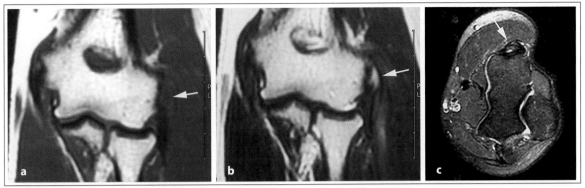

Fig. 24. Lateral epicondylitis. (**a**) Coronal T1-weighted MR image demonstrates increased signal and poor definition at the origin of the extensor tendon group (*arrow*). Normally this area is devoid of signal. (**b**) Coronal T2-weighted image of the same region demonstrates high signal intensity (*arrow*) equivalent to that of fluid, denoting severe inflammation. (**c**) Axial turbo STIR MR image shows high signal intensity adjacent to normal marrow in the lateral epicondyle (*arrow*)

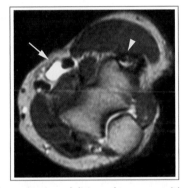

Fig. 25. Lateral epicondylitis and tenosynovitis of the distal biceps tendon. A T2-weighted axial MR image reveals large fluid collections within the bicipital tendon sheath (*arrow*) as well as mild thickening and increased focal signal intensity of the common extensor tendon (*arrowhead*) compatible with severe tendinitis

humeral epicondyle [55, 56]. The normal nerves are intermediate-to-low signal intensity in images obtained with both T1- and T2-weighted sequences. The nerves are best seen on the T1-weighted images particularly when large amounts of fat highlight them. The T2-weighted images are useful to assess edema and signal intensity changes within and around the nerves, as well as to accentuate soft tissue masses that displaced the nerves. Entrapment of radial and median nerve also may be evaluated with MR imaging [57-59]. Particularly MRI plays a role in narrowing the differential clinical diagnosis of nerve disease in case of a radial nerve entrapment that mimics or is associated with refractory lateral epicondylitis (Figs. 26, 27) [51, 52]. Unsuspected causes of neurologic disorders such as congenital or acquired bony, muscular, or ligamentous anomalies may also

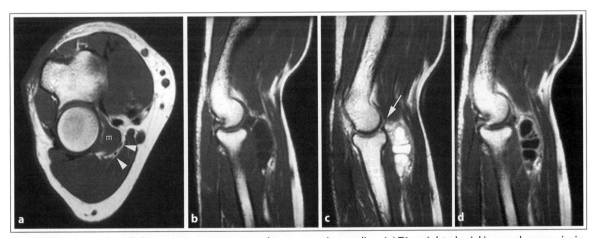

Fig. 26. Symptomatic radial nerve entrapment secondary to a cystic ganglion. (**a**) T1-weighted axial image shows an isointense mass (*m*) with muscle lying between the brachialis and brachioradialis muscles at the location of the branches of radial nerve (*arrowheads*). The lesion demonstrates low signal intensity on a T1-weighted sagittal image (**b**) and hyperintensity on T2-weighted sagittal image; the lesion communicates with the radiohumeral joint (*arrow*) (**c**). No significant enhancement of mass is present on T1-weighted sagittal image after administration of contrast material indicating the fluid nature (**d**)

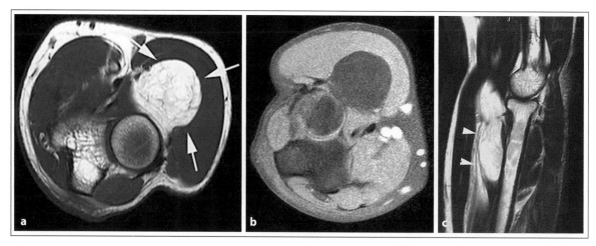

Fig. 27. Symptomatic radial nerve entrapment secondary to a lipoma. (**a**) A T1-weighted axial image demonstrates a mass with fat signal intensity (*arrows*) adjacent to the radius and the extensor musculature. The branches of the radial nerve are not visualized. (**b**) The signal of mass is typically suppressed on fat saturation T1-weighted SE axial image. (**c**) The extension of lipoma and the relationship to the superficial branche of radial nerve (*arrowheads*) are shown in the T2-weighted sagittal plane

be viewed. Moreover, the site and cause of entrapment may be discovered with MR imaging by following the nerve implicated from the distribution of abnormal muscle on MR imaging [60]. In subacute denervation, the affected muscles have prolongation of T1 and T2 relaxation times secondary to the muscle fiber shrinkage and associated increases in extracellular water [61]. These changes therefore cause increased signal within the muscles innervated on the T2-weighted or STIR images followed to resolution or progressive atrophy and fatty infiltration [62].

Radiographically occult or equivocal fractures may be assessed with MR imaging. MR imaging may identify or exclude supracondylar fractures in children when radiographic evidence of a joint effusion is present and a fracture is not visualized. CT scan is the best technique when additional information about the fracture morphology or degree of comminution is needed. MR imaging may detect and characterize radial head fractures and is useful to exclude associated collateral ligament injury (Fig. 28).

MRI can be useful in the assessment of osteochondral injury and intra-articular bodies [63, 64]. Osteochondral lesions appear as well-defined focal areas of abnormal marrow signal intensity in the subchondral bone of the capitellum (Fig. 29). MRI

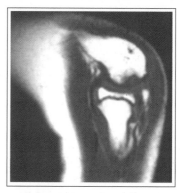

Fig. 29. Osteochondritis dissecans. Sagittal T1-weighted MR image reveals a low signal intensity lesion in the anterior aspect of the capitellum

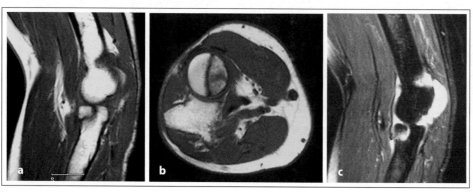

Fig. 28. Radial head fracture. T1-weighted sagittal (**a**) and axial (**b**) images reveal a minimally displaced fracture of the anterior aspect of the radial head. A STIR sagittal image (**c**) shows the radial head fracture as well as an effusion

can reliably detect and stage the lesions. Unstable lesions are characterized by fluid encircling the osteochondral fragment on T2-weighted images. The fragment may migrate throughout the joint as loose bodies. Small fragments, particularly those made only of cartilage, are difficult to identify without the surrounding fluid of an effusion. For this reason, STIR or T2-weighted fat suppression MR images are recommended. Large osseous fragment may contain fatty marrow and therefore may be easily seen on T1-weighted MR images. The accuracy of staging is improved by performing MR arthrography using dilute gadolinium [65, 66].

Injuries to the biceps and triceps tendons are well seen with MRI. Injury patterns may range from tendinitis to partial or complete disruptions [67, 68]. Distal biceps tendinosis is common and has been shown to precede spontaneous tendon rupture [69]. Tears usually involve the distal aspect of the tendon near its insertion on the radial tuberosity as a result of resisted elbow flexion [70]. MRI provides useful information regarding the degree of tearing, the size of the gap, and the location of the tear for preoperative planning [71]. Sagittal and axial T2-weighted or STIR MR images are the most specific for grading the extent of injury. The disrupted tendon can be seen along the expected course of the tendon sheath anterior to the brachial muscle. Large fluid collections or hematoma within the sheath aid diagnosis. The triceps tendon typically avulses from its attachment on the olecranon by falling an a flexed arm or secondary to forced hyperextension. Complete tears of the triceps tendon are thought to be much more common than partial tears [72].

The superior contrast discrimination provided by MR imaging has proved extremely useful in the evaluation of bone and soft tissue tumors [73, 74]. MR imaging of bone tumors and masses in the elbow follows the general caveats for imaging of tumors elsewhere in the musculoskeletal system. Di-

rect multiplanar imaging facilitates improved preoperative evaluation of the exact extent of a lesion. A combination of both T1- and T2-weighted MR sequences should be performed in at least two planes (Fig. 30). T1-weighted images provide excellent contrast for identification of marrow, cortical, and soft tissue involvement. Conventional fat-suppressed, T2-weighted images are valuable in distinguishing muscle from tumor and can increase diagnostic specificity in evaluating marrow infiltration. Images should be obtained before and after the intravenous administration of gadolinium DTPA to evaluate the vascularity of the lesion and to better define its characterization [75].

Articular Contrastographies

Contrastographic techniques are based on the injection of one or two contrast agents in the articular space and can be performed either through a radiographic study (conventional arthrography) or using modalities like CT (CT arthrography) or MR (MR arthrography).

Conventional arthrography of the elbow can be performed both with a single contrast agent, by injecting an iodinated solution in the articular cavity [76] or with double contrast, by injecting an iodinated contrast agent and air [77]. In this examination technique radiographs are performed in several projections (antero-posterior, lateral, and oblique) both before and after the injection procedure, which is usually carried out under fluoroscopic guidance. Usually the puncture is made with a lateral approach, at the level of the radial capitellum, with a needle of 21-23 gauge. In cases of resection of the radial capitellum the approach can be posteriorly.

Since the anatomic complexity of the elbow makes it difficult to represent the various profiles of

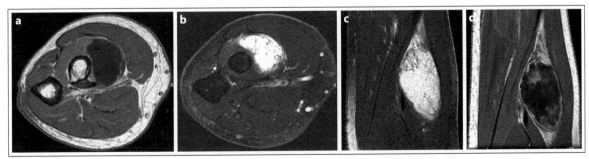

Fig. 30. Intramuscular hemangioma of the supinator muscle. The mass demonstrates hypointensity on T1-weighted axial image (**a**) and lobulated hyperintensity on fat suppressed T2-weighted axial (**b**) and coronal images (**c**). The mass shows inhomogenous enhancement after administration of intravenous gadolinium on T1-weighted coronal image (**d**)

the articular surfaces, arthrography can be effectively completed by arthrotomography [76].

Arthrotomography consists of a series of tomograms to be performed both before and after the injection of preferably two contrast agents. Usually tomograms are performed in antero-posterior and lateral projection with an interval of about 3 mm. Arthrography and arthrotomography in the past were employed to detect loose bodies and in the study of articular structures that were not visible with the radiographic examination. Now these modalities are rarely used, usually replaced by more recent imaging modalities like CT and MR.

CT arthrography can be performed both with a single iodinated contrast medium and with a double contrast [78]. In the latter case both an iodinated contrast agent and air are injected. The examination procedure consists, after the articular injection, of a high resolution CT study of the elbow (thin slices, low pitch, small field of view, etc.) and subsequent use of multiplanar imaging. CT arthrography is indicated for the visualization of intra-articular loose bodies, in capitellum osteochondrosis (Panner's Disease), in the study of the articular cartilage and to detect ligamental lesions in case of elbow instability.

In MR arthrography [79] a physiologic solution containing a paramagnetic contrast agent (gadolinium-DTPA) is injected into the articular space

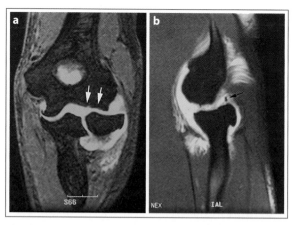

Fig. 32. Osteoarthritis of the elbow. MR arthrography on a fat-suppressed T1-weigthed coronal image (**a**) reveals irregular chondral surface of the trochlea with small foci of decreased signal (*arrows*) and minimal spurring of the medial margin of coronoid process. A fat-suppressed, T1-weighted sagittal image (**b**) depicts irregular aspect of capitellum and the radial head as well as a small loose body (*arrow*)

(Fig. 31). MR study consists of sequences obtained on the various planes (axial, coronal, and sagittal), using a surface coil to produce images of high quality. MR arthrography has proved very useful to detect pathologic abnormalities of the capsule and ligaments, such as capsular tears and partial or complete lesions of the ulnar collateral ligament. This methodology is also particularly indicated for the assessment of fragment stability in osteochondral fractures and in degenerative osteoarthritis (Fig. 32) [80].

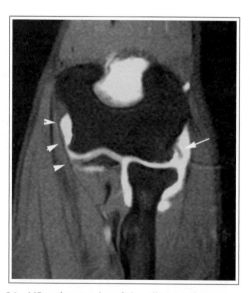

Fig. 31. MR arthrography of the elbow. A fat suppressed T1-weighted coronal image obtained after intra-articular injection of gadolinium shows the normal capsular anatomy of the joint. The anterior bundle of medial collateral ligament attaching to the medial margin of coronoid process (*arrowheads*). The contrast extends through a large distension of lateral capsule and annular recess. A lateral synovial fringe is seen (*arrow*)

References

1. Stoller DW (1997) Magnetic resonance imaging in orthopaedics & sports medicine, 2nd edn. Lippincott-Raven, Philadelphia
2. Stoller DW, Tirman PFJ (2004) Diagnostic imaging orthopaedics. Amirsys Elsevier Saunders, Philadelphia
3. Manaster BJ, Disler DG, May DA (2002) Musculoskeletal imaging: the requisites, 2nd edn. Mosby, St Louis
4. Berquist TH (2000) Diagnostic imaging of the elbow. In: Morrey BF (ed) The elbow and its disorders, 3rd edn. Saunders, Philadelphia, pp 84-101
5. Fritz RC, Steinbach LS, Tirman PFJ et al (1997) MR imaging of the elbow. An update Radiol Clin North Am 35:117-144
6. Sonin AH, Tutton SM, Fitzgerald SW et al (1996) MR imaging of the adult elbow. Radiographics 16:1323-1336
7. Steinbach LS, Schwartz ML (1998) Elbow arthrography. Radiol Clin N Am 36:635-649
8. Timmerman LA, Schwartz ML, Andrews JR (1994) Preoperative evaluation of the ulnar collateral ligament by mag-

netic resonance imaging and computed tomography arthrography. Am J Sports Med 22:26-31

9. Lynne SS, William EP, Mark ES (2002) Special focus session: MR arthrography. RadioGraphics 22:1223-1246

10. Munshi M, Pretterklieber ML, Chung CB et al (2004) Anterior bundle of ulnar collateral ligament: evaluation of anatomic relationships by using MR imaging, MR arthrography, and gross anatomic and histologic analysis. Radiology 231:797-803

11. Berquist TH (1993) Diagnostic radiographic techniques of the elbow. In: Morrey BF (ed) The elbow and its disorders, 2nd edn. Saunders, Philadelphia, pp 98-119

12. Bledsoe RC, Izenstark JL (1959) Displacement of fat pads in disease and injury of the elbow. A new radiographic sign. Radiology 73:717-724

13. Bohrer SP (1970) The fat pad sign following elbow trauma. Clin Radiol 21:90-94

14. Greenspan A, Norman A (1982) The radial head, capitellar view. Useful technique in elbow trauma. Am J Roentgenol 138:1186-1188

15. Dalinka MK, Boorstein JM, Zlatkin MB (1989) Computed tomography of musculoskeletal trauma. Radiol Clin North Am 27:933-944

16. Pretorius ES, Fishman EK (1995) Helical (spiral) CT of the musculoskeletal system. Radiol Clin North Am 33:949-979

17. Fishman EK, Kuszyk B (2001) 3D imaging: musculoskeletal applications. Crit Rev Diagn Imaging 42:59-100

18. Martinoli C, Bianchi S, Giovagnorio F et al (2001) Ultrasound of the elbow. Skeletal Radiol 30:605-614

19. Chiou HJ, Chou YH, Chiou SY et al (2003) Peripheral nerve lesions: role of high-resolution US. Radiographics 23:e15

20. De Smet AA, Winter TC, Best TM et al (2002) Dynamic sonography with valgus stress to assess elbow ulnar collateral ligament injury in baseball pitchers. Skeletal Radiol 31:671-676

21. Connell D, Burke F, Coombes P et al (2001) Sonographic examination of lateral epicondylitis. Am J Roentgenol 176:777-782

22. Dayna L, Levon NN, Theodore TM et al (2005) Lateral epicondylitis of the elbow: US findings. Radiology 237:230-234

23. Spina V, Montanari N, Romagnoli R (1998) Il Gomito. In: Simonetti G, Del Maschio A, Bartolozzi C, Passariello R (eds) Trattato Italiano di Risonanza Magnetica, Idelson-Gnocchi ed, vol. 3, pp 1305-1338

24. Stark DD, Bradley WG (1988) Magnetic resonance imaging. Mosby, St Louis

25. Berquist TH (1991) Imaging of orthopaedic trauma, 2nd edn. Raven, New York

26. Mallisee TA, Boynton MD, Erickson SJ et al (1997) Normal MR imaging anatomy of the elbow. Magn Reson Imaging Clin N Am 5:451-479

27. Bunnell DH, Fisher DA, Bassett LW et al (1987) Elbow joint: normal anatomy on MR images. Radiology 165:527-531

28. An KN, Morrey BF (2000) Biomechanics of the elbow. In: Morrey BF (ed) The elbow and its disorders, 3rd edn. Saunders, Philadelphia, pp 43-60

29. Callaway GH, Field LD, Deng XH et al (1997) Biomechanical evaluation of the medial collateral ligament of the elbow. J Bone Joint Surg Am 79:1223-1231

30. Morrey BF, An KN (1985) Functional anatomy of the ligaments of the elbow. Clin Orthop 201:84-89

31. Jordan SE (1996) Surgical anatomy of the elbow In: Jobe FW (ed) Operative techniques in upper extremity sports injury. Mosby, St. Louis, p 402

32. Morrey BF (2000) Anatomy of the elbow. In: Morrey BF (ed) The elbow and its disorders, 3rd edn. Saunders, Philadelphia, pp 13-42

33. O'Driscoll SW, Bell DF, Morrey BF (1991) Posterolateral rotatory instability of the elbow. J Bone Joint Surg Am 73:440-446

34. Cohen MS, Hastings H (1995) Rotatory stabilizers of the elbow: the lateral stabilizers. J Shoulder Elbow Surg 4:S10

35. Mirowitz SA, London SL (1992) Ulnar collateral ligament injury in baseball pitchers: MR imaging evaluation. Radiology 185:573-576

36. Hill NB, Bucchieri JS, Shon F et al (2000) Magnetic resonance imaging of injury to the medial collateral ligament of the elbow: a cadaver model. J Shoulder Elbow Surg 9:418-422

37. Conway JE, Jobe FW, Glousman RE et al (1992) Medial instability of the elbow in throwing athletes. J Bone Joint Surg Am 74:67-83

38. Joyce ME, Jelsma RD, Andrews JR (1995) Throwing injuries of the elbow. Sports Med Arthosc Rev 3:224-226

39. Fleisig GS, Andrews JR, Dillman C et al (1995) Kinetics of baseball pitching with implication about injury mechanisms. Am J Sports Med 23:233-239

40. Timmerman LA, Andrews JR.(1994) Undersurface tear of the ulnar collateral ligament in baseball players. A newly recognized lesion. Am J Sports Med 22:33-36

41. Timmerman LA, Schwartz ML, Andrews JR (1994) Preoperative evaluation of the ulnar collateral ligament by magnetic resonance imaging and computed tomography arthrography. Evaluation in 25 baseball players with surgical confirmation. Am J Sports Med 22:26-31

42. Schwartz ML, Al-Zahrani S, Morwessel RM et al (1995) Ulnar collateral ligament injury in the throwing athlete: Evaluation with saline-enhanced MR arthrography. Radiology 197:297-299

43. Conway JE, Jobe FW, Glousman RE et al (1992) Medial instability of the elbow in throwing athletes: Treatment by repair or reconstruction of the ulnar collateral ligament. J Bone Joint Surg Am 74:67-83

44. Mulligan SA, Schwartz ML, Broussard MF et al (2000) Heterotopic calcification and tears of the ulnar collateral ligament: Radiographic and MR imaging findings. Am J Roentgenol 175:1099-1102

45. Potter HG, Weiland AJ, Schatz JA et al (1997) Posterolateral rotatory instability of the elbow: Usefulness of MR imaging in diagnosis. Radiology 204:185-189

46. Bennett JB (1994) Lateral and medial epicondylitis. Hand Clin 10:157-163

47. Potter HG, Hannafin JA, Morwessel RM et al (1995) Lateral epicondylitis: correlation of MR imaging, surgical, and histopathologic findings. Radiology 196:43-46

48. Martin CE, Schweitzer ME (1998) MR imaging of epicondylitis. Skeletal Radiol 27:133-138

49. Miller TT, Shapiro MA, Schultz E et al (2002) Comparison of sonography and MRI for diagnosing epicondylitis. J Clin Ultrasound 30:193-202

50. Nirschl RP (1992) Elbow tendinosis/tennis elbow. Clin Sports Med 11:851-870

51. Wittenberg RH, Schaal S, Muhr G (1992) Surgical treatment of persistent elbow epicondylitis. Clin Orthop 278:73-80

52. Werner CO (1979) Lateral elbow pain and posterior interosseous nerve entrapment. Acta Orthop Scand 174:1-62
53. Rosenberg ZS, Beltran J, Cheung YY et al (1993) The elbow: MR features of nerve disorders. Radiology 188:235-240
54. Beltran J, Rosenberg ZS (1998) Nerve entrapment. Semin Musculoskelet Radiol 2:175-184
55. Folberg CR, Weiss APC, Akelman E et al (1994) Cubital tunnel syndrome: Part I. Presentation and diagnosis. Orthop Rev 23:136-144
56. Britz GW, Haynor DR, Kuntz C et al (1996) Ulnar nerve entrapment at the elbow: Correlation of magnetic resonance imaging, clinical, electrodiagnostic, and intraoperative findings. Neurosurgery 38:458-465
57. Spinner M, Linscheid RL (2000) Nerve entrapment syndromes. In: Morrey BF (ed) The Elbow and its disorders, 3rd edn. Saunders, Philadelphia, pp 839-869
58. Ogino T, Minami A, Kato H (1991) Diagnosis of radial nerve palsy caused by ganglion with use of different imaging techniques. J Hand Surg Am 16:230-235
59. Spinner RJ, Carmichael SW, Spinner M (1991) Partial median nerve entrapment in the distal arm because of an accessory bicipital aponeurosis. J Hand Surg Am 16:236
60. Uetani M, Hayash K, Matosunaga N et al (1993) Denervated skeletal muscle: MR imaging. Radiology 189:511-515
61. Polak JF, Jolesz FA, Adams DF (1988) Magnetic resonance imaging examination of skeletal muscle prolongation of T1 and T2 subsequent to denervation. Invest Radiol 23:365-369
62. Fleckenstein JL, Watumull D, Conner KE et al (1993) Denervated human skeletal muscle: MR imaging evaluation. Radiology 187:213-218
63. Quinn SF, Haberman JJ, Fitzgerald SW (1994) Evaluation of loose bodies in the elbow with MR imaging. J Magn Reson Imaging 4:169-172
64. Mesgarzadeh M, Sapega AA, Bonakdarpour A et al (1987) Osteochondritis dissecans: analysis of mechanical stability with radiography, scintigraphy, and MR imaging. Radiology 165:775-780
65. Peiss J, Adam G, Casser R et al (1995) Gadopentetate-dimeglumine-enhanced MR imaging of osteonecrosis and osteochondritis dissecans of the elbow: initial experience. Skeletal Radiol 24:17-20
66. Kramer J, Stiglbauer R, Engel A et al (1992) MR contrast arthrography (MRA) in osteochondrosis dissecans. J Comput Assist Tomogr 16:254-260
67. Falchook FS, Zlatkin MB, Erbacher GE et al (1994) Rupture of the distal biceps tendon: evaluation with MR imaging. Radiology 190:659-663
68. Fitzgerald SW, Curry DR, Erickson SJ et al (1994) Distal biceps tendon injury: MR imaging diagnosis. Radiology 191:203-206
69. Kannus P, Jozsa L (1991) Hisptopathological changes preceding spontaneous rupture of a tendon: a controlled study of 891 patients. J Bone Joint Surg Am 73:1507-1525
70. Morrey BF (2000) Injury of the flexors of the elbow: biceps in tendon injury. In: Lampert R (ed) The elbow and its disorders, 3rd edn. Saunders, Philadelphia, pp 468-478
71. Chew ML, Giuffrè B (2005) Disorders of the distal biceps brachii tendon. RadioGraphics 25:1227-1237
72. Tarsney FF (1972) Rupture and avulsion of the triceps. Clin Orthop 83:177-183
73. Zlatkin MB, Chao Ph, Kricun ME et al (1990) The use of magnetic resonance imaging in the evaluation of bone and soft-tissue tumors. Radiol Clin North Am 28:461-470
74. LH Wetzel, E Levine, MD Murphey (1987) A comparison of MR imaging and CT in the evaluation of musculoskeletal masses. Radiographics 7:851-874
75. Benedikt RA, Jelinek JS, Kransdorf MJ et al (1994) MR imaging of soft-tissue masses: role of gadopentate dimeglumine. JMRI 4:485-490
76. Eto RT, Anderson PW, Harley JD (1975) Elbow arthrography with application of tomography. Radiology 115:283-288
77. Pavlov H, Ghelman B, Warren RF (1979) Double-contrast arthrography of the elbow. Radiology 130:87-95
78. Singson RD, Feldman F, Rosenberg ZS (1986) The elbow joint: Assessment with double-contrast CT arthrography. Radiology 160:167-173
79. Grainger AJ, Elliott JM, Campbell RS et al (2000) Direct MR arthrography: a review of current use. Clin Radiol 55:163-176
80. Kramer J, Stiglbauer R, Engel A et al (1992) MR contrast arthrography (MRA) in osteochondrosis dissecans. J Comput Assist Tomogr 16:254-260

CHAPTER 4

Elbow Surgical Approaches

A. CELLI, L. CELLI

Introduction

This is a review of the basic procedures in the surgical management of acute and chronic elbow lesions. The following approaches are generally the most used in elbow surgery and they allow the practicing orthopedic surgeon to treat any injury or disorder.

Surgeons should have a deep knowledge of functional and surgical anatomy in order to avoid injury to nervous and vascular structures.

In the last century, after the Kocher's first description in the "Textbook of Operative Surgery" [1], many authors described elbow approaches with the purpose to improve surgical outcome as well as to reduce complications. Every approach should consider primarily the relationship between the elbow and neurovascular structures (the relevant anatomy is discussed in Chap. 1).

When we perform surgery in the elbow medial or lateral aspect, the forearm-sensitive terminal branches of the skin are at risk, hence their injury causes the postsurgical symptomatic paresthesia, the formation of a painful neuroma, or a significant rate of sensory loss in the lateral or medial skin of the elbow and forearm.

A histological study [2] confirms that there are less and smaller cutaneous nerves in the posterior region of the elbow than in the lateral and medial region.

The midline posterior skin incision can be considered a safe skin incision if full-thickness fascio-cutaneous flaps are elevated at the level of the deep fascia, because it preserves the lateral and medial cutaneous nerves and the subcutaneous vascular plexus [3].

The anterior approach through the cubital fossa between the borders of the brachioradialis and pronator teres muscles (as extensile Henry's approach) is less used in the recent years because of the frequent neurovascular complications that can often occur in this approach.

All the reconstructive procedures of the elbow lesions can be done through a lateral, medial, or posterior extensile or limited skin incision in the safe internervous plane. The internervous plane is the intermuscular space where the two facing muscles receive supply from two different nerves.

The Posterolateral and Lateral Exposure

The indications include:
- fractures of the radial head or capitellum;
- fractures of the lateral column of the distal humerus and coronal sheer fracture;
- repair or reconstruction of the lateral collateral ligament and annular ligament;
- lateral tennis elbow debridement;
- release or reconstruction of the posterior interosseous nerve (PIN);
- release of post-traumatic elbow contracture with or without arthritis;
- radial head resection or replacement;
- resurfacing arthroplasty.

Patient's Position

The patient is in a supine position, his arm is placed on the table with a tourniquet. The elbow

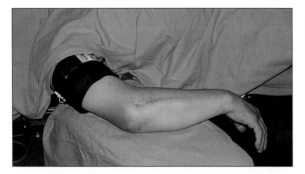

Fig. 1. Patient is in supine position with the arm on the table

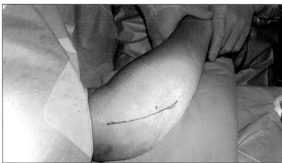

Fig. 3. The Kocher's skin incision runs from the supra-condylar ridge towards the lateral epicondyle over the radial head until the posterior border of the ulna

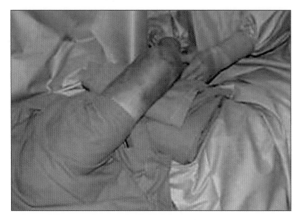

Fig. 2. Patient is in supine position with the elbow across the chest

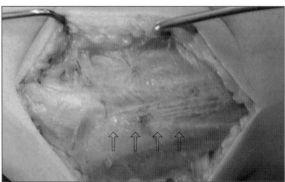

Fig. 4. The Kocher's interval is identified as a thin strip between the anconeus muscle and the extensor carpi ulnaris

is flexed while the patient's forearm is pronated (Fig. 1). If the surgeon chooses the extensive exposure option to approach the elbow anteriorly and posteriorly, it is useful to bring the elbow across the chest with the patient in a supine position (Fig. 2).

The Kocher's Approach

This extensile deep exposure [4] needs a straight posterolateral skin incision (about 16 cm): the incision runs from the humerus supracondylar ridge (about 8 cm) towards the lateral epicondyle, over the radial head, until the posterior border of the ulna (about 8 cm) (Fig. 3).

In the subcutaneous tissues the terminal branches of the lateral cutaneous nerve need protection.

The landmarks below the subcutaneous tissues are:
- proximally, the lateral column between the extensor carpi radialis longus and the triceps insertion on the posterior aspect of the humerus;
- distally from the epicondyle, the Kocher's interval (between the anconeus muscle and the ex-

tensor carpi ulnaris) can be identified as a thin strip of fat below the deep fascia (Fig. 4).

In the proximal half of Kocher's skin incision a deep dissection is performed between triceps muscle posteriorly and the brachioradialis muscle and extensor carpi radialis longus anteriorly. In the distal half of the Kocher's skin incision the deep dissection is made in the Kocher's interval.

The posterolateral approach can be performed, for specific purpose, only as a limited proximal approach, or a distal limited lateral approach or extensile posterolateral approach.

The posterolateral approach described by Kocher is realized by combining the two limited exposures [4].

The Proximal Limited Kocher's Approach (Lateral Column Approach)

This approach [5] is useful in the surgical treatment of the extension or flexion-extension elbow contracture without any intrinsic lesion.

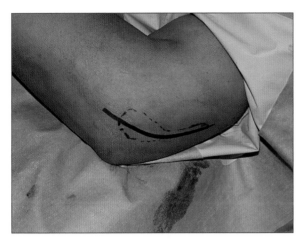

Fig. 5. The lateral column approach is the proximal half of the Kocher's skin incision

The supracondylar bone proximal to the lateral epicondyle, both anteriorly and posteriorly, is called "column" [5].

The proximal half of the Kocher's skin incision is performed about 6-8 cm in length (Fig. 5).

The insertion of the brachioradialis and extensor carpi radialis longus are elevated from the supracondylar ridge (Fig. 6a) and the brachialis muscle too is detached with a periosteal elevator from the anterior aspect of the lateral column (Figs. 6b, c).

The anterior capsule is isolated and a Homann retractor can be used to protect and retract the anterolateral muscles and nerve structures: the excision of the thick anterior capsule can be executed (Fig. 7a, b).

If the range of movement (flexion and extension) is not complete, the capsule is released posteriorly. If the triceps is elevated from the posterolateral column, the posterior capsule is excised, the olecranon fossa is cleaned off the tissue, and the tip of the olecranon is osteotomized (Fig. 8).

The Distal Limited Kocher's Approach

In the distal half of Kocher's approach, the skin incision runs from the lateral epicondyle to the posterior border of the ulna.

In the deep dissection, the interval between the anconeus and the extensor carpi ulnaris (ECU) is recognizable: these are the major landmarks for the direct deep approach (Fig. 9).

The fascia is opened and the anconeus muscle and the extensor carpi ulnaris are retracted, then

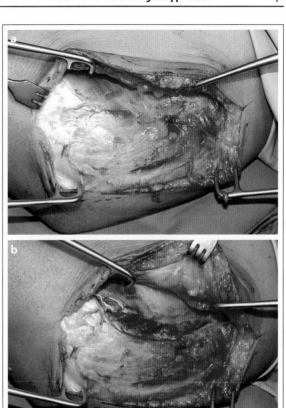

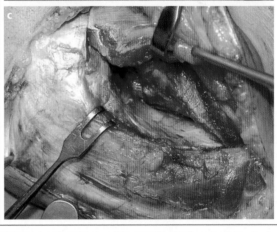

Fig. 6 a-c. The proximal limited Kocher's approach: the insertion of the brachioradialis and extensor carpi radialis longus are elevated from the supracondylar ridge and the brachialis muscle is detached from the anterior aspect of the lateral column

we coagulate the little branches of the recurrent interosseous artery and vein: thus, the joint capsule, the lateral collateral ligament (LCL) complex, and the posterior origin of the supinator muscle are exposed (Fig. 10).

Care must be taken to recognize the posterior bundle of the lateral collateral ligament complex

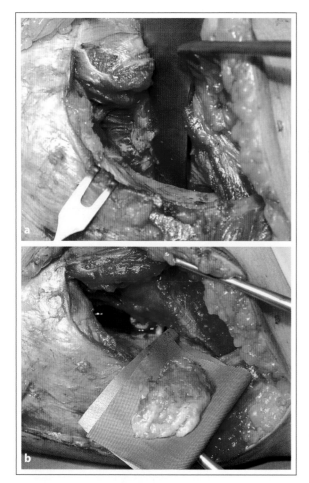

Fig. 7 a, b. The proximal limited Kocher's approach: the anterior capsula is exposed and its excision is performed

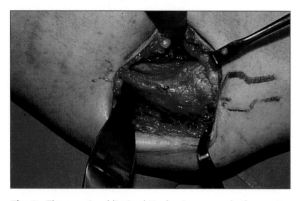

Fig. 8. The proximal limited Kocher's approach: the posterior capsula can be released, elevating the triceps from the posterior-lateral column

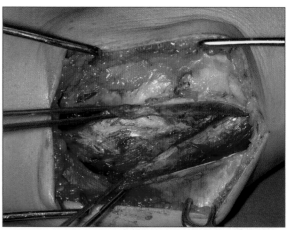

Fig. 9. The distal limited Kocher's approach: the Kocher's interval is identified between the anconeus and the extensor carpi ulnaris and the lateral collateral ligament is exposed

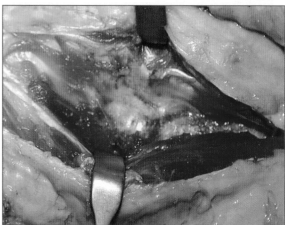

Fig. 10. The distal limited Kocher's approach: the little branches of the recurrent interosseous artery and vein are identified in the Kocher's interval

(LCL) and the annular ligament. In acute trauma with postero lateral rotatory instability, the LCL is disrupted. Afterwards it is recognized as the LCL complex: the exposure runs through the site of the

disruption. The radial head is exposed. In case of unrecoverable fractures the surgical management has to consider the correct level of the radial head resection for replacement with metallic implant and the anatomical reconstruction of the lateral ligament complex and muscle origins back to the lateral epicondyle (Fig. 11a, b).

If the LCL is not disrupted in acute trauma in radial head fractures without instability or in chronic lesions with radial head malunions or nonunions, the posterior bundle of the LCL and the annular ligament are recognizable.

The incision of the annular ligament is performed anteriorly in relation to the LCL (Fig. 12a, b) to prevent posterolateral rotatory instability: the back-to-origin reinsertion can be easily done pre-

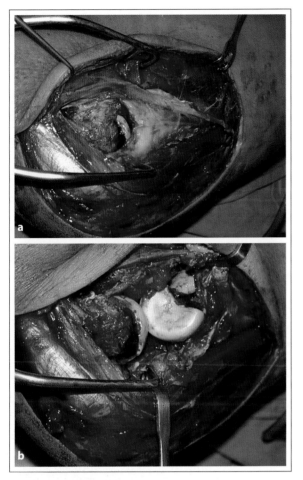

Fig. 11 a, b. The distal limited Kocher's approach: if the lateral collateral ligament is disrupted, the exposure runs through the site of the disruption

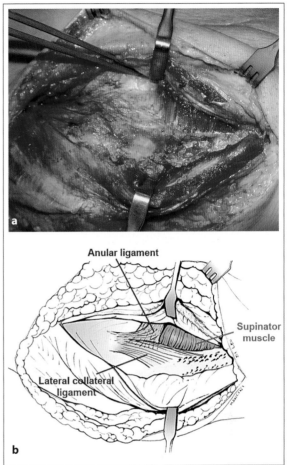

Fig. 12 a, b. The distal limited Kocher's approach: through the Kocher's interval the lateral collateral ligament and the annular ligament are recognizable

serving the function of the anterior bundle of the LCL and the annular ligament.

If a metallic radial head prosthesis has to be inserted, the proximal ulnar insertion of the supinator muscle is detached for 2-3 cm and thus the radial neck is exposed.

This approach offers more protection to the PIN, which usually emerges at 5,9 cm [6], that is, the mean distance from the radial head articular surface. In order to reduce the risk of nerve injury it is possible to remove the PIN away from the surgical field through full forearm pronation and also the release of the supinator muscle close to the ulna and the medial reflection of the two heads of this muscle (Fig. 13) [6].

In this way the neck of the radius is exposed and the nerve is at safe distance: thanks to a fit technique of radial head prosthesis implant, the correct resection of the radial neck is performed safely (Fig. 14a, b).

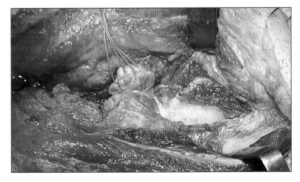

Fig. 13. The distal limited Kocher's approach: if the radial neck must be exposed the supinator muscle is detached close to the ulna

If the radial head fracture is not associated with elbow instability after the limited dissection of the extensor carpi ulnaris, the anterior capsule is opened anteriorly to the lateral complex: the frac-

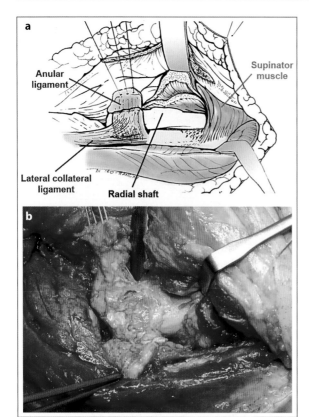

Fig. 14 a, b. The medial reflection of the two heads of the supinator muscle allows the exposure of the radial neck, avoiding damage to the posterior interosseous nerve

ture is reduced and stabilized with miniscrews. The screws can be applied through the nonarticular portion of the edge of the radial head that does not articulate with the ulna either in full pronation or in full supination.

The Extensile Kocher's Approach

The limited proximal and distal Kocher's exposure have been already described above.

For a more extensile approach the surgeon performs both the limited proximal and distal exposure (about 16 cm) [1].

The skin incision begins at 8 cm proximally to the joint and it goes on distally along the Kocher's interval, ending at the edge of the ulna.

The deep dissection allows the surgeon to divaricate proximally the triceps muscle from the brachioradialis and the extensor carpi radialis longus as well as to diverge distally the anconeus muscle from the common extensor tendon insertion.

The common extensor tendon is released from the lateral epicondyle of the humerus as it is necessary to expose the anterior capsule and the anterolateral joint compartment. The anconeus is reflected subperiostally from the ulna and it is separated from the lateral ligament, preserving its fascial attachment to triceps. When the posterior capsula has to be excised the triceps muscle is elevated from the posterior aspect of the humerus.

The extensile Kocher's approach is used in case of joint stiffness complex release, complex fractures, synoviectomy, fracture-dislocation, and debridement-arthroplasty.

The Posteromedial and Medial Exposure

These approaches are indicated in case of:
- contracture release in a stiff elbow;
- posteromedial osteophytes or heterotopic ossification;
- delayed treatment of the elbow subluxation or dislocation;
- the ulnar nerve lesion or compression in the cubital tunnel;
- the treatment of medial collateral ligament lesion;
- open reduction, internal fixation (ORIF) of the coronoid fracture;
- the treatment of the medial epicondylitis.

Patient's Position

The patient is in a supine position on the operating table, his upper limb is externally rotated and lies on a hand table. The tourniquet should be applied.

The Skin Incision

The skin incision can be either limited direct medial or extensile posteromedial. It is usually centered on the medial epicondyle, then it extends 4-5 cm long in a proximal and distal direction (total length: 8-10 cm).

In the subcutaneous tissue it is very important to identify and protect the arm and forearm medial cutaneous nerve branches that cross the incision.

The injury may lead to painful neuroma formation. Once divaricated, the cutaneous tissue of many structures are visible: the medial epicondyle, the flexor pronator mass and brachialis muscles tendon anteriorly, the triceps tendon, and the olecranon posteriorly.

The Medial "Over the Top" Approach

This extensile deep exposure described by Hotchkiss [7] allows access to the anterior, the posterior, and the medial aspect of the elbow joint.

The skin incision runs 15-20 cm long in the posterior medial region of the elbow (Fig. 15).

The bone landmarks are the humerus supracondylar bridge, the medial epicondyle, and the posterior and medial edge of the olecranon and ulna.

In the subcutaneous tissue the terminal branches of the medial antebrachial cutaneous nerve and the ulnar nerve in the cubital tunnel are isolated and protected.

It is possible to recognize distally, under the deep fascia, between both heads of flexor carpi ulnaris (FCU), the arcuate fibrous bands of Osborn's fascia: the ulnar nerve lies below it (cubital tunnel retinaculum).

The nerve can be palpated proximally at its supracondylar level before its entry in the cubital tunnel.

It is important to know the average distance of the neurovascular structures (brachial artery and median nerve) from the medial epicondyle, that is, 3-4 cm, and from the coronoid process, that is, 1.5 cm (Fig. 16) [7].

The landmarks for a deep dissection are proximally the intermuscular septum between the triceps and the brachialis muscle, and distally between the flexor pronator mass and the FCU humeral head (Fig. 17).

The ulnar nerve should be identified, released, and mobilized anteriorly over the medial flexor pronator mass in order to reduce the risk of lesion during the surgery (Fig. 18).

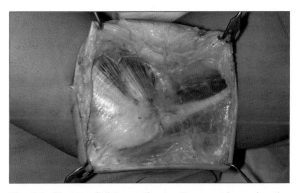

Fig. 16. The medial "over the top" approach: under the deep fascia the flexor-pronator muscles and the ulnar nerve are identified

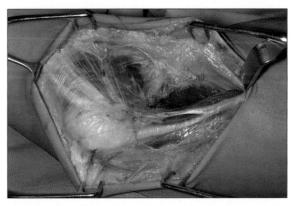

Fig. 17. The medial "over the top" approach: the deep dissection runs between the triceps and the brachialis muscle and distally between the flexor pronator mass and the flexor carpi ulnaris

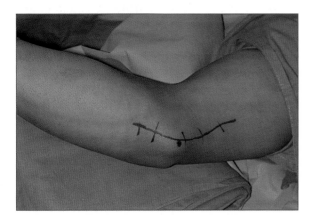

Fig. 15. The medial "over the top" approach: the skin incision runs 15-20 cm long in the posterior medial region of the elbow

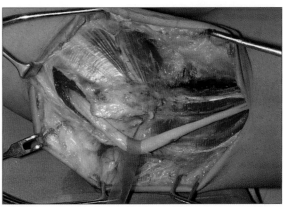

Fig. 18. The medial "over the top" approach: the ulnar nerve is released and mobilized anteriorly over the flexor pronator muscle

JET LIBRARY

The medial intermuscular septum can be excised proximally, taking care to clip the large vessel branches from the ulnar collateral artery that cross its base. The brachialis muscle is detached by a periosteal elevator from the humerus anterior cortex, and lifted by a wide Cobb retractor.

Distally, the splitting of the flexor-pronator mass is performed between the FCU (innervated by the ulnar nerve) and the flexor carpi radialis or palmaris longus, if present (innervated by the median nerve). This interval is identified by the pres-

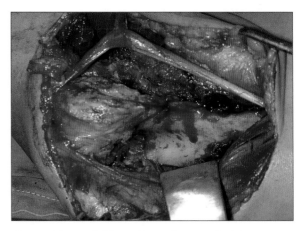

Fig. 20. The medial "over the top" approach: this approach can be extended posteriorly in order to expose the posterior capsula

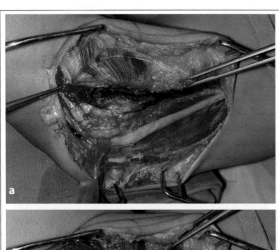
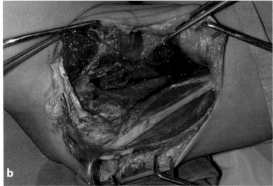
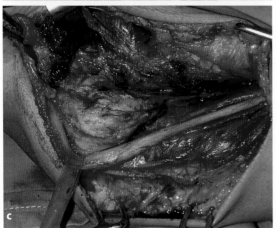

Fig. 19 a-c. The medial "over the top" approach: the anterior capsula and the medial collateral ligament are exposed

ence of the small vessels that pierce the fascia. These two muscles are split respecting their innervation. The palmaris longus, flexor carpi radialis, and pronator teres are dissected carefully 2 cm from their origin on the medial epicondyle. The elevation of the flexor-pronator mass allows the surgeon to see the anterior capsule. The lateral retraction of the muscle mass protects the median nerve and the brachial artery (Fig. 19a, b). The anterior capsule is excised, preserving the anterior bundle of the medial collateral ligament, and allowing the removal of heterotopic bone, the treatment of trochlea, and coronoid fractures, and also the reconstruction in case of medial collateral ligament deficiency (Fig. 19c).

This approach can be extended posteriorly in order to see the posterior capsule after raising the triceps from the humerus posterior surface, allowing the excision of the retracted periarticular soft tissue and posterior capsule (Fig. 20).

The Medial Column Procedure

This approach is performed with limited medial skin incision (6-8 cm long) for the treatment of:
- the contracture release and stiff elbow with or without heterotopic ossification or the ulnohumeral joint degenerative osteoarthritis;
- medial collateral ligament reconstruction.

The aim of the medial column procedure [5] is to release the anterior capsule and to remove safely with limited exposure the coronoid or olecranon osteophytes or heterotopic ossification when the bone osteo-articular anatomy is preserved.

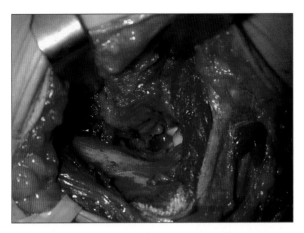

Fig. 21. The medial column procedure enables the exposure of the anterior capsula and of the coronoid process

The skin incision follows the medial humerus border proximally to the medial epicondyle.

The subcutaneous nerves and the intermuscular septum are exposed and the ulnar nerve is released, if necessary.

Once excised from the intermuscular septum, the anterior muscles are lifted up from the humerus anterior aspect with a Cobb elevator and a wide retractor allows the surgeon to see the anterior capsule, as well as the coronoid and the medial collateral ligament (Fig. 21). The extra-articular or intra-articular procedure can be carefully addressed.

If an interior capsulectomy is needed, a part of the common flexor tendon is reflected from the medial epicondyle, giving access to the anterior capsule: the brachialis muscle is easily retracted aside with a retractor and both the median nerve and the brachial artery are well protected with this approach.

The release of the Medial Collateral Ligament (MCL) posterior bundle is performed when the elbow movement is restricted in flexion and the posterior oblique bundle of the MCL is scarred and thickened: the correction of the flexion loss is obtained by excising the posterior part of the MCL and the posterior joint capsule [8, 9]. The origin of the humeral head flexor pronator muscle with the anterior part of the MCL are preserved.

The Posterior Exposure

The longitudinal posterior skin incision, made just lateral or just medial to the tip of olecranon, should be considered a universal skin incision for elbow surgery.

The posterior approach is extensible and it allows the exposition of all deep medial lateral and anterior structures of the elbow and most elbow surgery can be performed.

"The front door to the elbow is the back" [10, 11].

We can treat any disorder or injury in the posterior lateral and medial side of the elbow if a full thickness subcutaneous dissection is carried out: laterally through the Kocher's interval, and medially through Hotchkiss "over the top".

The indications include:
- reduction and fixation of distal humeral fractures;
- treatment of nonunion or malunion fractures;
- the operative reduction of the unreduced elbow subluxation or dislocation;
- the post-traumatic stiff elbow surgical treatment;
- the complex elbow instability with terrible triad and varus posteromedial instability;
- triceps tendon lesion;
- the Monteggia lesion with posterior olecranon fracture and radial head dislocations;
- the debridement of the osteoarthritic elbow;
- total elbow arthroplasty.

Position of the Patient

The patient is positioned:
- supine with the arm across the chest;
- prone with the arm abducted 90° and the elbow flexed with the forearm hanging vertically;
- controlateral decubitus with the upper arm supported on a bolster and the forearm hanging vertically free.

Surgical Landmarks

The posterior aspect of the olecranon and its relationship to the medial and lateral epicondyles should be identified.

The ulnar nerve can be palpated posteriorly to the supracondylar ridge.

The radial nerve lies about 20 cm proximally from the medial epicondyle and 12 cm from the lateral epicondyle [26].

Skin Incision

The posterior skin incisions (midline or posterolateral or posteromedial) are so flexible that all deep posterior, medial, and lateral exposures can be performed (Fig. 22).

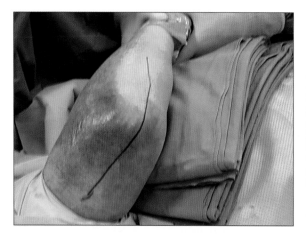

Fig. 22. The posterior skin incision is so flexible that the majority of the elbow approaches can be performed

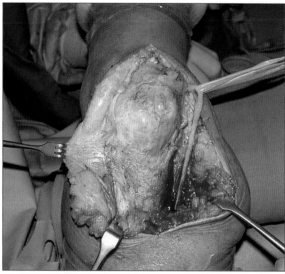

Fig. 24. The posterior exposure: the ulnar nerve is identified and dissected from the margin of the triceps until the first motor branch to the flexor carpi ulnaris

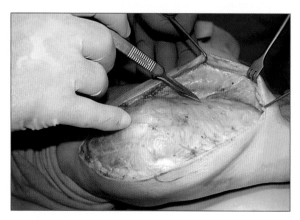

Fig. 23. The posterior exposure: the full thickness medial and lateral fascia-cutaneous flap is elevated

Currently, a straight midline linear incision centered at the level of the olecranon is usually preferred: it should avoid the tip of the olecranon.

The incision begins in the midline from 8 to 10 cm above the tip of the olecranon and it bends gently, medially or laterally, around the olecranon, finishing 8-10 cm below, over the midline subcutaneous tissue of the ulna.

The fascia overlying the triceps is incised and a full-thickness medial and/or lateral fascia cutaneous flap is elevated (Fig. 23).

The ulnar nerve is identified and carefully dissected from its bed and from the margin of the triceps in the cubital tunnel until the first motor branch to the FCU (Fig. 24).

In the posterior approach to the elbow the management of the triceps muscle tendon unit allows an adequate exposure.

In particular, when we perform the elbow arthroplasty it is advisable to use an approach that

removes the triceps off the ulna, giving the best exposure of the joint. This condition is essential in all revision arthroplasties. Otherwise, the triceps can be left inserted in the olecranon with elbow replacement for distal humerus fracture and nonunion.

The olecranon osteotomy is a surgical exposure that is useful in the treatment of complex intra-articular fractures of the distal humerus because it allows the best exposure of the humeral articular surface.

Different surgical managements of the extensor apparatus of the elbow could be performed, such as:
- triceps splitting;
- triceps reflecting;
- triceps preserving;
- triceps splitting and tendon reflection;
- triceps reflecting anconeus pedicle (TRAP);
- olecranon osteotomy.

Triceps Splitting (Campbell's Posterior Approach)

The midline split incision is made through the triceps muscle tendon unit and down to the tip of the olecranon where the dissection is continued subperiosteally.

The triceps insertion is released from the olecranon by reflecting the forearm muscles laterally (anconeus) and medially (FCU), allowing the exposure of the posterior distal humerus and elbow joint [13].

Indications:
- total elbow arthroplasty;

- unreduced elbow dislocation and supracondylar humerus fracture;
- elbow ankylosis;
- distal humerus malunion or nonunion.

    The surgical steps:

- A straight skin incision (about 10-15 cm) is performed and large and thick skin flaps are elevated medially and laterally.
- The ulnar nerve is identified and mobilized from its bed; the intermuscular septum is removed. The triceps extensor apparatus is visible. The triceps is split by excising from the proximal to the distal part of the muscle.
- The tendon insertion is peeled from the tip of the olecranon subperiosteally and the FCU and anconeus are released from the ulna (Fig. 25a, b).
- The splitting is extended by removing part of the tendon insertion from the medial and lateral epicondyle.
- The capsular release can be performed and the tip of the olecranon is excised to expose the trochlea (Fig. 26a, b).

    Simple sutures can repair the splitting of the tri-

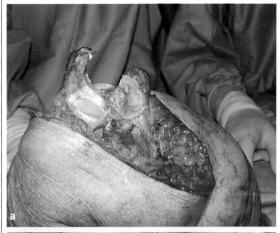
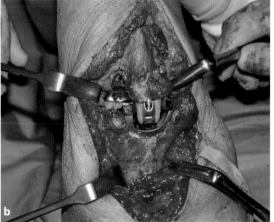

Fig. 26 a, b. Triceps Splitting: the elbow replacement can be performed using this approach

ceps: the tendon is attached to the tip of the olecranon through drill bone holes with a nonabsorbable suture number 5.

Triceps Reflecting or Triceps Sparing Approach (The Bryan-Morrey Approach)

The aim of an extensile triceps reflecting procedure is to preserve the continuity of the triceps and the anconeus with the forearm fascia and ulnar periosteum after detaching the extensor mechanism from the humerus and the olecranon. The Bryan-Morrey technique [14] reflects the triceps in continuity from the medial to the lateral side (Fig. 27).

Otherwise in the Kocher-modified Mayo technique the anconeus and the triceps are elevated from the olecranon and translocated from the lateral to the medial side.

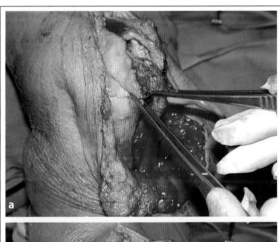
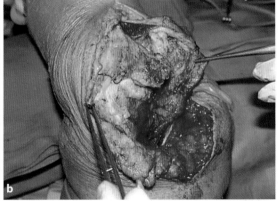

Fig. 25 a, b. Triceps Splitting: the tendon insertion is peeled from the tip of the olecranon subperiosteally and the flexor carpi ulnaris and the anconeus are elevated from the ulna

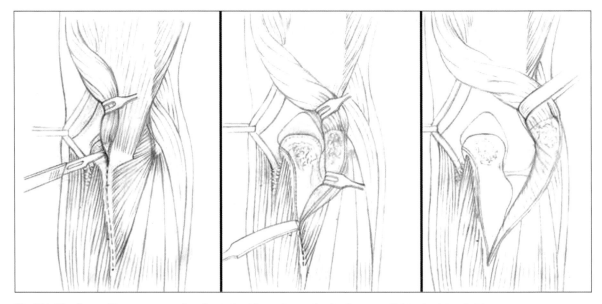

Fig. 27. The Bryan-Morrey approach reflects the triceps in continuity from medial to the lateral side

Indications:
- joint arthroplasty;
- unreduced dislocation;
- supracondylar fractures;
- elbow synoviectomy;
- joint stiffness.

The surgical steps:
- A straight skin incision in made between the medial epicondyle and the tip of olecranon (about 12-15 cm long).
- The ulnar nerve is isolated from the triceps edge and it is dissected so that it lies free from the cubital tunnel after removing the intermuscular septum.
- The medial aspect of the triceps is elevated subperiosteally from the humerus, and the fascia of the forearm is incised along the medial aspect of the proximal ulna (Fig. 28).
- In the periosteal plane the triceps is elevated from the olecranon and the ulna, maintaining the continuity of the extensor mechanism with the anconeus muscle as a single unit from the medial to the lateral side and from the proximal to the distal side.
- The capsule is excised and the tip of the olecranon is osteotomized if we have to implant the semiconstrained total elbow arthroplasty (TEA) both collateral ligament are resected. The elbow is fully flexed and the humerus is externally rotated; the joint is exposed (Fig. 29).

At the end the extensor apparatus can be reattached at the proximal ulna with a heavy nonabsorbable suture in the drill holes placed in the olecranon and the ulna.

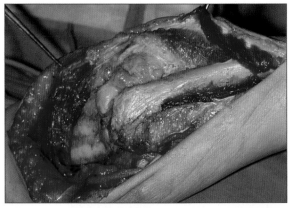

Fig. 28. The triceps reflecting: the medial aspect of the triceps is elevated subperiosteally from the humerus and the fascia of the forearm

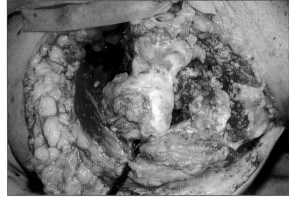

Fig. 29. The triceps reflecting: after the excision of the capsula, the elbow is fully flexed and the humerus is externally rotated; the joint is exposed

Triceps Preserving or "Triceps on" Approach (The Alonso-Llames Approach)

In certain circumstances the triceps attachment can not be released from the olecranon insertion. This surgical technique is not often indicated but it can be performed to implant an elbow prosthesis in older patients with articular comminute fractures [15].

In recent years we have implemented this technique in order to reduce the risk of triceps failure after elbow arthroplasty in patients with rheumatoid arthritis. Alonso-Llames [16] described a surgical approach called the "bilateral tricipital approach" that preserves the triceps attachment for the treatment of the supracondylar fractures in children.

Pierce and Herndon [17] and Boorman et al. [18] have reported the implant of the semiconstrained TEA without detaching the triceps.

Indications:
- ORIF in the supracondylar or noncomminute "T" intercondylar distal humerus fractures;
- TEA in elderly patients with osteopenic bone;
- TEA in the patients with rheumatoid or inflammatory arthritis and with fragile bone and soft tissues.

The surgical steps:
- The patient is in supine position with the arm over the chest. A straight posteromedial skin incision (about 15-20 cm long) is performed.
- The ulnar nerve is released from its bed and gently retracted with a rubber band.
- The full subcutaneous flap is elevated from the triceps aponeurosis from the lateral to the medial side (Fig. 30).
- The medial capsular release is performed, including the medial collateral ligament, the capsule, and the flexor pronator insertion. The posterolateral aspect of the joint is exposed.
- Through the Kocher's interval the lateral ligaments and the anterior capsule are released and the triceps and anconeus muscle are lifted up from the distal humerus and the ulna and translated medially (Fig. 31).
- The triceps is mobilized from the distal humerus in both lateral and medial sides, exposing the olecranon fossa, the medial and the lateral humerus column, and the lateral and medial collateral ligaments: the ligament attachments are resected completely if a semiconstrained prosthesis has to be implanted (Fig. 32).
- The lateral dislocation of the elbow is possible by hyperpronating the forearm. The ulnar nerve is

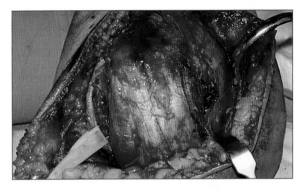

Fig. 30. The triceps preserving: the full subcutaneous flap is elevated from the triceps, from the lateral to the medial side; the ulnar nerve is released and gently retracted with a rubber band

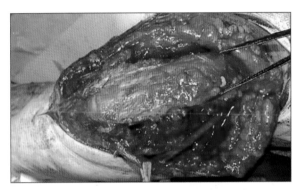

Fig. 31. The triceps preserving: through the Kocker's interval, the anconeus and the triceps are lifted up from the distal humerus

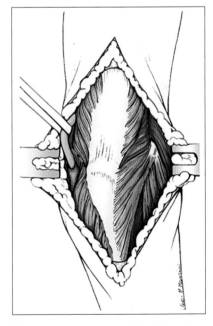

Fig. 32. The triceps preserving: the triceps is mobilized from the distal humerus in both lateral and medial side

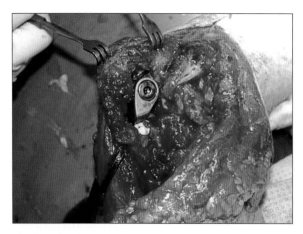

Fig. 33. The triceps preserving: the elbow replacement can be performed through this approach without detaching the triceps tendon from the olecranon

carefully protected during this manoeuvre, avoiding the axial traction caused by the forearm manipulation. After implanting TEA, the ulnar nerve is transposed anteriorly in the subcutaneous tissue (Fig. 33).

The Triceps Splitting and Tendon Reflection (The Van Gorder "Turn Down Procedure")

Campbell [13], Van Gorder [19], and Wadsworth [20] described this approach as the elevation of a 10-cm long, inverted V-shaped flap of the triceps aponeurosis which is then reflected distally just as a tongue ("turn down procedure").

The remaining part of the triceps (the medial head) is split and then reflected.

This technique can increase the elbow flexion but many authors reported triceps weakness [21] or triceps devascularization, rupture, or adhesions, although this approach is very useful in case of a triceps contracture.

Before starting a turn-down procedure the surgeon has to master the anatomy of the distal insertion of the triceps tendon and muscle on the olecranon.

The long and lateral heads are superficial and blend in the midline to form a common superficial tendon that is inserted into the posterior surface of the proximal olecranon.

The deep medial head is fleshy and it is inserted mainly into the olecranon and joint capsule. The muscular fibers of the medial head are also inserted in the deep surface of the common tendon.

The turn-down procedure splits and reflects the common tendon-like a "tongue" preserving the insertion on the olecranon, while the deep medial head is split by many authors in different ways:

- obliquely (from the medial and proximal side to the lateral and distal side);
- midline, by reflecting the split portions medially and laterally.

In order to reduce the risk of denervation of the deep head of the triceps, we advise a superficial technique where at the triceps tendon reflection the underlying muscle is split in the medial third, detaching the muscular insertion on the olecranon.

The muscular flap of the medial head ("L-shaped portion") is divaricated laterally allowing the surgeon to see the posterior aspect of the joint.

The surgical steps:

- The patient should be positioned in the contro-lateral decubitus or supine with the arm on the chest.
- The straight posterolateral skin incision is performed.
- The subcutaneous tissue is divaricated and the triceps tendon is exposed.
- The posterior tendon of the triceps is incised transversally along the medial and the lateral border leaving the distal rim attached to the olecranon (Fig. 34a, b).
- During the superficial tendon flap dissection care must be taken in separating the superficial tendinous plane from the fleshy deeper one.
- The deep muscular exposition of the medial head is split longitudinally along the medial third of the muscle without separating it laterally from the superficial tendon: the muscular distal portion is detached from the olecranon insertion (Fig. 35a, b).
- The lateral part of the medial head flap and lateral superficial triceps tendon are reflected outwards, leaving continuity with the anconeus muscle. The anconeus nerve supply is preserved with the medial head flap.
- During this dissection the olecranon fat pad is carefully separated from the underlying synovium in the olecranon fossa and it is reflected in continuity with the overlying medial head of triceps. In this way the fat pad is preserved and the postoperative adhesions between triceps and humerus can be avoided (Fig. 36).
- In the closure of the surgical field the deep muscular lamina of the triceps is sutured on the olecranon and on the medial edge of the dorsal musculotendinous lamina (Figs. 37a, b).
- The dorsal tendon lamina of the triceps is sutured in its original position (Fig. 37c).

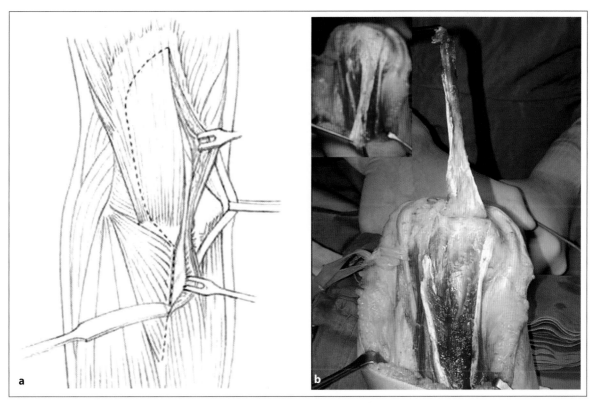

Fig. 34 a, b. The "Turn Down Procedure": the triceps tendon is incised along the medial and lateral border leaving the distal rim attached to the olecranon. The superficial tendinous plane is separated from the fleshy deeper one

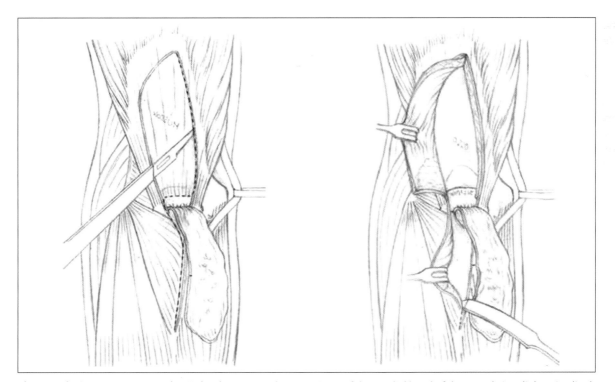

Fig. 35. The "Turn Down Procedure": the deep muscular exposition of the medial head of the muscle is split longitudinally along the medial third; the distal portion of the muscle is detached from the olecranon insertion. The anconeous muscle is detached from the ulna leaving continuity wit the triceps muscle

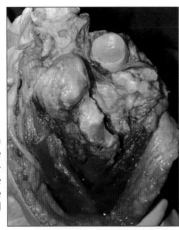

Fig. 36. The "Turn Down Procedure": the elbow can be exposed preserving the continuity with the overlying medial head of the triceps

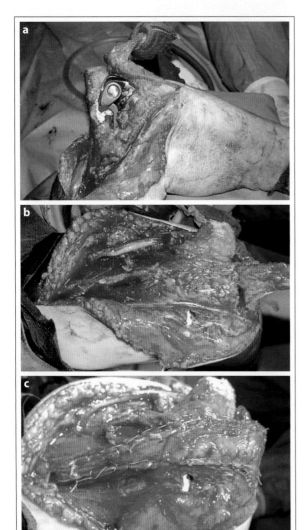

Fig. 37 a-c. The "Turn Down Procedure": after the total elbow replacement the deep lamina of the triceps is sutured on the olecranon and on the medial edge of the dorsal musculo-tendinous lamina

The Olecranon Osteotomy

This deep approach to the elbow was described by Mac Ausland [22] as a transverse transarticular osteotomy on the posterior portion of the sigmoid notch. Muller [23] proposed an extra-articular osteotomy, involving only the triceps attachment.

In recent years the most common modification is achieved by orthopedic surgeons with a chevron osteotomy [24].

A V-shaped osteotomy is made at the midportion of the olecranon "in the void region" that is not covered by hyaline cartilage. The advantages of this type of osteotomy are:

- a larger bone surface contact adds stability to the osteotomized olecranon, allowing improved bone healing;
- the morphology of the bone section should be placed in the void region just distally to the midarticular level;
- in this region slight incongruities of the osteotomy reduction are well tolerated.

Indications:

- the surgical treatment of the "T" and "Y" condylar fractures;
- the intra-articular comminuted fractures of the distal humerus;
- the intra-articular malunion management.

The surgical steps:

- The patient should be positioned in the controlateral decubitus.
- A straight midline posterior skin incision is performed slightly laterally from the olecranon.
- After divaricating the subcutaneous tissue the ulnar nerve should be isolated and released and the posterior humero-olecranon capsule can be seen. Once the capsule is opened the surgeon can identify and mark with a pin (Fig. 38a) the "void region" of the sigmoid notch and the level of the intra-articular chevron osteotomy (Fig. 38b). It is useful to distract the joint with a bone holding forceps.
- The chevron osteotomy should be made so that its apex point is distal, and the osteotomy involves the olecranon articular surface which is violated at the precise level identified before.
- The saw is used to perform the osteotomy and the final breakthrough is performed with a thin osteotome. The olecranon fragment with attached triceps muscle is then reflected proximally. In this way the humeral fractures and trochlea comminution can be manipulated allowing a fit anatomical reduction and stabilization (Fig. 39).

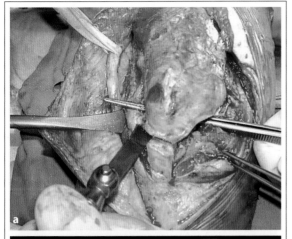

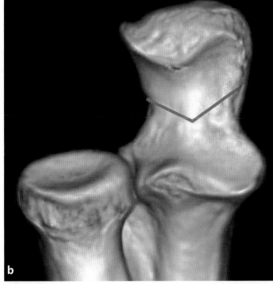

Fig. 38 a, b. The olecranon osteotomy: the chevron osteotomy should be made in the "void region" of the sigmoid notch

- The final osteotomy fixation can be performed by a tension band, an olecranon plate, or a large cancellous screw and tension band wire.

The olecranon osteotomy enables an excellent exposure of the distal humerus and the anterior aspect of the trochlea and capitellum, but the complications include:

- 5% incidence of olecranon osteotomy non-unions [24];
- denervation of the anconeus muscle for the dissection between triceps and olecranon;
- intra-articular adhesions and osteoarthritis if the osteotomy is not reduced anatomically.

The Olecranon Osteotomy Modification "Combined Olecranon Osteotomy with Anconeus Reflection"

From several years in our institution we modified the Mac Ausland olecranon osteotomy, preserving the relationship between triceps and anconeus muscle: we defined this approach as "Combined olecranon osteotomy with anconeus reflection". Recently, this approach is described as "the anconeous flap transolecranon approach to the distal humerus" [25]. This surgical modified approach avoids damage to the anconeus nerve and vascular supply. In this way we preserve the muscle innervation and the vascularity of the olecranon proximal fragment so that the risk of olecranon nonunion is reduced.

The surgical steps:
- The deep dissection starts proximally from the lateral epicondyle; it runs along the Kocher's interval until the anconeus ulnar insertion, and finally it turns proximally along the periosteal ulnar posterior border (Fig. 40).

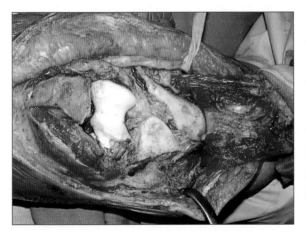

Fig. 39. The olecranon osteotomy: the olecranon osteotomy enables a wide exposure of the distal humerus fracture

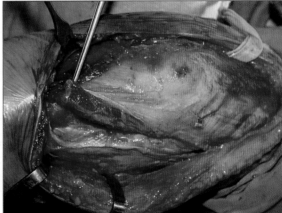

Fig. 40. The combined olecranon osteotomy with anconeus reflection. Laterally: the Kocher's interval is identified

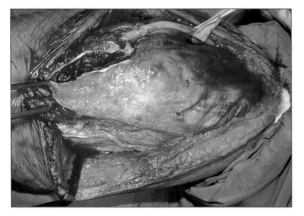

Fig. 41. The combined olecranon osteotomy with anconeus reflection. Medially: an incision is made in the periosteum in the subcutaneous border of the ulna

- The anconeus muscle is elevated subperiosteally from the ulna and from the lateral epicondyle until the supracondylar ridge insertion. Medially, an incision is made in the periosteum in the subcutaneous border of the ulna (Fig. 41). The periosteum is elevated with the ulnar insertion of the anconeus muscle until the olecranon osteotomy is at the correct level (Fig. 42a-d).
- The olecranon fragment with periosteal flap is reflected proximally (including the anconeus muscle in continuity with the triceps muscle) (Fig. 43).

The Triceps Reflecting Anconeus Pedicle (Trap Approach)

A deep exposure combining medial Brian Morrey and lateral modified Kocher's approach allows the detachment of the triceps olecranon and anconeus pedicle insertion and the ulnar periosteum (TRAP), with proximal reflection. This approach, described by O'Driscoll [26] enables an adequate exposure of the joint, when the elbow is fully flexed.
Indications:
- open reduction and internal fixation of comminuted intra-articular fractures;
- nonunion of the distal humerus fractures;
- the open treatment of humerus fractures in elderly patients, keeping the olecranon intact so that the total elbow arthroplasty, the open reduction, and the internal fixation are practicable.
The surgical steps:
- The patient is placed in a supine position with the arm on the chest or in the lateral decubitus position.
- A longitudinal posterior skin incision (about 15 cm long) is placed just laterally to the tip of the olecranon.

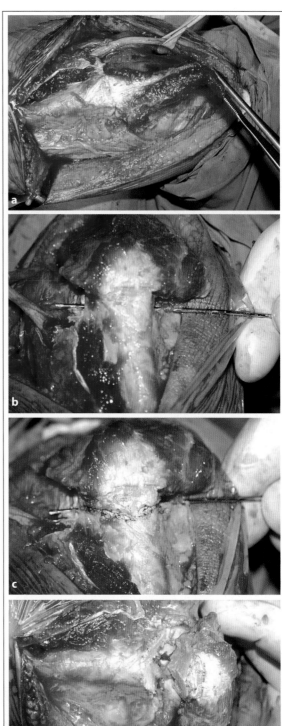

Fig. 42 a-d. The combined olecranon osteotomy with anconeus reflection: the periosteum is elevated with the ulnar insertion of the anconeus muscle until the olecranon osteotomy is at the correct level

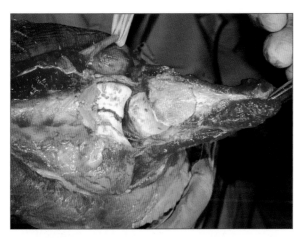

Fig. 43. The combined olecranon osteotomy with anconeus reflection: the olecranon fragment with the periosteal flap is reflected proximally (the anconeus is in continuity with the triceps muscle)

- The deep exposure involves combined approaches from the medial and lateral sides of the elbow.
- In the medial side the ulnar nerve is exposed and released.
- Laterally, in the Kocher's interval, the anconeus is elevated subperiosteally from the ulna, preserving the lateral collateral ligament, the annular ligament, the common origin of the extensor tendons, and the extensor carpi radialis longus and brachioradialis tendons.
- The dissection is carried out proximally between the triceps and the posterior aspect of the humerus on the supracondylar ridge.
- Medially, the exposure lies in reflecting the triceps to the posterior surface of the elbow joint as described by Bryan and Morrey.
- An incision is made about 10 cm distally from the olecranon in the periosteum and in the subcutaneous border of the ulna along the FCU (Fig. 44).
- The periosteum is elevated from the posterior surface of the ulna from the medial to the lateral side, continuing beneath the anconeus, which is elevated subperiosteally (Fig. 45a, b).
- The triceps tendon insertion is released at the tip of the olecranon and a marking suture is placed on the tendon area insertion: this allows reattaching the triceps at the precise point in order to restore the fit length tension.
- The flap of the triceps and anconeus pedicle are detached from the ulna and reflected proximally.
- The full flexion of the elbow allows the exposure of the distal humerus, as an olecranon osteotomy usually permits, but the articular surface of the anterior trochlea is very difficult to expose.

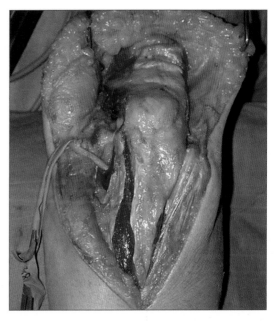

Fig. 44. The Trap approach: the deep incision is made about 10 cm distally from the olecranon in the periosteum and in the subcutaneous border of the ulna along the flexor carpi ulnaris

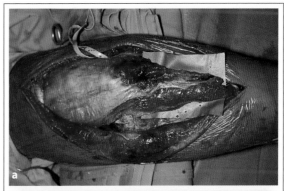

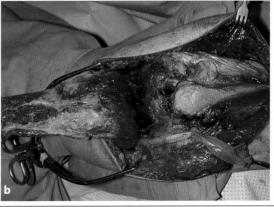

Fig. 45 a, b. The Trap approach: the periosteum is elevated from the posterior surface of the ulna from the medial to the lateral side. The flap of the triceps and the anconeus pedicle are detached from the ulna and reflected proximally

- The triceps tendon reattachment on the olecranon is particularly important: a heavy nonabsorbable suture (5) is placed through the triceps, in the area marked by the suture, and afterwards the suture is brought in. The main complication of the suture concerns the secondary triceps weakness caused by a partial or complete detachment of the triceps tendon from the olecranon. In our experience we also had muscle tendon degeneration for over-tension of the reattached triceps tendon.
- The tendon is sutured with two criss-cross drill holes made through the ulna from the proximal side to the distal one. The suture is tied tightly and pulled down the tendon to the bone.

The Global Approach (The Combined Medial and Lateral Approach)

The midline extensile posterior skin incision allows the wide, deep access at each compartment of the elbow. This approach was called "Global Approach" [27] because it involves the elevation of a full-thickness, fascio-cutaneous flap, medially and laterally.

The indications include:
- complex elbow contractures;
- extensive heterotopic ossification;
- elbow fracture dislocation with associated radial head and coronoid process fractures and elbow instability (Terrible Triad);
- complex fractures of the olecranon with associated fractures or dislocation of the radial head (Monteggia injuries);
- transolecranon fracture-dislocation or posterior fracture dislocation;
- unreduced chronic elbow subluxation or dislocation.

Position of the Patient

The patient is in a supine position and the arm is brought on the chest. A sterile tourniquet is applied in the most proximal arm.

Bone Landmarks

Bone landmarks include the subcutaneous profile of the olecranon and posterior borders of the ulna, and the lateral and medial epicondyle.

The surgical steps:
- A posterior midline longitudinal skin incision is made just medially or laterally from the tip of

the olecranon to avoid the wound-healing complication when the underlying tissue is exposed.
- The skin incision has to be taken directly down through the subcutaneous tissue to the deep fascia of the triceps tendon and the posterolateral and medial aspect of the joint to the posterior border of the ulna.
- A full-thickness medial and lateral fascio-cutaneous flap is elevated, preserving the subcutaneous arterial plexus and cutaneous nerves.
- The ulnar nerve is released and retracted after excision of the medial intermuscular septum, and the fibrous arcade in the cubital tunnel allows the ulnar nerve to become free for anterior subcutaneous transposition at the end of the surgery.

References

1. Kocher T (1911) Text book of operative surgery, 3rd edn. Adam and Charles Black, London
2. Dowdy P, Bain G, King G, Patterson SD (1995) The midline posterior elbow incision. J Bone Joint Surg Br 77:696-699
3. Pearl RM, Johnson D (1983) The vascular supply to the skin: An anatomical and physiological reappraisal. Ann Plast Surg 11:99-105
4. Kocher T (1911) Operations at the elbow. In: Kocher T (ed) Text book of operating surgery, 3rd edn. Adam and Charles Black, London, pp 313-318
5. Mansat P, Morrey BF (1998) The column procedure: A limited surgical approach for the treatment of the stiff elbow. J Bone Joint Surg Am 80:1603-1615
6. Witt JD, Kaminemi S (1998) The posterior interosseous nerve and the posterolateral approach to the proximal radius. J Bone Surg Br 80:240-242
7. Hotchkiss RN, Kasparyon G (2000) The medial "Over the top" approach to the elbow. Tech Orthop 15(2) 105-112
8. Wada T, Ishii S, Usui M et al (2000) The medial approach for operative release of post traumatic contracture of the elbow J Bone Joint Surg Br 1:68-73
9. Dutta A, Henry M, Levoro F (2003) Limited medial approach elbow capsulectomy with active assist split rehabilitation. Tech Shoulder Elbow Surg 4:185-194
10. O'Driscoll SW (1993) Elbow arthritis: Treatment options. J Am Acad Orthop Surg 1:106-116
11. O'Driscoll SW (2000) The triceps reflecting anconeus pedicle (TRAP) approach for distal humeral fractures and non union. Orthop Clin North Am 31:91-101
12. Gerwin M, Hotckiss RN, Weiland A (1996) Alternative operative exposure of the posterior aspect of the humeral diaphysis with reference to the radial nerve. J Bone Joint Surg 7Am 8:1690-1695
13. Crenshaw AH (1987) Surgical approaches. In: Crenshaw AH (ed) Campbell's operative orthopaedics. Mosby, St. Louis, p 88-94
14. Bryan RS, Morrey BF (1982) Extensive posterior exposure of the elbow: A triceps sparing approach. Clin Orthop 116:188-192

15. Morrey BF (2000) Surgical exposure of the elbow. In: Morrey BF (ed) The elbow and its disorders, 3rd edn. Saunders, Philadelphia, pp 109-134

16. Alonso Llames M (1972) Bilaterotricipital approach to the elbow. Acta Orthop Scand 43:479-490

17. Pierce TD, Herndon JH (1998) The triceps preserving approach to total elbow arthroplasty. Clin Orthop 354:144-152

18. Boorman RS, Page WT, Weldon III EJ, Lippitt S, Matsen FA (2003) A triceps-on approach to semi constrained total elbow arthroplasty. Tech Shoulder Elbow Surg 4:139-144

19. Van Gorder GW (1940) Surgical approaches insupracondylar "T" fractures of the humerus requiring open reduction. J Bone Joint Surg 22:278-292

20. Wadsworth TG (1979) A modified postero-lateral approach to the elbow and proximal radioulnar joints. Clin Orthop 144:151-153

21. Morrey BF, Bryon RS, Dobyns JH et al (1981) Total elbow arthroplasty: A five years experience at the Mayo Clinic. J Bone Joint Surg Am 63:1050-1063

22. Mac Ausland WR (1915) Ankylosis of the elbow with report of four cases treated by arthroplasty. JAMA 64:312-318

23. Muller ME, Allgower M, Willenegger H (1979) Manual of internal fixation: Technique recommended by the AD group, 2nd edn. Springer, Heidelberg Berlin New York

24. Jupiter JB (2002) The surgical management of the intra-articular fractures of the distal humerus. In: Morrey BF (ed) The elbow: Master techniques in orthopaedics surgery. Lippincott, New York, pp 65-81

25. Athwal GS, Rispoli DN, Steinmann SP (2006) The anconeus flap transolecranon. Approaches to the distal humerus. J Orthop Trauma 20:282-285

26. O'Driscoll SW (2000) The triceps reflecting anconeus pedicle (TRAP) approach for distal humeral fractures and non unions. Orthop Clin North Am 31(1):91-101

27. Patterson SD, King GJW, Bain G (1995) A posterior global approach to the elbow (abstract). J Bone J Surg Br 77:316

CHAPTER 5

The Treatment of Distal Humerus Fractures

S.W. O'DRISCOLL

Introduction

The goal of restoring normal, pain-free elbow function after a fracture of the distal humerus requires anatomic reconstruction of the articular surface, restitution of the overall geometry of the distal humerus and stable fixation of the fracture fragments to allow early and full rehabilitation [1-7]. Although these goals are now widely accepted by the orthopedic community, they may be technically difficult to achieve, especially in the presence of substantial osteoporosis or comminution [7].

Until recently, the standard technique for fixation of distal humerus fractures has been that proposed by the AO/ASIF group [5, 7]. Their recommended technique includes fixation of the articular fragments with screws and column stabilization with two plates at a 90° angle to one another [5, 8, 9]. The limiting factor of this technique unquestionably is fixation of the distal fragments to the shaft. When this method fails, it does so because of nonunion at the supracondylar level or stiffness resulting from prolonged immobilization that has been used in an attempt to avoid failure of inadequate fixation [7]. Using these fixation techniques, different authors have reported unsatisfactory results in 20%-25% of the patients [1-6].

We have found that optimal function after fixation of distal humerus fractures can be achieved by stable fixation, even in the presence of osteoporosis or comminution, using a philosophy and technique based on principles that maximize fixation in the distal fragments and compression at the supracondylar level. The stability achieved has allowed us to routinely commence an intensive rehabilitation program 36 hours post-operatively including full active motion with no external protection.

The following discussion expands on the general principles of our current approach to these fractures, the specific technical details, the post-operative program and the potential complications.

Principles

Exposure

Accurate reduction of the articular surface of the distal humerus requires good exposure, which can be achieved with either an olecranon osteotomy or the TRAP (triceps reflecting anconeus pedicle) approach [10]. Osteotomy provides the best exposure, while the TRAP approach allows adequate exposure without the need for an olecranon osteotomy. This is especially important in older patients when elbow replacement may be necessary. With the TRAP approach, the intact proximal ulna and radial head can be used as a template against which the distal humerus can be reconstructed. In addition, the potential complications associated with olecranon osteotomies are avoided [2, 11] and the innervation of the anconeus is preserved [10].

Reconstruction

Articular Surface

The articular surface of the distal humerus should be reconstructed anatomically unless bone is missing. If bone is missing, two important principles should be taken into consideration. Firstly, the anterior aspect of the distal humerus is the critical part of the articulation that needs to be fixed in order to have a functional joint; reconstruction of the posterior half is important but not as critical. Secondly, stability of the articulation requires the medial trochlea and either the lateral half of the trochlea or the capitellum. Thus, the medial trochlea is essential in order to obtain a stable and well-aligned joint.

The articular surface is fixed provisionally with small smooth Kirschner wires. In addition, or alternatively, very small (0.035 or 0.045) threaded Kirschner wires can be placed in the subchondral bone and left in place for definitive fixation after cutting them off. No screws are placed in the distal fragments before applying the plates.

Metaphyseal Region

The metaphyseal region of the distal humerus can be fixed in two different ways. An anatomic reconstruction is desirable whenever possible. However, adequate bony contact with interfragmentary compression is necessary to ensure the stability of the construct and eventually fracture union at this level. If metaphyseal comminution precludes an anatomic reconstruction with satisfactory bony contact, the humerus can be shortened at the metaphyseal fracture site, provided that the overall alignment and geometry of the distal humerus are restored. We call this alternative reconstructive technique supracondylar shortening. This technique is especially useful in cases of combined soft-tissue and bone loss. Shortening by 1 cm or less creates no apparent loss of function, and up to 2 cm of shortening can be tolerated without serious disturbance of elbow biomechanics [12]. The details of this technique of supracondylar shortening have been published [13].

Fixation

By far the majority of fixation failures after a distal humerus fracture occur at the supracondylar level, whereas the articular fragments typically unite. Based on current practice and recommendations, this should not be surprising. Many of the fractures are dependent on only two or three screws for stability at the supracondylar level. The fixation strategy should concentrate on maximizing stability between the distal fragments and the shaft of the humerus at the metaphyseal level. These "principles" are achieved by the successful execution of the following set of eight technical objectives, each of which contributes to maximizing fixation in the articular segment and the stability between it and the shaft.

Technical objectives

Concerning screws in the distal fragments (articular segment):
- Every screw should pass through a plate.
- Each screw should engage a fragment on the opposite side that is also fixed by a plate.
- Each screw should be as long as possible.
- Each screw should engage as many articular fragments as possible.
- As many screws as possible should be placed in the distal fragments.
- The screws in the distal segment should lock together by inter digitations, thereby creating a fixed-angle structure and linkage between the two columns.

Concerning the plates used for fixation:
- Plates should be applied such that compression is achieved at the supracondylar level for both columns.
- Plates used must be strong enough and stiff enough to resist breaking or bending before union occurs at the supracondylar level.

The practical application of these principles involves "parallel" (in this case is a figure-of-speech, as both plates are actually rotated slightly posteriorly) plates that permit a total of at least four long screws to be placed in the distal fragments, from one side across the other (the plates are placed with a slight offset, postero-medially and postero-laterally) (Fig. 1). The screws placed at the epiphyseal level interlock, which links the two columns together and greatly increases the stability of the construct just as the keystone provides stability to an arch (Fig. 2). The plates must be contoured or pre-contoured to the normal geometry of the distal humerus in order to allow screw placement at the appropriate places and also not to be too prominent under the skin. We use

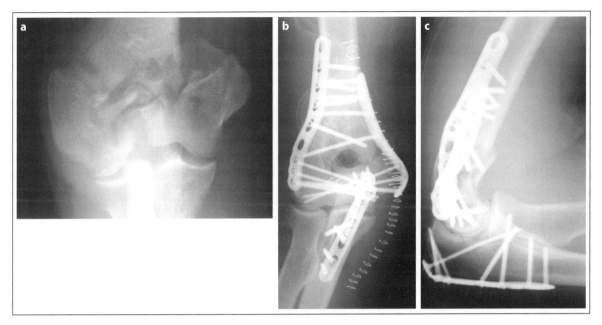

Fig. 1. (**a**) Comminuted intra-articular fracture of the distal humerus with both intra-articular and supercondylar comminution. (**b**) The fracture was fixed with the "parallel" plating technique. A total of six long screws fixed the distal articular segment to the shaft via the plates. The screws interdigitate in the articular segments giving ridged fixation, and a structure against which to fix small articular fragments as well (small threaded K-wires as seen in the X-ray). This technique is facilitated by the use of pre-contoured Mayo Clinic Congruent Elbow Plate System (Acumed, Beaverton, OR). (**c**) Fixation of the olecranon osteotomy can be performed with a plate especially designed for olecranon osteotomies and fractures. This permits interdigitation of four screws in the proximal fragment, compression across the osteotomy site, and a specially contoured plate that minimizes hardware irritation by virtue of its low profile shape and the fact that the screw heads are contained within the plate. (Figures reproduced with permission, Mayo Foundation)

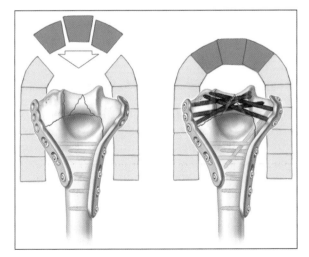

Fig. 2. Locking the screws together by interdigitation within the distal segment links the two columns, thereby creating a stable construct around and within the bone that is analogous to the means by which the keystone confers stability to an arch. Thus, it is the arch itself (the linkage of hardware from medial to lateral columns) that renders the distal humerus stable. (Figures reproduced with permission, Mayo Foundation)

the Mayo Congruent Elbow Plates (Acumed, Hillsboro, OR) that are precontoured to the geometry of the distal humerus and also designed to permit placement of multiple long screws (2.7 or 3.5 mm) in the distal fragments by clustering the distal screw holes. Locking screws can be used and may decrease the need for as many screws to be used. However, these principles and technical objectives can be achieved without the use of locking screws. From an engineering perspective, the best way to create a fixed-angle screw is not to lock it in the plate, but to fix it at the opposite end (objectives number 2 and 6).

Interfragmentary compression is obtained both between articular fragments and at the metaphyseal level through the use of large bone clamps that provide compression during the insertion of the screws. This is done instead of using lagscrews to provide maximum thread purchase for each screw. Additional compression at the metaphyseal level results from slight undercontouring of the plates and the use of dynamic compression holes in the plates.

Technique

The patient is placed in the supine position and the affected upper extremity is prepared and draped in the usual fashion. The lateral position with the arm on a support can be used, but hyperflexion, which is necessary with the TRAP approach [10], is easier in the supine position. A sterile tourniquet can be used for the initial ulnar nerve dissection, but we prefer to avoid the use of the tourniquet. The ulnar nerve is routinely identified, isolated and transposed subcutaneously to avoid irritation by the hardware or swelling-induced nerve compression that can cause ulnar neuropathy or limit flexion postoperatively.

Anatomic reconstruction

Assembly of the Articular Surface
Once the fracture is exposed, the first step is the anatomic reconstruction of the articular surface. The intact ulna and radial head can be used as a template for the reconstruction of the distal humerus. The articular fragments are assembled paying attention to their rotational alignment and are held in place provisionally with smooth Kirschner wires (Fig. 3). Fine threaded wires (0.035 or 0.045) are used in cases with extensive com-

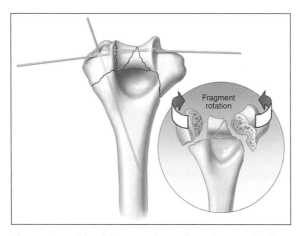

Fig. 3. Assembly of the Articular Surface. The articular fragments, which tend to be rotated towards each other in the axial plane, are reduced anatomically and provisionally held with 0.035 or 0.045 smooth Kirschner wires. It is essential that the wires be placed close to the subchondral level to avoid interference with later screw placement, and away from where the plates will be placed on the lateral and medial columns (Fig. 4). One or two strategically placed pins can be used to provisionally hold the distal fragments aligned with the shaft. (Figure reproduced with permission, Mayo Foundation)

minution, cut-off and left in as definitive adjunct fixation. The articular fragments are fixed in the following order:
- anterior trochlea and capitellum;
- medial trochlea;
- posterior fragments.

As stated above, in cases with severe intra-articular comminution all efforts should be directed to reconstruct the anterior half of the distal humerus articular surface and the condyle and medial trochlea. It is necessary that all wires be placed at the subchondral level so as not to interfere with plate application or with passage of screws from the plates into the distal fragments. No screws are placed in the distal fragments until the plates are applied. This is very important, as every major screw in the distal fragments should pass through a plate so that it contributes to stability at the supracondylar level as well.

Plate Placement and Provisional Reduction
The next step is to contour plates to fit the distal humerus medially and laterally or to choose medial and lateral precontoured plates from the Mayo Congruent Elbow Plate System (Acumed, Hillsboro, OR). One-third tubular plates are not strong enough although 3.5 mm pelvic reconstruction plates usually are. The medial plate can be extended to the articular margin in very distal or comminuted fractures and is contoured to the shape of the medial epicondyle. Both plates should be slightly undercontoured to provide additional compression at the metaphyseal region when applied. The length of the plates is selected so that at least three screws are placed both medially and laterally proximal to the metaphyseal component of the fracture. Ideally, the plates should end at different levels to avoid the creation of a stress riser. The Mayo Congruent Plates are designed to always stop at different levels regardless of how they are combined. The plates are then provisionally applied according to the following steps (Fig. 4):
- two 2.0 mm smooth Steinmann pins are introduced at the medial and lateral epicondyles through holes in the plates while they are held accurately against the bone; the most commonly used holes are the second one laterally and the third medially;
- the appropriate reduction of the distal fragments to the humeral shaft at the supracondylar level is confirmed;
- one cortical non-locking screw is loosely introduced into a slotted hole to hold each plate in place. Use of slotted holes for these screws facilitate later adjustments in plate positioning.

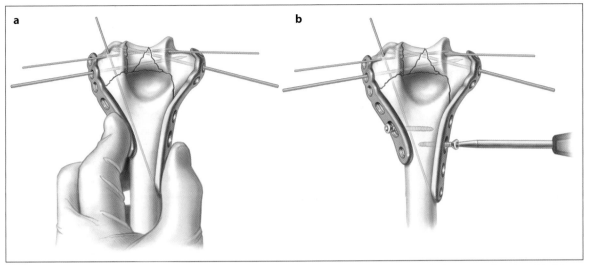

Fig. 4. Plate Placement and Provisional Reduction. (**a**) Medial and lateral precontoured plates are placed and held apposed to the distal humerus, while one smooth 2.0 mm Steinmann pin is inserted through hole #2 (numbered from distal to proximal) of each plate through the epicondyles and across the distal fragments, to maintain provisional fixation of the plates to the distal fragments. (**b**) A screw is placed in the slotted hole (#5) of each plate, but not fully tightened, leaving some freedom for the plate to move proximally during compression later. Because the undersurface of each plate is tubular in the metaphyseal and diaphyseal regions, the screw in the slotted hole only needs to be tightened slightly to provide excellent provisional fixation of the entire distal humerus. (Figures reproduced with permission, Mayo Foundation)

Articular and Distal Fixation

Once the plates are provisionally applied, medial and lateral screws are introduced distally to provide stable fixation of the intra-articular fragments and rigid anchorage of the plates distally (Fig. 5).

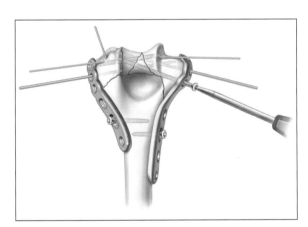

Fig. 5. Articular and Distal Fixation. Screws are inserted through hole #1 of the lateral plate and across the distal articular fragments from lateral to medial, and tightened. This step is repeated on the medial side, using hole #3. In young patients 3.5 cortical screws are used (to prevent breakage) while long 2.7 screws are used in patients with osteoporotic bone. The distal screws should be as long as possible, passing through as many fragments as possible, and engaging the condyle or epicondyle of the opposite column. (Figure reproduced with permission, Mayo Foundation)

Two distal non-locking screws, one medial and one lateral, are inserted. As stated above, the screws should be as long as possible, pass through as many fragments as possible and engage in the opposite column. Prior to their application, a large bone clamp is used to compress the intra-articular fracture lines unless there is a gap in the articular surface. This ensures interfragmentary compression without the need of lag screws.

Two proximal non-locking screws, one medial and one lateral, are inserted in compression mode to fix the plates to the diaphysis proximally and to obtain some interfragmentary compression at the supracondylar level.

Supracondylar Compression and Proximal Plate Fixation

The plates are then fixed proximally under maximum compression at the supracondylar level (Fig. 6-8).

The proximal screw on one side is backed out and a large bone clamp is applied distally on that side and proximally on the opposite shaft cortex to eccentrically load the supracondylar region. Care should be taken to ensure correct varus-valgus or rotational alignment of the articular surface. A non-locking screw is then placed in dynamic compression mode in a proximal hole. The initial screw in the slotted hole is then tightened.

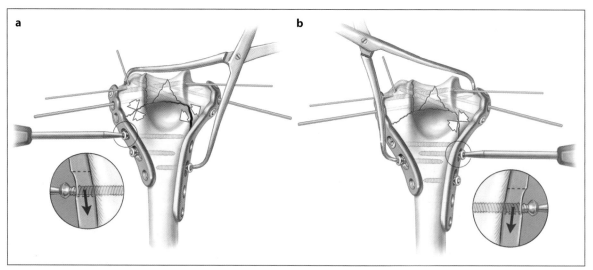

Fig. 6. Supracondylar Compression and Proximal Plate Fixation. (**a**) Using a large tenaculum to provide interfragmentary compression across the fracture at the supracondylar level, the lateral column is first fixed. A screw is placed in dynamic compression mode (inset) in hole #4 of the lateral plate. Tightening this further enhances interfragmentary compression at the supracondylar level (converging arrows) to the point of causing some distraction at the medial supracondylar ridge (diverging arrows). (**b**) The medial column is then compressed in a similar manner using the large tenaculum and a screw is inserted in the medial plate in dynamic compression mode. If the plates are slightly undercontoured, they can be compressed against the metaphysis with a large bone clamp, giving further supracondylar compression. (Figures reproduced with permission, Mayo Foundation)

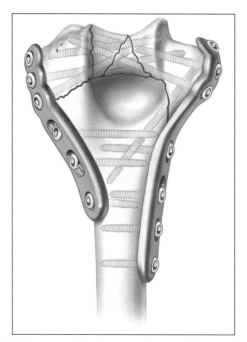

Fig. 7. The smooth Steinmann pins are all removed and the remainder of the screws is inserted. The distal screws interdigitate for maximum fixation in the distal articular fragments. (Figure reproduced with permission, Mayo Foundation)

The same steps are followed on the opposite side. Following this step the fixation is already quite stable.

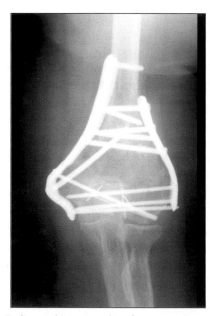

Fig. 8. Radiographic example of a comminuted distal humerus fracture fixed with this principle-based technique. Using this approach, fixation is virtually always adequate to commence an intensive early rehabilitation program consisting of active and passive motion without fear of failure of fixation. (Figure reproduced with permission, Mayo Foundation)

The remaining diaphyseal screws are then introduced providing additional compression as a result of the undercontoured plates being pulled down to the underlying bone. To avoid screws stripping the bone, this last step is best performed by squeezing the plates against the bone with a large clamp rather than relying on the screws to deform the plates.

Final screw insertion

The various K-wires are removed and the remaining screws inserted, generally using locking screws.

The intra-operative motion should be full unless significant swelling has already developed. One deep and one subcutaneous drain are placed and the type of approach used dictates the closure. The skin should be closed with staples or interrupted sutures.

Post-operative Treatment

Immediately after closure, the elbow is placed in a bulky non-compressive Robert-Jones dressing with an anterior plaster slab to keep the elbow in extension. The upper extremity is kept elevated for 2-3 days to lessen the soft tissue response to the trauma and surgery. After that, the Robert-Jones dressing is removed, an elastic nonconstrictive sleeve is applied over an absorbent dressing placed on the wound. Active and gentle passive motion (CPM), and sometimes continuous passive motion, are started with the goal of avoiding swelling as much as possible.

If the fracture unites with the normal anatomic relationships restored and heterotopic bone formation does not occur, any limitation of the range of motion will be secondary to the response of the soft tissues to the traumatic and surgical insults and/or the post-operative immobilization. An intensive program of CPM is a reliable method to achieve a satisfactory range of motion. The CPM is used to avoid fluid accumulation at the elbow. Experimental and clinical data support the use of CPM for this purpose [14]. The fluid that would tend to accumulate at the surgical site as part of the inflammatory response is literally squeezed out of the elbow region by the high hydrostatic pressures generated when maximally flexing and extending the elbow. The stability of the bony reconstruction allows such motion without fear of failure of fixation. The only factors limiting motion immediately after the operation are the amount of swelling, the response of the overlying skin and any problems with pain control. However, avoiding infection or serious wound complications are the highest priority in the first week or two, and may preclude or delay the use of CPM.

The CPM program is labor-intensive. The CPM machine is adjusted so that the elbow is higher than the shoulder. To use CPM most effectively, the patient works on progressively stretching the end ranges of flexion and extension. Full extension is normally easier to achieve because the elbow was initially splinted in extension. The patient lets the machine extend the elbow to the point at which it feels tight, backs it into flexion a few degrees and keeps the elbow in that position for about 1 or 2 minutes while the fluid is being squeezed from the tissues. After that couple of minutes, the patient will tolerate further extension and continues working with several stops and starts until full extension is achieved. The same sequence is then repeated for flexion.

As part of the post-operative management, the patient is also encouraged to work on passive and active-assisted pronation and supination exercises. Finally, thorough massage of the elbow by the patient or a relative will help in squeezing the fluid out of the elbow region and also partially desensitize it to pain. Close attention should be paid to the neurovascular status and the condition of the skin while the patient is in the CPM machine. The patient should be encouraged to continuously readjust his position in the machine to avoid nerve palsies secondary to prolonged pressure. Some discoloration of the posterior skin is to be expected with elbow motion, but if the integrity of the skin is in doubt the CPM should be stopped and the arm elevated in a Robert-Jones dressing until the status of the skin improves. Large subcutaneous hematomas are washed out and drained to avoid excess tension on the posterior wound and to lessen the chance of infection.

The CPM program is continued at home for 3 to 4 weeks. If by the fourth week motion is still substantially less than what was achieved intra-operatively, formation of heterotopic ossification should be investigated and a program of patient-adjusted static flexion and extension splints used up to 3 to 4 months after surgery. With adequate internal fixation, there is no need to wait for bone union before commencing a therapy or splinting program.

Potential Complications

The main complications that have been reported after internal fixation of distal humerus fractures are residual decreased range of motion, fixation failure with nonunion or malunion, nerve dysfunction, extensor mechanism dysfunction, post-traumatic degenerative changes, wound and skin problems, and avascular necrosis [11, 15, 16].

As stated above, the neurovascular status and the condition of the skin should be followed carefully during the post-operative period. Anterior subcutaneous transposition of the ulnar nerve prevents many of the ulnar nerve complications [16]. Neurapraxias may develop secondary to sustained pressure on the arm if the patient does not readjust his position while using the CPM machine. Serious skin problems can be avoided if motion is stopped and the elbow elevated in a compressive dressing in extension as soon as a skin problem is apparent. The combination of ischemic skin and a subcutaneous hematoma is an indication for surgical lavage and re-closure of the wound.

With the internal fixation technique described above we have experienced only one case of fixation failure. A 3.5 reconstruction plate experienced fatigue fracture 6 months after surgery in a patient with a severe open injury treated by supracondylar shortening and coverage with a latissimus dorsi flap and skin graft. The lateral column had healed, necessitating only refixation and bone grafting of the medial column, which did result in union. His final range of motion was 20°-120°. Decreased range of motion may occur secondary to heterotopic ossification, intra-articular adhesions or capsular contracture. If improved motion does not occur in response to a program of splinting, the patient may require a capsular release that can be performed as early as 3-4 months after the surgery. If the capsular release is performed later, the hardware can be removed if the fracture is completely healed.

Dysfunction of the extensor mechanism may occur if the triceps tendon was elevated or detached from the olecranon. Should discontinuity or subluxation of the extensor mechanism occur, it can be surgically treated by primary repair or augmentation with an Achilles tendon allograft. Olecranon non-union can be treated by plate fixation and bone grafting.

Joint deterioration may be secondary to the cartilage damage sustained at the initial injury or avascular necrosis secondary to the devascularization of some articular fragments in severely comminuted injuries. We have had one case of severe osteonecrosis in a severe multifragmentary fracture. To minimize the likelihood of this complication, it is necessary to leave all soft tissues attached to the distal fragments during surgery.

The single biggest impediment to successful application of this principle-based technique is the misconception that plates must be applied in two perpendicular planes. While that may have been true when very weak 3.5 one-third tubular plates were used, it most certainly is not true when strong plates are used. The "parallel" double-plate construct has been shown to provide excellent stability even in the presence of supracondylar gaps [17]. In zero of the five biomechanical studies of distal humeral fixation in the literature, three compared "90-90" plating to parallel plating in the sagittal plane [8, 9, 17-19]. Two of those studies found a significant improvement with parallel plating [9, 17], while one found no difference [18]. The other two did not compare these two techniques [8, 19]. Thus, there is no evidence in the published literature to support the claim that "90-90" or perpendicular plating is more stable than parallel plating in the sagittal plane. In fact, Schemitsch et al. [17], showed that the combination of a medial reconstruction and lateral DuPont plate in parallel planes was stronger than two reconstruction plates placed in two planes 90° to each other, as is recommended by the AO/ASIF group and currently employed by most surgeons. We strongly recommend the use of this technique for comminuted distal humerus fractures, and prefer its use routinely for less complex fractures as well, because the stability is such that intensive rehabilitation is possible. However, for non-comminuted fractures in good quality bone, either technique can be used reliably.

Currently, there is much interest in locking screws. While there are advantages to locking screws, there are also some disadvantages. For the distal humerus, there is significant risk of screw malplacement and penetration into the radial or coronoid fossae, which are hidden from view or even the joint. Korner et al., in a biomechanical evaluation of locking screw/plates, stated, "We consider the inability to change the direction of the screws a disadvantage" [19]. At our Institution, we agree with this opinion. It is our belief that the solution for this dilemma is to position the plate optimally, drill the screw holes for optimal position in the distal segment, then tap the plate in situ with a special device designed for that purpose and insert locking screws that will lock properly into the plate at the chosen angle (Fig. 9). We have successfully employed this technique using The Mayo Clinic Congruent Elbow Plates (Acumed, Hillsboro, OR). We would emphasize, however, that the principles and technical objectives that ensure stability even in severely comminuted fractures or osteoporotic bone do not require locking screws.

In summary, this philosophy and technique for fixing distal humerus fractures have many advantages. Complex fractures are able to fixed with sufficient stability to permit immediate intensive rehabilitation. Some fractures that have been thought to be unfixable have been very satisfactorily fixed by applying the principles outlined in this paper. More straightforward fractures are easily fixed using the same techniques. In our experience, the stability achieved with this approach is so

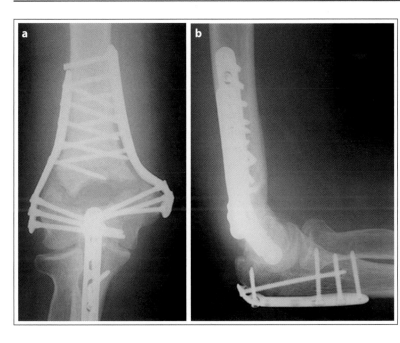

Fig. 9 a, b. Optimal use of locking screws in the peri-articular region would not only permit those screws to achieve all of the technical objectives in the principle-based approach described in this technique, but also permit the screws to be placed in optimal screw position and the plates in optimal plate position. As a result, the angle between the screw and the plate will not be constant and requires that it be able to be varied. The plate design used by the author, The Mayo Clinic Congruent Elbow Plates (Acumed, Hillsboro, OR), permits the screws to be inserted at an angle to the plate and then locked in place after having tapped the plate in situ with a special tapping device. In this example, the patient has multiple locking screws in the distal segment at various angles to the plates. (Figures reproduced with permission, Mayo Foundation)

much greater than that with traditional methods of fixing distal humerus fractures that bone graft has only very rarely been required, despite the severity of injuries so typical of the tertiary referral nature of our practice.

References

1. Gabel GT, Hanson G, Bennett JB et al (1987) Intra-articular fractures of the distal humerus in the adult. Clin Orthop 216:99-108
2. Henley MB, Bone LB, Parker B (1987) Operative management of intra-articular fractures of the distal humerus. J Orthop Trauma 1:24-35
3. Holdsworth BJ, Mossad MM (1990) Fractures of the adult distal humerus. J Bone Joint Surg Br 72:362-365
4. John H, Rosso R, Neff U, Bodoky A et al (1994) Operative treatment of distal humeral fractures in the elderly. J Bone Joint Surg Br 76:793-796
5. Jupiter JB, Neff U, Holzach P, Allgower M (1985) Intercondylar fractures of the humerus. J Bone Joint Surg 67-A:226-239
6. Letsch R, Schmit-Neuerburg KP, Sturmer KM, Walz M (1989) Intra-articular fractures of the distal humerus. Surgical treatment and results. Clin Orthop 241:238-244
7. Ring D, Jupiter JB (2000) Fractures of the Distal Humerus. Orthop Clin North Am 31:103-113
8. Helfet DL, Hotchkiss RN (1990) Internal fixation of the distal humerus: A biomechanical comparison of methods. J Orthop Trauma 4:260-264
9. Self J, Viegas SF, Buford WL, Patterson RMA (1995) Comparison of double-plate fixation methods for complex distal humerus fractures. J Shoulder Elbow Surg 4:11-16
10. O'Driscoll S (2000) The triceps-reflecting anconeus pedicle (TRAP) approach for distal humeral fractures and nonunions. Ortho Clin North Am 31:91-101
11. Sodergard J, Sandelin J, Bostman O (1992) Post-operative complications of distal humeral fractures. 27/96 adults followed up for 6 (2-10) years. Acta Orthop Scand 63:85-89
12. Hughes RE, Schneeberger AG, An KN, Morrey BF, O'Driscoll SW (1997) Reduction of triceps muscle force after shortening of the distal humerus: a computational model. J Shoulder Elbow Surg 6:444-448
13. O'Driscoll SW, Sanchez-Sotelo J, Torchia ME (2002) Management of the smashed distal humerus. Orthop Clin North Am 33:19-33
14. O'Driscoll S, Giori N (2000) Continuous passive motion (CPM): theory and principles of clinical application. J Rehabil Res Dev 37:179-188
15. Ackerman G, Jupiter JB (1988) Non-union of fractures of the distal end of the humerus. J Bone Joint Surg Am 70:75-83
16. Wang KC, Shih HN, Hsu KY, Shih CH (1994) Intercondylar fractures of the distal humerus: routine anterior subcutaneous transposition of the ulnar nerve in a posterior operative approach. J Trauma 36:770-773
17. Schemitsch EH, Tencer AF, Henley MB (1994) Biomechanical evaluation of methods of internal fixation of the distal humerus. J Orthop Trauma 8:468-475
18. Jacobson SR, Glisson RR, Urbaniak JR (1997) Comparison of distal humerus fracture fixation: a biomechanical study. J South Orthop Assoc 6:241-249
19. Korner J, Diederichs G, Arzdarf M et al (2004) A biomechanical evaluation of methods of distal humerus fracture fixation using locking compression plates versus conventional reconstruction plates. J Orthop Trauma 18:286-293

CHAPTER 6

The Fractures of the Olecranon

J.E. ADAMS, S.P. STEINMANN

Introduction

The subcutaneous location of the olecranon makes it vulnerable to trauma [1]. Isolated fractures of the olecranon comprise approximately 10% of fractures about the elbow [2, 3], with an estimated incidence of 1.08 per 10,000 person-years [3]. Most result from low energy trauma such as a fall from a height of less than 2 m, a direct blow to the elbow, or from forced hyperextension [2-7]. A fall on a partially flexed elbow may generate an avulsion fracture of the olecranon from the pull of the triceps [1]. Amis et al. [7] investigated variable impact mechanisms and the resultant fracture patterns in a cadaveric model. A trend was noted in which radial head and coronoid fractures tended to occur with forearm impacts with the elbow in up to 80° of flexion [7]. Olecranon fractures occurred with direct blows at 90° of flexion, while injuries occurring with the elbow in > 110° of flexion tended to result in distal humerus fractures [7].

Fractures of the olecranon are generally amenable to treatment and have a favorable prognosis following treatment [1, 3-5, 8, 9]. Ninety-six percent of patients have a good to excellent long term outcome with only rare subjective complaints [3, 8].

Anatomic Considerations

The olecranon, together with the coronoid process, forms the semilunar or greater sigmoid notch of the ulna [1]. This articulates with the trochlea of the humerus and confers stability and facilitates motion in the anterior-posterior plane [1]. A transverse "bare area" devoid of cartilage is found at the midpoint between the coronoid and the tip of the olecranon. The unwary surgeon may inadvertently discard structurally significant portions of the olecranon if this is not considered when reconstructing the fractured olecranon [1]. The ossification center of the olecranon generally appears by 9 to 10 years of age, and fuses to the proximal ulna by age 14 years [1, 10]. Persistence of the physis in adulthood may occur, and is usually bilateral and familial [1]. In addition, patella cubiti, an accessory ossicle embedded in the distal triceps may be present and likewise be confused with a fracture [1].

Evaluation

Because the fracture by nature is intra-articular with the exception of some avulsion-type fractures of the olecranon, hemarthrosis is frequently present in conjunction with olecranon fracture [1]. Although this sign may be obfuscated by pain due to the injury, inability to actively extend the elbow against gravity may be an important indication of triceps discontinuity [1]. Because of the proximity of the ulnar nerve, the first and each subsequent examination should document the status of the ulnar nerve [1]. Anteroposterior and true lateral radiographs should be obtained to aid in diagnosis and treatment considerations [1]. The true lateral film should be examined to determine the extent and nature of the fracture pattern and to evaluate for the presence of other lesions such as a radial head fracture or dislocation, or distal humerus or coronoid fractures [1].

Classification of Olecranon Fracture

Colton [11] classified olecranon fractures according to the amount of displacement and fracture pattern. Undisplaced fractures, Colton Type I, are characterized by displacement of less than 2 mm, with separation remaining less than 2 mm with flexion of the elbow to 90° or with extension against gravity, and the patient is able to actively extend the elbow against gravity [1, 11]. Type II, displaced fractures, may be further subtyped into avulsion fractures, oblique and transverse fractures, comminuted fractures, and fracture-dislocations [11].

Horne and Tanzer [4] proposed a classification system and treatment algorithm for olecranon fractures based upon their experience and review of 100 cases. In this system, Type I fractures are either transverse intra-articular fractures of the proximal third of the olecranon or extra-articular fractures involving the point of the olecranon. Type II fractures are oblique or transverse intra-articular fractures involving the middle third of the olecranon fossa with IIA representing those with a single fracture line and IIB representing those with a second more distal and posteriorly oriented fracture line. Type III fractures include those intra-articular fractures of the distal third of the olecranon fossa. From their review of these one hundred cases, Horne and Tanzer made treatment recommendations, including favoring the use of plate and screw with tension band fixation in cases of delay of greater than one week to decrease the risk of nonunion. Extra-articular Type I fractures were best treated with excision, while intra-articular Type I and Type II fractures should be treated with open reduction and internal fixation with tension band wiring. Recommendations for Type IIB fractures involved elevation of the depressed intra-articular fracture and buttressing with bone graft followed by tension band wiring. Type III fracture were best treated with plate and screw fixation to provide optimum rigidity to the construct as tension band wiring was less effective at this location.

Morrey classified olecranon fractures according to criteria regarding stability, comminution, and displacement (Fig. 1) [12, 13]. The Mayo Classification thus divides olecranon fractures into three types, facilitating classification and providing an algorithm for treatment. Type I, undisplaced fractures as defined by the Colton criteria above, may be subdivided into Type IA, noncomminuted fractures and Type IB, comminuted fractures. Due to the fact that these are by definition undisplaced, the practical significance of the degree of comminution is not significant and Types IA and IB may essentially be regarded and treated as the same lesion [12].

Mayo Type II fractures are the most common type [2, 6, 12]. These fractures, which are stable frac-

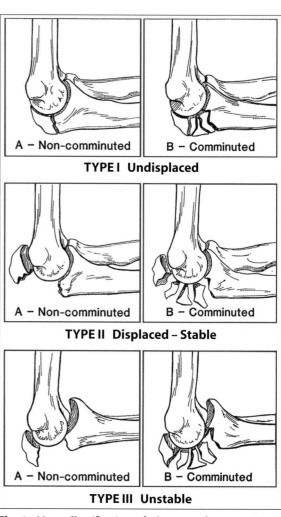

Fig. 1. Mayo Classification of olecranon fractures. Type I fractures are nondisplaced, non-comminuted (IA) or comminuted (IB) fractures. Type II fractures are stable displaced fractures, and may be non-comminuted (IIA) or comminuted (IIB). Type III fractures are unstable, displaced fractures, and may be non-comminuted (IIIA) or comminuted (IIIB). (Figures reproduced with permission, [13])

tures with greater than 3 mm of displacement, may be noncomminuted (Type IIA) or comminuted (Type IIB) [12]. Because the collateral ligaments are intact, the forearm is stable relative to the humerus [12]. Mayo Type III fractures are unstable, displaced fractures and represent a fracture-dislocation. Like Types I and II, Type III fractures may be subclassified into noncomminuted (IIIA) or comminuted (IIIB) types [12,13].

Complex Olecranon Fracture-Dislocations

Olecranon fractures associated with subluxation of the radial head and/or fracture of the coronoid process are typically multifragmentary, complex injuries [14-16]. Anterior fracture dislocations are often referred to trans-olecranon fracture-dislocations, as the mechanism of injury appears to involve anterior displacement of the forearm resulting in the trochlea being driven through the olecranon process. The radial head is displaced anteriorly, and this injury is differentiated from the Bado Type I Monteggia fracture by the presence of ulnohumeral joint destabilization with preservation of the radioulnar relationship [14,15]. Posterior fracture dislocations of the olecranon are more similar to Type II Monteggia fractures, with posterior dislocation of the radial head, an apex posterior fracture of the ulna, and similar implications for the stability and function of both the ulnohumeral joint as well as the forearm [14,16]. These fractures may be considered a variant of the posterior Monteggia lesion [16]. Both posterior and anterior variants are commonly associated with fractures of the coronoid, which are usually basal fractures involving 50%-100% of the height of the coronoid [14]. In anterior olecranon fracture-dislocations, reduction of the olecranon and coronoid fracture fragments results in restoration of stability with little implications for forearm dysfunction. Posterior olecranon fracture-dislocations, in contrast, have important implications with elbow instability and forearm dysfunction is common despite fracture reduction.

Treatment

The Mayo Classification provides a basis for a rational treatment algorithm by fracture type and subtype and conveys prognostic value [2,12].

Nondisplaced fractures (Mayo and Colton Types I) may be treated symptomatically and non-operatively with 7-10 days of immobilization followed by an active range of motion program [5,12,13,17]. Restrictions upon active resisted elbow extension and weightbearing should be maintained for 6-8 weeks with gradual increases in these activities as tolerated [17]. Close follow up with radiographs at 1 week, 2 weeks, and 4 weeks is recommended to assess for displacement and possible need for further intervention [1]. Rarely, in select patients, Type I fractures may benefit from open reduction and internal fixation to allow immediate motion and stability [12, 13]. Some Type I fractures may be treated with immobilization in a long arm cast at 90° of flexion for 3-4 weeks [1]. Thereafter, protected range of motion with avoidance of flexion greater than 90° until radiographic evidence of bony healing occurs, usually at 6-8 weeks, is recommended. Range of motion exercises may be commenced at an earlier time point in select patients, such as the elderly, in whom stiffness occurs more frequently.

Displaced fractures usually require surgical intervention [5,13,17]. Goals of surgical management include restoring the articular congruity and stability of the elbow, maintaining extension power, and providing stable anatomic fixation such that early range of motion is possible, thereby lessening the risk of post-operative stiffness [1, 5, 18, 19]. Options include tension band wiring, intramedullary screw placement, plate and screw constructs, bioabsorbable pins, or excision [2, 5, 6, 12, 17, 20, 21]. Tension band wiring is generally accepted and widely used as treatment for most olecranon fracture types (Fig. 2) [2,12].

Mayo Type IIA fractures, displaced noncomminuted stable fractures, are the most common type of olecranon fracture, and are usually adequately treated with tension band wiring [12, 13]. Intramedullary fixation has also been described for selected patients, although reported outcomes have been variable and biomechanical data is less supportive of this technique [6, 22, 23]. Type IIB frac-

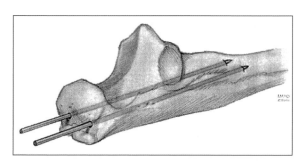

Fig. 2. Line drawing demonstrating optimal AO technique for placement of K-wires engaging the anterior cortex to assure maximal stability for tension band wiring. (Figure reproduced with permission, [13])

tures, displaced, comminuted, stable fractures are treated according to the age and activity level of the patient [12, 13]. In patients younger than age 60, anatomic reduction of fracture fragments followed by plate and screw fixation is the treatment of choice [12]. Care should be taken to avoid shortening the articular groove of the ulna between the olecranon process and the coronoid process, as doing so may lead to early arthritis.

In older patients, or when comminution is severe, excision of proximal fragments with advancement and re-insertion of the triceps tendon may be preferred [9, 12, 21, 24, 25].

Mayo Type III fractures, displaced, unstable fractures, represent the most difficult treatment challenge of all olecranon fractures and are associated with the highest complication rates and less satisfactory outcomes [2, 6, 12, 13, 26]. Again, goals of surgical management include anatomic reduction of the articular surface and stable fixation to allow for early motion as well as preservation of the extensor mechanism [1, 5, 18, 19, 26]. Type III fractures are associated with a high incidence of concomitant pathology, such as ligamentous trauma or bony injuries of the radial head or coronoid or distal humerus [6]. These associated injuries should be addressed at time of olecranon fixation. Type III olecranon fractures typically require plate fixation and ligamentous reconstruction [12, 13]. One may consider application of a hinge fixator if stability is not restored [12].

Non-comminuted (Type IIIA) fractures may be treated with a plate and screw construct and anatomic reduction [12]. Comminuted (Type IIIB) fractures may likewise be treated with plate osteosynthesis or preferentially be treated with excision of fracture fragments. In addition, excision of fracture fragments is indicated in cases of nonunion, patients who are elderly, or who have poor soft tissue viability, and in cases with severe comminution [1, 9].

Avulsion type fractures do not fit into the Mayo Classification well, but are common in the elderly, and may result from forces generated by the triceps [1]. Generally, these fractures have little comminution present, making tension band wiring the treatment of choice. In cases in which the fracture fragments are small, excision with triceps advancement and repair to bone may be considered.

Olecranon fracture-dislocations require special considerations for treatment. Because of inherent instability of these fracture patterns, they are best treated with plate and screw osteosynthesis. O'Driscoll et al. [14] and others [16] recommend a dorsal midline approach to the olecranon and use of a contoured plate. One-third tubular plates lack the stiffness necessary to withstand early range of motion and have been associated with early loosening or fatigue fractures [15]. Medial and or lateral flaps may be raised to access other pathology to bone or ligamentous structures, or concomitant radial head or coronoid fractures may be treated through the window created by the olecranon fracture [14]. The plate may be applied over part of the triceps insertion without muscle or periosteal elevation to optimize bone healing or the triceps may be split longitudinally and mobilized. If a concomitant anteromedial coronoid fracture fragment is present, it should be fixed to optimize stability of the elbow. When comminution is extensive, a skeletal distractor or temporary external fixation device may be helpful to facilitate reduction; after satisfactory reduction is obtained, definitive fracture fixation using plate and screws with or without augmentation with tension band wiring is usually possible [14, 15]. If extensive comminution is present such that plate and screw fixation does not provide sufficient fracture stability, augmentation with tension band wiring through the triceps insertion may facilitate stable fixation [14].

Range of motion exercises are ideally initiated within the first 1-2 days post-operatively if fracture stability allows [14]. More tenuous fixation or fractures in osteoporotic bone, particularly the inherently less stable posterior fracture-dislocation patterns, may require support with splinting for up to 4 weeks after surgery. The integrity of the lateral collateral ligament (LCL) and the anteromedial coronoid are important factors in stability of the fracture. Ring et al. [15] noted mostly good to excellent elbow scores following fixation of transolecranon fractures and attributed their low incidence of post-traumatic arthrosis to the nature of the articular surface of the olecranon. Restoration of the olecranon and coronoid facets is key as the intervening segment, the transverse ridge of the olecranon, contributes little surface contact area to the articular interface.

Specific Treatment Options

Excision

Excision of fracture fragments with advancement and re-insertion of the triceps tendon may be indicated in cases of nonunion, patients who are elderly or who have poor soft tissue viability, avulsion-type extra-articular fractures, and in cases with severe comminution as in Mayo Type IIB or IIIB fractures (Fig. 3) [1, 9, 12, 21, 24, 25]. Disadvantages

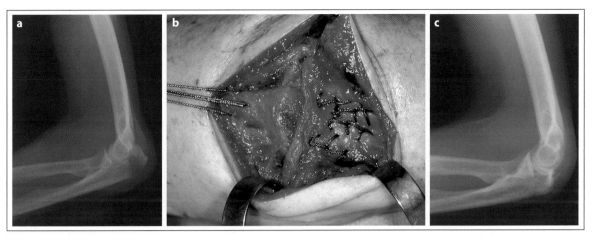

Fig. 3. (**a**) This 69-year-old man with poorly controlled Type I diabetes fell sustaining this Type IIA olecranon fracture. (**b**) He was subsequently treated with excision of fracture fragments and by suturing the triceps down to the remaining distal fragment. (**c**) At 4 years follow-up, the patient had no complaints, no instability, and range of motion was pronation-supination 80-80, full flexion and a 25° extension lag. Radiographs were satisfactory

of excision include subsequent risks of triceps weakness, instability, stiffness, and a theoretical risk for increased arthrosis [1, 24, 27-29].

Many authorities recommend re-attachment of the triceps at the level of the articular surface [1, 24]. However, doing so may result in decreased extension strength [24]. Didonna et al. [24] studied variable positions for triceps re-attachment following partial olecranon (50%) excision for simulated olecranon fracture in a cadaveric model. Loads were applied along the triceps mechanism at 45°, 90° and 135° and the resultant forces recorded. A significant decrease in extension strength with anterior placement of the triceps relative to normal and relative to posterior placement was noted, with the differences greatest with increasing extension. In contrast, posterior reattachment was noted to result in decreased extensor strength only at 90°. The authors therefore recommended more posterior re-attachment site to minimize loss of extension strength.

Fern et al. [21] described reconstruction of the ulna with osteotomy and excision of comminuted proximal segments with advancement and repair of the remaining proximal fragment to the remaining distal fragment. This may be useful in cases in which the degree of articular involvement is too great to preserve stability if the fragments were simply excised and the triceps tendon advanced only.

McKeever and Buck determined that one may excise up to 80% of the olecranon without sacrificing stability if the coronoid and anterior soft tissues are intact [1, 21, 30]. If anterior damage is present, instability is a sequelae if too much proximal ulna is excised [1]. In addition, An et al. [29] noted increasing instability of the elbow with olecranon excision. Kamineni et al. [27] investigated the results of olecranon resection upon stability to posteromedial stresses in a cadaveric model to simulate resection of osteophytes and proximal ulna as in treatment of posteromedial osteophytes such as in throwing athletes. The investigators noted a clinically significant level of instability to valgus stresses following resection of as little as 6 mm of posteromedial olecranon. The authors speculated that this may not be clinically relevant in low demand, elderly patients, but may be problematic in higher demand athletes or active patients or laborers. The increased instability may place increased stress upon the medial collateral ligament (MCL), predisposing to possible failure [27]. However, satisfactory clinical outcomes (Fig. 3) have been described for treatment of olecranon fracture by excision when used in appropriate patient populations [5, 9, 21, 25]. Gartsman [5] noted equivalent range of motion, functional status, extensor strength, pain, stability, and incidence of degenerative changes in cases of olecranon fracture treated by open reduction and internal fixation or primary excision. In addition, local complications (23% *vs* 4%) and requirements for additional procedures (an additional 23%), such as hardware removal, were more common in the patients treated with open reduction and internal fixation.

Despite documented satisfactory outcomes with excision, some speculate that excision may lead to development of arthrosis [28]. In a cadaveric model with 50% olecranon osteotomy to simulate an olecranon fracture, peak forces across the ulnohumeral joint were measured following either excision of the proximal fragment or open reduction and internal fixation with tension band wiring. Elbows fixed with tension band wiring had no significant difference in peak ulnohumeral pressures when compared to the intact elbow joint. In contrast, elbows with excision of the proximal fragment were noted to have significant increases in joint forces over the medial and lateral articular surfaces. The authors theorized that open reduction and internal fixation with tension band wiring restores the normal biomechanics of the elbow while excision results in abnormal joint forces, which may predispose to arthrosis. As such, Moed et al. favored open reduction and internal fixation in cases in which a large proximal fragment is present.

Options for Fracture Fixation Following Open Reduction

Tension Band Wiring

Tension band wiring is a widely accepted and used fixation technique for osteosynthesis of olecranon fractures. Tension band wiring converts tensile forces across the fracture to compressive forces, that with motion, exert compression across the fracture site [1]. It may be favored over plate and screw fixation due to requirements for less soft tissue dissection and less periosteal stripping [4]. However, this fixation technique may have technical challenges and be associated with undesirable post-operative sequelae [2]. Due to the subcutaneous nature and location of the elbow, prominent hardware may be problematic with large numbers

of patients in one series reporting hardware-related pain (24%) and functional difficulties (32%) relieved by hardware removal (13% and 15% pain and functional difficulties post removal, respectively) [2]. Nevertheless, up to 97% good to excellent results have been widely reported with use of tension band wiring using the proper technique [31].

Some have proposed modifications of the AO technique for tension band wiring of olecranon fractures, citing an increased load to failure, technically easier insertion and fewer complication with these modifications [32]. Biomechanical studies have suggested that these claims may not be accurate. Wu et al. found no difference in the rate of K-wire extrusion or load to failure in a series of cadaveric simulated transverse olecranon fractures fixed either with the traditional AO technique or the new modifications. Furthermore, results suggested that < 5.5 kg loads could be borne post-operatively during activities of daily living, with single loads to not exceed 8 kg, without adverse consequences. Paremain et al. [33] investigated biomechanics of tension band wiring for fixation of olecranon fractures. In a cadaveric model, transverse olecranon fractures were repaired using two techniques of tension band wiring: the tightening knot AO technique espoused by Weber and Vasey [34], and the modification to this technique proposed by Rowland and Burkhart [33]. Similar mechanism of failure occurred in both groups with no statistical significance in load to failure between the groups [33].

Intramedullary Nail *vs* Tension Band Wiring

Others have reported on unlocked intramedullary screw fixation for olecranon fractures, but higher rates of fixation loss than in tension band wiring have been noted (Fig. 4) [22, 23]. Some have uti-

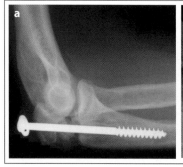 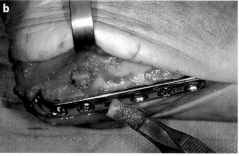 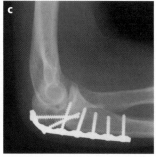

Fig. 4. (**a**) This 74-year-old man presented with a symptomatic and painful nonunion of the olecranon six months following failed treatment with an intramedullary screw. (**b**) He underwent open reduction and internal fixation with autogenous iliac crest bone graft. (**c**) Post-operative radiographs were satisfactory, and the patient experienced complete pain relief and return of

lized tension band wiring in conjunction with un-locked intramedullary screws [22].

Molloy et al. [22] investigated biomechanical features of tension band wiring *vs* intra-medullary nail fixation of transverse olecranon fractures. Both tension band wiring and plate-and-screw fixation have high success and union rates; however, due to painful or prominent hardware, 80% of tension band wiring and 20% of plate-and-screw constructs require removal. In addition, some fracture patterns, particularly oblique and distal fractures, may be less amenable to tension band wiring, and require plate-and-screw osteosynthesis. Accordingly, some have espoused the use of locked in-tramedullary nail fixation to enhance fracture fixation with minimal hardware prominence. Molloy et al. studied biomechanical features of olecranon fracture fixation with tension band wiring or with intramedullary nail in a cadaveric model. Tension band wiring was performed ac-cording to the AO technique. Cannulated 75 mm × 75 mm long intramedullary nails were inserted in the olecranon until flush with the bone, and then locking screws were placed. Specimens un-derwent mechanical testing to failure. Intrame-dullary nail fixation was stiffer and had a higher maximum load to failure than did tension band wiring fixation. However, the authors note that this *in vitro* study fails to replicate important *in vivo* considerations, such as the potential for damage to the triceps, the ulnar nerve during locking screw placement, and the effect of cycli-cal loading as well as union rate. In addition, with intramedullary nailing, the potential exists for fracture malreduction secondary to off-axis placement of the nail [22].

Plate-and-Screw Fixation

Multiple plate-and-screw constructs have been described for the treatment of olecranon frac-tures [26]. Advantages of plate fixation include favorable biomechanics which can act as a ten-sion band and as a buttress. In addition, hard-ware prominence is less problematic in plate-and-screw constructs relative to tension band wiring fixation [6]. Nowinski et al. [26] de-scribed results of treatment of comminuted ole-cranon fractures with an AO limited contact dy-namic compression plate formerly used for wrist fusion. They noted the low-profile but rigid char-acteristics of this plate were favorable for adap-tation to olecranon fracture fixation, and de-scribed satisfactory clinical outcomes. Bailey et al. [20] retrospectively reviewed outcomes of plate fixation of olecranon fractures in 25 pa-tients. All of these patients were Mayo Type II or III, and satisfactory anatomic reduction was maintained to bony union. Only supination was statistically poorer in the fractured side relative to the normal side; side to side differences in range of motion and strength were not statisti-cally significantly different between the fractured and unfractured sides. Mayo Elbow Performance Index (MEPI) scores were 88% good to excellent and the DASH scores were consistent with almost normal upper extremities. SF-36 demonstrated no impairment relative to the average American population. Twenty percent of patients required hardware removal due to plate prominence, but outcomes were satisfactory with minimal pain and a high degree of patient satisfaction in most cases (Fig. 4, 5).

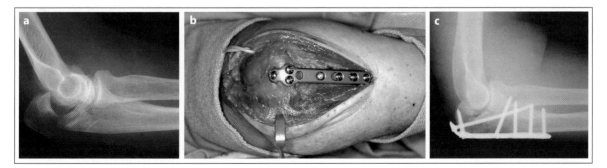

Fig. 5. (**a**) This 62-year-old female goat farmer fell on her left elbow sustaining a Type IIB olecranon fracture, (**b**) which was treated with plate-and-screw osteosynthesis. At just one month post-operatively, her range of motion was 15-115 degrees in the flexion-extension arc, with 80 degrees of pronation and 80 degrees of supination

Plate-and-Screw Fixation *vs* Tension Band Wiring

Hume et al. [35] studied outcomes of displaced olecranon fractures treated with either plate or tension
band wiring fixation in a prospective randomized
trial. Plate fixation was superior with respect to
maintenance of reduction without step off or gap
(95% *vs* 47%), radiographic outcomes (86% *vs* 47%
good) and clinical outcomes (63% *vs* 37% good).
Range of motion at 6 months was equivalent. Plate
fixation required longer operative times but was associated with no increase in complication rates. Tension band wiring was complicated with symptomatic hardware prominence in 42%.

Horner et al. [19] investigated use of tension
band wiring *vs* one-third tubular plate and screws
for fixation of simulated fractures of the most distal
portion of the olecranon (Colton Type III and
Horne Type III) in a cadaveric model. These fractures, due to the deforming forces of the forearm
flexors, tend to be more unstable than their more
proximal counterparts. The study demonstrated
increased fixation stiffness in those fractures treated with one-third tubular plate fixation (163 N/mm
vs 53 N/mm) *vs* tension band wiring and the authors concluded that fixation with plate and screws
would better counteract forces exerted by the brachioradialis and the biceps than tension band
wiring in this fracture pattern.

Fyfe et al. [18] investigated rigidity of various
methods of fixation of transverse, oblique, and simulated comminuted olecranon fractures in a cadaveric model. Tension band wiring with two knots was
the most stable fixation construct for simulated
transverse fractures, whereas intramedullary screw
fixation with or without tension banding was unreliable in restoring stability. Oblique osteotomies
were best repaired with one-third tubular plate fixation or tension band wiring with two knots, whereas
the comminuted fractures were most rigidly fixed
with five-hole AO plate and screw fixation. In all cases, either tension band wiring or plate-and-screw
fixation yielded fixation sufficiently rigid to withstand forces equivalent to those experienced *in vivo*
with active mobilization of the elbow. For comminuted fractures, plate-and-screw fixation was recommended due to the greater stability noted in this *in
vitro* study.

Bioabsorbable Fixation

Bioabsorbable fixation may be desirable because of
the potential to avoid future operations for hard-

ware removal [36]. Patients treated with conventional metal fixation devices have a high likelihood
of requiring and additional procedure for removal
of bothersome and/or prominent hardware. Bostman et al. explored costs associated with the need
for hardware removal. Savings averaged $410 for
use of bioabsorbable implants in olecranon fractures when total costs for metallic fixation and subsequent removal were considered. The break-even
point was 46% of fractures requiring removal, so
that only at > 46% removal rate would use of bioabsorbable implants be financially favorable. Juutilainen et al. [37] found equivalent outcomes in patients with olecranon fracture treated with either
bioabsorbable implants (poly-L-lactide wire with
self-reinforced polyglycolide screws or self-reinforced poly-L-lactide plugs) *vs* metallic implants
(tension band wiring or K-wire plus cerclage wire
fixation) and noted cost savings due to avoiding a
second operation for hardware removal. Further
clinical experience is needed to determine the role
that bioabsorbable fixation techniques will assume
in the future.

Results

Complications of olecranon fracture include
nonunion (Fig. 4), infection, loss of motion, ulnar
nerve symptoms, arthrosis, and need for additional procedures, such as hardware removal [2, 3,
5, 6, 12, 38]. Loss of motion may be problematic,
and a 10°-15° extension lag is particularly common [12]. This appears to be related to immobilization. Radiographic evidence of degenerative
changes in the ulnohumeral joint has been documented in 20%-50% of patients up to 15-25 years
following olecranon fracture [3, 5].

The need for hardware removal of tension band
fixation may be obviated if wires are bent 180° and
impacted into bone with the triceps securely sutured over wires [6, 12]. Mullett et al. [38] noted the
effect of K-wire position on backing out of the wire
in a clinical series. They noted an increased risk of
back-out when wires were placed down the long
axis of the ulna as opposed to crossing the anterior
cortex with a concomitant increase in symptomatic
hardware, requiring hardware removal (42% *vs*
11.4%). In addition, Mullett found a higher pullout
strength in a cadaveric investigation in those
K-wires placed according to optimal AO specifica-
tion with transcortical contact (122.7 N *vs* 56.3 N).
These clinical and biomechanical data reinforce
the importance of use of proper transcortical

rather than shaft K-wire placement and adherence to the AO technique to avoid potential hardware complications.

Rommens et al. [2] described outcomes of surgical fixation of 95 consecutive olecranon fractures treated from 1992 to 2000. By type and subtype, 14% were Type IA, 8% Type IB, 20% Type IIA, 29% Type IIB, 11% Type IIIA, 19% Type IIIB. About one third of patients had concomitant upper extremity fractures. Ninety-five percent were treated with tension band wiring constructs, and the remainder were treated with plate osteosynthesis. Approximately 10% experienced implant migration and 3.2% had delayed union, 2.1% infection, and 14.7% required additional surgical procedures for complications. In addition, two-thirds underwent hardware removal at an average of 12 months post-operatively. Radiographic changes included intra-articular stepoff without frank arthrosis in 7%; mild-moderate arthrosis in 20%, severe arthrosis in 12%, and pseudoarthrosis in 1%. Most patients experienced little or no limitations in pronation or supination (>90% had normal or less than a 10° deficit) or flexion (81% had no or less than 10° of deficit); but 46% of patients had a > 10° extension deficit. In addition, many patients experienced decreased strength in extension (50%) or flexion (37%). Patients with Mayo Type III fractures or coexisting lesions of the ipsilateral upper extremity were more likely to have larger deficits in the flexion extension arc than patients with Type I or II lesions. Likewise, suboptimal fixation was noted to be a risk factor for development of arthrosis; although this may be a confounding factor as both were more commonly seen in more complex fracture patterns.

Karlsson et al. [8] investigated long-term outcomes of tension band wiring and figure of eight wiring techniques for fixation of olecranon fractures. With respect to all fractures, 96% of patients had a good or excellent outcome up to 25 years post injury and fracture fixation. No significant difference between fracture fixation type and subjective outcome was noted. Fractures fixed with figure-of-eight wiring were more likely to have impaired pronation but contralateral reduced pronation was also noted in this group, indicating a possible difference between the groups unrelated to the surgical technique. No significant differences in other parameters of range of motion were noted between the groups. Follow-up radiographs demonstrated degenerative changes in most of the injured elbows, with subchondral cysts in 45%, subchondral sclerosis in 73%, osteophyte formation in 45%, and joint incongruity in 36%. Frank osteoarthritis was noted in 7%. When the two groups were compared, subchondral cyst formation (50% *vs* 39%), subchondral sclerosis (93% *vs* 54%), and radiographic frank arthrosis (16% *vs* 5%) were more common in the figure of eight wiring group, whereas osteophyte formation (61% *vs* 50%) and joint incongruity (43% *vs* 29%) were more common in the tension band group. Hardware removal was performed in 81% of those elbows treated by tension band wiring and 43% of elbows treated with figure-of-eight fixation. Because there were no significant clinical differences between the groups regarding outcome, Karlsson et al. recommended use of figure-of-eight wiring for fixation of olecranon fractures as the hardware removal rate was half that of elbows treated with tension band wiring.

Authors' Preferred Techniques

For Mayo Type I fractures, conservative non-operative management is preferred. The patient is placed in sling immobilization for comfort with early active gentle range of motion exercises. Close follow-up (weekly) with radiographs is essential to rule out displacement and need for alternative treatment.

Type II and III fractures are best treated surgically, with either excision or open reduction and internal fixation (Figg. 3 and 5). For fractures with fragments distal to the coronoid, plate-and-screw osteosynthesis is preferred, as these more distal fragments are usually not adequately fixed by tension band wiring. Likewise, more comminuted fractures or oblique patterns are best treated with plate-and-screw fixation to optimize stability [18, 19].

Excision of fracture fragments is preferred for elderly, low demand patients (Figg. 3) or those with extensive fracture comminution, or for treatment of nonunions. Tension band wiring using the standard AO technique may be performed for selected patterns amenable to this fixation technique. Otherwise, in the Authors' experience, plate-and-screw osteosynthesis provides the optimal fixation stability with minimal complications. Intramedullary screw or nail fixation or figure-of-eight wiring are generally not recommended due to their less reliable fixation stability (Fig. 4).

Technique for Excision or Open Reduction and Internal Fixation

We recommend a midline longitudinal incision curving over the olecranon to avoid placing the incision over the subcutaneous bone [5]. Excision may be performed by sharp dissection of fracture fragments from the triceps aponeurosis, and longitudinal drill holes made through the proximal ulna to secure the triceps tendon down to bone. Tension band wiring or plate-and-screw osteosynthesis may be performed using the standard AO technique. The wound is then closed in the standard fashion and a posterior plaster dressing is applied in full extension. The arm should be elevated overnight and the initial dressing changed on the second day. Active and passive motion is then initiated. Alternatively, if for any reason the operative fixation was felt to be less than optimal, splinting may be continued for 3 to 4 weeks to allow for some bony healing. Protected use of the extremity is maintained with minimal weightbearing and no resistance greater than that of gravity for 6 weeks or until radiographic evidence of healing is seen.

In conclusion, olecranon fractures are commonly seen in orthopedic practice and with appropriate treatment, generally have good to excellent outcomes with little adverse sequelae. Decreased range of motion, radiographic evidence of degenerative changes, and requirement for hardware removal are common but generally are not devastating complications, and may be obviated by attention to proper technique, anatomic reduction, and proper post-operative management.

References

1. Bucholz RW, Heckman JD (2001) Rockwood and Green's Fractures in Adults, 5th ed. Lippincott, Williams & Wilkins
2. Rommens PM, Schneider RU, Reuter M (2004) Functional results after operative treatment of olecranon fractures. Acta Chir Belg 104:191-197
3. Karlsson MK, Hasserius R, Karlsson C, Besjakov J, Josefsson PO (2002) Fractures of the olecranon: a 15- to 25-year follow-up of 73 patients. Clin Orthop 403:205-12
4. Horne JG, Tanzer TL (1981) Olecranon fractures: a review of 100 cases. J Trauma 21:469-472
5. Gartsman GM, Sculco TP, Otis JC (1981) Operative treatment of olecranon fractures. Excision or open reduction with internal fixation. J Bone Joint Surg Am 63:718-721
6. McKay PL, Katarincic JA (2002) Fractures of the proximal ulna olecranon and coronoid fractures. Hand Clin 18:43-53
7. Amis AA, Miller JH (1995) The mechanisms of elbow fractures: an investigation using impact tests in vitro. Injury 26:163-168
8. Karlsson MK, Hasserius R, Besjakov J et al (2202) Comparison of tension-band and figure-of-eight wiring techniques for treatment of olecranon fractures. J Shoulder Elbow Surg 11:377-382
9. Compton R, Bucknell A (1989) Resection arthroplasty for comminuted olecranon fractures. Orthop Rev 18:189-192
10. Evans MC, Graham HK (1999) Olecranon fractures in children: Part 1: a clinical review. Part 2: a new classification and management algorithm. J Pediatr Orthop 19:559-569
11. Colton CL (1973) Fractures of the olecranon in adults: classification and management. Injury 5:121-129
12. Morrey BF (1995) Current concepts in the treatment of fractures of the radial head, the olecranon, and the coronoid. Instr Course Lect 44:175-185
13. Cabenela ME, Morrey BF (2000) Fractures of the olecranon. In: BF Morrey (ed.) The Elbow and its Disorders, WB Saunders Co, Philadelphia
14. O'Driscoll SW et al (2003) Difficult elbow fractures: pearls and pitfalls. Instr Course Lect 52:113-134
15. Ring D et al (1997) Transolecranon fracture-dislocation of the elbow. J Orthop Trauma 11:545-550
16. Doornberg J, Ring D, Jupiter JB (2004) Effective treatment of fracture-dislocations of the olecranon requires a stable trochlear notch. Clin Orthop 429:292-300
17. Boyer MI et al (2003) Intra-articular fractures of the upper extremity: new concepts in surgical treatment. Instr Course Lect 52:591-605
18. Fyfe IS, Mossad MM, Holdsworth BJ (1985) Methods of fixation of olecranon fractures. An experimental mechanical study. J Bone Joint Surg Br 67:367-372
19. Horner SR, Sadasivan KK, Lipka JM, Saha S (1989) Analysis of mechanical factors affecting fixation of olecranon fractures. Orthopedics 12:1469-1472
20. Bailey CS, MacDermid J, Patterson SD, King GJ (2001) Outcome of plate fixation of olecranon fractures. J Orthop Trauma 15:542-548
21. Fern ED, Brown JN (1993) Olecranon advancement osteotomy in the management of severely comminuted olecranon fractures. Injury 24:267-269
22. Molloy S, Jasper LE, Elliott DS et al (2004) Biomechanical evaluation of intramedullary nail versus tension band fixation for transverse olecranon fractures. J Orthop Trauma 18:170-174
23. Helm RH, Hornby R, Miller SW (1987) The complications of surgical treatment of displaced fractures of the olecranon. Injury 18:48-50
24. Didonna ML, Fernandez JJ, Lim TH et al (2003) Partial olecranon excision: the relationship between triceps insertion site and extension strength of the elbow. J Hand Surg Am 28:117-122
25. Estourgie RJ, Tinnemans JG (1982) Treatment of grossly comminuted fractures of the olecranon by excision. Neth J Surg 34:127-129
26. Nowinski RJ, Nork SE, Segina DN, Benirschke SK (2000) Comminuted fracture-dislocations of the elbow treated with an AO wrist fusion plate. Clin Orthop Relat Res 378:238-244
27. Kamineni S, Hirahara H, Pomianowski S et al (2003) Partial posteromedial olecranon resection: a kinematic study. J Bone Joint Surg Am 85:1005-1011
28. Moed BR, Ede DE, Brown TD (2002) Fractures of the olecranon: an in vitro study of elbow joint stresses after tension-band wire fixation versus proximal fracture fragment excision. J Trauma 53:1088-1093
29. An KN, Morrey BF, Chao EY (1986) The effect of partial removal of the proximal ulna on elbow restraint. Clin Orthop 209:270-279
30. McKeever FM, Buck RM (1947) Fracture of the olecranon process of the ulna: treatment by excision of fragment and repair of triceps tendon. JAMA 135:1-5

31. Wolfgang G, Burke F, Bush D et al (1987) Surgical treatment of displaced olecranon fractures by tension band wiring technique. Clin Orthop 224:192-204

32. Wu CC, Tai CL, Shih CH (2000) Biomechanical comparison for different configurations of tension band wiring techniques in treating an olecranon fracture. J Trauma 48:1063-1067

33. Paremain G, Novac VP, Jinnah RH, Belkoff S (1997) Biomechanical evaluation of tension band placement for the repair of olecranon fractures. Clin Orthop Relat Res 335:325-330

34. Weber BG, Vasey H (1963) Osteosynthesis in olecranon fractures. Z Unfallmed Berufskr 56:90-96

35. Hume MC, Wiss DA (1992) Olecranon fractures. A clinical and radiographic comparison of tension band wiring and plate fixation. Clin Orthop 285:229-235

36. Bostman OM (1996) Metallic or absorbable fracture fixation devices. A cost minimization analysis. Clin Orthop 329:233-239

37. Juutilainen T, Patiala H, Rokkanen P, Tormala P (1995) Biodegradable wire fixation in olecranon and patella fractures combined with biodegradable screws or plugs and compared with metallic fixation. Arch Orthop Trauma Surg 114:319-323

38. Mullett JH, Shannon F, Noel J et al (2000) K-wire position in tension band wiring of the olecranon – a comparison of two techniques. Injury 31:427-431

CHAPTER 7
The Radial Head Fractures

M.W. HARTMAN, S.P. STEINMANN

Introduction

Radial head fractures represent the most common fracture of the elbow in the adult population, accounting for 1.7%-5.4% of all adult fractures. Approximately 85% of these fractures occur in young, active individuals ranging in age from 20 to 60 years-old. Radial head fractures may occur in isolation or may be part of a more extensive traumatic elbow injury. An estimated 20% of all acute elbow injuries have an associated radial head fracture (Fig. 1). In elbow dislocations, a radial head fracture is commonly associated with other traumatic pathologies including medial collateral ligament (MCL) rupture, olecranon fracture, and/or coronoid fracture. Therefore, in the setting of trauma, the elbow must be carefully evaluated to rule out associated ligamentous and bony pathology.

Radial head fractures usually result from a fall onto the outstretched hand with the elbow slightly flexed and the forearm in a pronated position. Biomechanical studies have demonstrated that the greatest amount of force is transmitted from the wrist to the radial head when the elbow and forearm are oriented in this position. During a fall, the body rotates internally on the elbow, the weight of the body contributes an axial load to the radius, and a valgus moment is applied to the elbow since the hand becomes laterally displaced from the body. The resultant combination of axial, valgus,

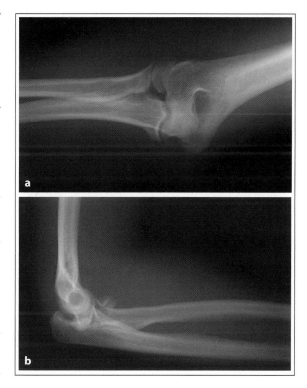

Fig. 1. Type III radial head fracture. (**a**) Anteroposterior view; (**b**) Lateral view

and external rotatory loading mechanisms forces the anterolateral margin of the radial head to come into contact with the capitellum, resulting in a fracture of the radial head and/or capitellum.

Surgical Indications and Other Options

The modified Mason classification proposed by Hotchkiss [4] is useful in predicting the surgical management of radial head fractures. Type I fractures include nondisplaced or minimally displaced fractures of the head and neck, fractures with intra-articular displacement of <2 mm, or marginal lip fractures. There should be no mechanical block to forearm rotation, however rotation may be limited by acute pain and swelling. The mainstay of treatment of Type I fractures involves non-operative measures that encourage early elbow and forearm range of motion. In the acute setting, the elbow hemarthrosis should be aspirated and injected with local anesthetic to allow a better assessment of forearm rotation, improve patient discomfort, and encourage earlier range of motion. The patient is placed into a sling for comfort and instructed to begin active and passive range of motion as tolerated within seven days. Protected weightbearing of the upper extremity for a period of six weeks is encouraged to prevent fracture displacement. Serial X-rays are obtained on a weekly basis to assess for fracture displacement. Open reduction internal fixation (ORIF) is indicated if the fracture displacement subsequently occurs. Good to excellent results are expected in the majority of Type I fractures managed non-operatively with a program of early elbow and forearm range of motion.

Type II fractures include displaced (>2 mm) fractures of the radial head or neck without severe comminution. These fractures may have mechanical block to motion or be incongruous. Nonoperative management of Type II fractures should be considered only if elbow stability is not dependent on fracture fixation and no significant block to elbow motion is present. In the absence of comminution, these fractures are usually amenable to ORIF (Fig. 2). Recent data suggest that ORIF should be reserved for minimally comminuted fractures with three or fewer articular fragments [5]. These data also suggest that fracture-dislocations of the elbow or forearm managed with ORIF result in less optimal results, especially with regard to forearm rotation. Other surgical options for Type II fractures include fragment excision, head excision, and radial head replacement arthroplasty. Fragment excision alone may be indicated when a fracture fragment blocks forearm rotation but is too small, comminuted, or osteoporotic to adequately gain fixation (Fig. 3). The fracture fragment should not involve the lesser sigmoid notch or involve more than 1/3 of the circumference of the head's articular surface. Most elbow surgeons discourage fragment excision due to the possibility of subsequent radial head subluxation.

Type III fractures include severely comminuted radial head or neck fractures that are deemed unreconstructable based on radiographic and/or intra-

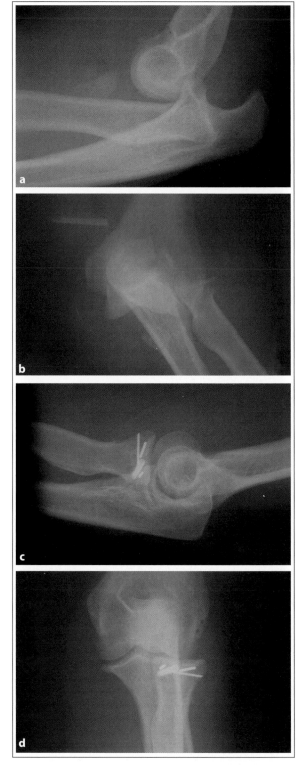

Fig. 2. (a) Lateral radiograph of fracture dislocation of elbow Type II fracture radial head. (b) Anteroposterior radiograph Type II fracture radial head. (c) Postoperative view: pin and screw fixation of radial head fracture (lateral view). (d) Postoperative view: pin and screw fixation of radial head fracture (anteroposterior view)

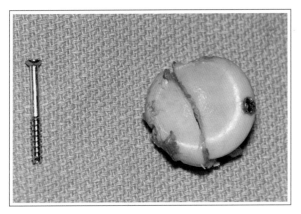

Fig. 3. Attempted screw fixation of radial head fracture

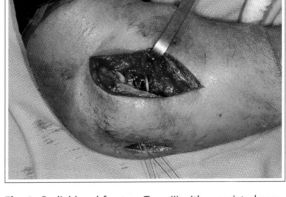

Fig. 4. Radial head fracture Type III with associated coronoid fracture. The radial head was replaced with a prosthesis and the coronoid fracture repaired with suture (second smaller, posterior incision)

operative appearance. Surgical options include radial head excision with or without radial head replacement arthroplasty. Prosthetic head replacement is indicated under associated conditions of instability such as complex elbow instability, Essex-Lopresti lesion, Monteggia lesion with instability, or a fracture of a major portion of the coronoid (Fig. 4).

Radial head excision alone may be indicated in elderly, low-demand patients without ligamentous instability. Numerous series report good to excellent results in terms of pain relief and elbow range of motion after head excision alone. The potential disadvantages of head excision include decreased grip strength, weak forearm rotation, and radial shortening with resultant wrist pain. Altered load transfer at the elbow joint may also lead to the development of early ulnotrochlear arthrosis and el-

bow pain. When compared to head excision, results of metal prosthetic radial head replacement demonstrate similar range of motion, better clinical scores, less proximal radial migration, and decreased elbow arthritis (Fig. 5).

Surgical Techniques

Pre-operative planning is essential in the surgical management of radial head fractures. A full selection of internal fixation and reconstructive options should be available to the surgeon. Options for internal fixation include various combinations of threaded K-wires (for provisional fixation), screws (bioabsorbable, Accutrak, Herbert, or Minifrag-

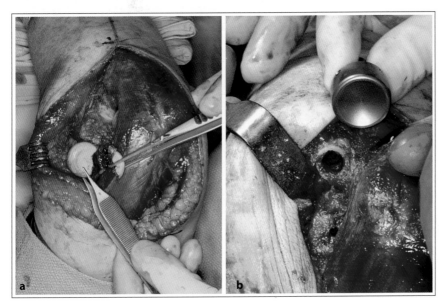

Fig. 5. (**a**) Type III radial head fracture. Attempt at open reduction internal fixation was unsuccessful. (**b**) Radial neck has been prepared for implantation of radial head prosthesis

ment screws), and plates (T-plate, L-plate, condylar blade plate, modular hand set). The ultimate goal of these hardware devices is to obtain rigid fixation and hence, allow early post-operative range of motion. The surgeon should be prepared to replace the radial head if indicated, preferably with a metallic prosthesis. The patient is positioned supine on the operating table, and general or regional anesthesia is administered. A sandbag is placed under the ipsilateral scapula to facilitate positioning of the upper extremity across the chest. Prophylactic antibiotics are administered 30 minutes prior to making the incision. An examination under anesthesia is performed prior to prepping and draping the involved extremity. Examination under anesthesia is absolutely essential in evaluating elbow and forearm stability and range of motion prior to proceeding. A skin incision is centered laterally over the lateral epicondyle and extended distally over the radial head and neck. Alternatively, a posterior elbow incision just lateral to the tip of the olecranon may be utilized in complex injuries in which access to the radial head, coronoid, medial collateral ligament, and/or lateral collateral ligament may be required (Fig. 6). Full-thickness flaps are developed down to the level of the fascia. The classic approach to the radial head utilizes Kocher's interval between the anconeus and extensor carpi ulnaris. This approach is disadvantageous for two reasons. First, the approach tends to expose the radial head too posteriorly, making internal fixation of the commonly fractured anterolateral head difficult, if not impossible. Second, iatrogenic injury to the lateral ulnar

collateral ligament is difficult to avoid, and may lead to posterolateral rotatory instability. An alternative approach that splits the extensor digitorum comminus is the preferred approach. This approach is more anterior and hence avoids disruption of the posterolateral collateral ligamentous complex (Fig. 7). The lateral epicondyle is identified, and the elbow capsule is elevated subperiosteally off its anterior aspect. Anterior capsular elevation is continued distally to the level of the capitellum and elbow joint taking care to avoid the collateral ligamentous complex posteriorly. Dissection next proceeds through the annular ligament exposing the radial head. If the fracture involves only the radial head, minimal distal (1-2 cm) dissection is usually necessary. If the radial neck is involved, further distal exposure is required. The forearm is fully pronated and the posterior portion of the extensor digitorum communis is divided. To avoid placing the posterior interosseous nerve at risk, distal dissection should not proceed more than two fingerbreadths from the radial head. If the location of the posterior interosseous nerve is in doubt,

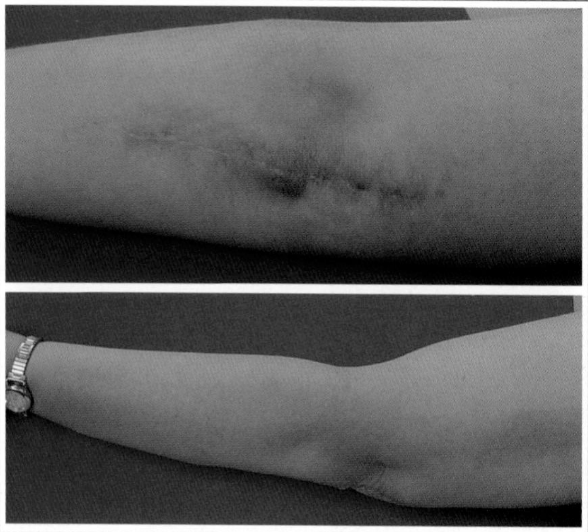

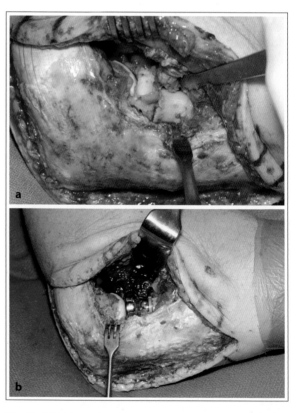

Fig. 7. (**a**) Type III fracture. Severe comminution noted at surgery. Surgical approach involved posterior skin incision with split of the EDC tendon origin to gain exposure. (**b**) Radial head prosthesis. Note metallic head centered on capitellum

Fig. 6. Post-operative photograph of posterior incision for radial head fracture. This is the standard approach used by the Authors due to the pleasing cosmetic result

definitive identification of the nerve may be required. Once sufficient exposure is obtained, the character of the fracture is thoroughly assessed. The capitellum is also visually assessed for the presence of an associated chondral injury or osteochondral fracture. The decision to proceed with fragment excision, head excision, ORIF, or radial head replacement arthroplasty can be made at this point. At the time of closure, the annular ligament and the posterolateral collateral ligament complex (if disrupted) are repaired. The fascial layer over the common extensor group is closed to augment lateral elbow stability. Elbow and forearm range of motion and stability are carefully assessed and recorded.

Open Reduction Internal Fixation

The concept of an anatomic "safe zone" must be understood when attempting hardware placement into the radial head. Hardware may be placed into this zone without causing impingement of the proximal radioulnar joint. The safe zone is defined by a 110° arc centered anterolaterally over the equator of the radial head with the forearm in neutral rotation. Alternatively, one may identify the safe zone as a 90° arc defined by the right angle from the radial styloid to Lister's tubercle. Surface anatomy can also help to identify the proper location for hardware placement. Once the fracture has been reduced, K-wires may be used for provisional fixation. K-wires should be absolutely avoided for definitive fixation given their tendency for migration post-operatively. For fractures that do not involve the radial neck, definitive fixation is typically obtained by using small screws such as Herbert mini-screws, mini-Acutrak screws, mini-fragment screws (sizes 1.5, 2.0, or 2.7 mm), and 3.0 mm cannulated screws. Screws should be countersunk beneath the articular surface but not protrude through the opposite cortex. Fractures involving the radial neck are often impacted and require bone grafting to elevate the radial head. These fractures may be amenable to screw and/or plate fixation. One technique that has been successful in the Authors' experience avoids the inherent problems associated with plate fixation for impacted neck fractures. In this technique, the radial head is first elevated to its anatomic position and temporarily secured using threaded K-wires. Screws are then placed obliquely from the radial head proximally to the opposite cortex of the radial neck distally. This arrangement may be likened to a bar stool in which the seat (the radial head) is supported by the eccentrically arranged legs (the screws). The resultant bony defect in the radial neck secondary to impaction is filled with autogenous bone graft or bone graft substitute. This technique has several advantages over plate fixation for radial neck fractures. First, screws are less bulky than plates and may decrease annular ligament impingement. Second, placement of screws generally requires less dissection and periosteal stripping, which may lessen the amount of blood supply disruption to the neck and decrease risk of injury to the posterior interosseous nerve. These advantages should theoretically result in decreased post-operative stiffness, painful hardware, heterotopic ossification, proximal radioulnar synostosis, and nonunion rates. If plate fixation is chosen, low-profile plates are necessary given the close proximity of the annular ligament and paucity of overlying soft tissues. Mini-condylar L-plates, T-plates, and fixed-angled blade plates are all available for radial head and neck fixation. There are few studies comparing internal fixation devices. A recent biomechanical study compared the average stiffness of several radial neck fracture plate fixation constructs axially loaded in compression [6]. The study demonstrated significantly greater stiffness with a 2.7 mm T-plate modified with a fixed angle blade compared to a 2.0 mm T-plate and 2.0 mm fixed angle blade. The investigators also noted increased proximal screw hole toggle when a fixed-angle device was not utilized. Contouring of the plate to the radius was observed to be the most important factor affecting overall construct stiffness. In another biomechanical study, investigators found no statistically significant difference in fixation stiffness when a low-profile blade plate and 3.0 mm cannulated screws were compared, but both constructs were significantly stiffer compared to a 2.7 mm T-plate [7].

Radial Head Replacement Arthroplasty

For all practical purposes, metal radial head prostheses have replaced silicone radial heads as the implant of choice in radial head replacement arthroplasty. Compared to metal radial heads, silicone implants are associated with worse clinical scores, increased elbow arthritis, and increased radial shortening. Furthermore, silicone implants are associated with increased failure secondary to fracture, fragmentation, and production of silicone synovitis. Both monoblock and modular radial head prostheses are now available. Anthropometric studies of cadaver proximal radii demonstrate that the head is inconsistently elliptical in shape, the head is variably offset from the axis of the neck, and the head diameter correlates poorly with the diameter of medullary canal of the neck [8]. These findings may support the use of modular implants that allow improved sizing options that more closely approximate the anatomy of the proximal radius.

The radial head is approached in the manner previously described. The annular ligament is incised transversely to expose the radial head. The appropriate radial head resection guide is utilized to determine proper alignment and resection level. The neck should be osteotomized proximal to the bicipital tuberosity. The medullary canal of the proximal radius is then prepared with a starter awl, burrs, and broaches to accept the implant. Exposure may be improved by applying varus stress and placing the forearm in supination. Serial-sized broaches are used until a snug fit is obtained in the canal at the appropriate depth. The appropriate-sized trial stem is inserted assuring that the collar of the prosthesis is flush with the resected neck. In modular designs, the trial head is secured to the trial stem, and the elbow and forearm are placed through a full arc of motion. Tracking as well as the relationship between the prosthesis and the capitellum are carefully assessed. Once acceptable alignment and tracking are determined, the trial components are removed, and the final prosthesis is inserted. The stem may be press-fit or cemented in place depending on the design and stability of the stem in the medullary canal. The head is inserted over the taper of the stem and secured using an impactor. Final assessment of motion and stability of the elbow and forearm is performed.

Conclusions

Radial head and neck fractures are common injuries that require a thorough understanding of elbow anatomy and biomechanics for proper management. The goals of current management are aimed at restoring the normal anatomical and biomechanical relationships of the elbow in an effort to prevent the development of elbow stiffness, instability, and arthritis. Preservation of the radial head should be attempted in fractures that are amenable to internal fixation. Severely comminuted fractures that are not salvageable should be managed with radial head replacement. Regardless of the type of fracture and chosen method of management, a program of early range of motion should be incorporated.

References

1. Boyer MI, Galatz L, Borrelli J Jr et al (2003) Intra-articular fractures of the upper extremity: new concepts in surgical treatment. Instr Course Lect 52:591-605
2. Parasa RB, Maffulli N (2001) Surgical management of radial head fractures. J R Coll Surg Edinb 46:76-85
3. Van Glabbeek R, Van Riet R, Verstreken J (2001) Current concepts in the treatment of radial head fractures in the adult. A clinical and biomechanical approach. Acta Orthop Belg 67:430-441
4. Hotchkiss R (1997) Displaced fractures of the radial head: internal fixation or excision? J Am Acad Ortho Surg 5:1-10
5. Ring D, Quintero J, Jupiter J (2002) Open reduction and internal fixation of fractures of the radial head. J Bone Joint Surg Am 84:1811-1815
6. Patterson J, Jones C, Glisson R et al (2001) Stiffness of simulated radial neck fractures fixed with 4 different devices. J Shoulder Elbow Surg 10:57-61
7. Griffin J, Rath D, Chess D et al (1998) Internal fixation of radial neck fractures: in-vitro biomechanical analysis. Trans ORS 23:731
8. King G, Zarzour Z, Patterson S, Johnson J (2001) An anthropometric study of the radial head: implications in the design of a prosthesis. J Arthroplasty 16:112-116
9. O'Driscoll S, Jupiter J, Cohen M et al (2003) Difficult elbow fractures: pearls and pitfalls. Instr Course Lect 52:113-134

CHAPTER 8

The Treatment of Coronoid Fractures and their Complications

A.G. SCHNEEBERGER

▶ **Introduction**
▶ **Classification**
▶ **Diagnosis of Coronoid Fractures**
▶ **Treatment**
▶ **Complications**
▶ **Conclusions**
▶ **References**

Introduction

Fractures of the coronoid process often occur as combined injuries with ligamentous tears and various osseous lesions. Previously, the treatment of such injuries was often focused on the associated lesions such as the fractured radial head. This was due in part to the rather difficult approach to the coronoid. In addition, the importance of the coronoid process has been rather underestimated.

In 1989, Regan and Morrey [1] published a series of coronoid fractures. They reported poor outcome for large coronoid fractures. In 1996, Hotchkiss introduced the term "terrible triad" injury as a combined injury with fractures of the coronoid process and radial head, and dislocation of the elbow. The prognosis of such a complex injury has been found to be poor due to a high risk of persistent instability and early arthrosis [2, 3]. More recently, the importance of even small coronoid fracture fragments for causing instability was pointed out [4]. A recent *in vitro* study by this Author and others outlined the important role of the coronoid process in conditions after radial head resection [5]. Identification and accurate treatment of coronoid fractures are therefore essential to restore articular stability.

Classification

Classification by Regan and Morrey

The classification published in 1989 received wide acceptance [1]. On the basis of lateral plain radiographs, Regan and Morrey classified coronoid fractures into three types (Fig. 1): Type I, fracture of the tip of the coronoid; Type II, a fragment involving 50% of the coronoid, or less; and Type III, a fragment involving more than 50% of the coronoid.

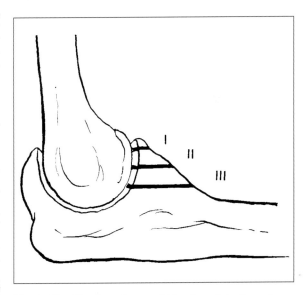

Fig. 1. Classification of coronoid fractures into three types by Regan and Morrey: Type I, fracture of the tip of the coronoid; Type II, a fragment involving 50% of the coronoid, or less; and Type III, a fragment involving more than 50% of the coronoid. (Figure reproduced with permission from [1])

Classification by O'Driscoll and Co-Authors

The classification by O'Driscoll and co-authors [6] was introduced in 2003. It considers in addition to the Regan and Morrey classification an anteromedial fracture pattern (Fig. 2, Table 1). It is based on the anatomic location with subtypes according to the severity of the coronoid involvement. It consists of three types: coronoid tip fractures, anteromedial fractures, and basal fractures.

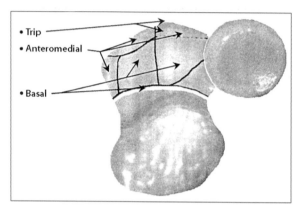

Fig. 2. Classification of coronoid fractures into three types and subtypes by O'Driscoll and co-authors. (Figure reproduced with permission from [6])

Table 1. O'Driscoll et al. classification of coronoid fractures

Fracture	Subtype	Description
Tip	1	≤2 mm of coronoid bony height (i.e. flake fractures)
	2	> 2 mm of coronoid height
Anteromedial	1	anteromedial rim
	2	anteromedial rim and tip
	3	anteromedial rim and sublime tubercle (± tip)
Basal	1	coronoid body and base
	2	transolecranon basal coronoid fractures

Coronoid Tip Fractures

Fractures of the coronoid tip have a fracture line in the coronal plane. They correspond to the coronoid Type I fractures of the Regan and Morrey classification. These fractures indicate a shear fracture by way of a joint subluxation or dislocation. This is not a capsular avulsion, because the el-

bow joint capsule inserts 4-6 mm distal to the tip of the coronoid. Subtype 1 is a small flake fracture, typically found after a posterior dislocation of the elbow. Subtype 2 fractures involve more than 2 mm of the tip, but they do not extend more than one-third of the coronoid or past the sublime tubercle medially. These subtype 2 fractures are often seen after a posterolateral rotatory dislocation of the elbow in association with a radial head fracture, the so-called terrible triad injury [7]. Typically, the lateral collateral ligament complex is torn after such injuries while the medial collateral ligament can be intact.

Anteromedial Coronoid Fractures

Subtype 1 of the anteromedial fractures involves an area between the tip of the coronoid and the sublime tubercle in an oblique plane between the coronal and the sagittal planes (Fig. 3). Medially, the fracture line usually exits the cortex in the anterior half of the sublime tubercle, i.e. in the anterior portion of the anterior bundle of the medial collateral ligament. The medial collateral ligament usually remains sufficient without causing medial joint space opening on valgus stress. Laterally, the fracture line exits just medial to the tip of the coronoid.

The anteromedial fractures can be comminuted and also include the tip of the coronoid (subtype 2)

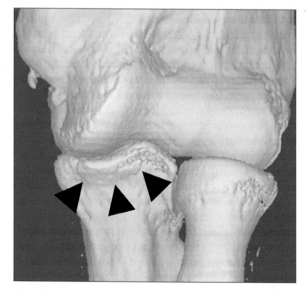

Fig. 3. A 3D reconstruction of CT scan of slightly displaced, anteromedial coronoid fracture subtype 1 (O'Driscoll et al. [6] classification) of a 48-year-old patient 8 weeks after a fall. He presented with severe pain and marked stiffness of the elbow. The fracture had been missed on plain radiographs

(Fig. 4), or they may include, besides the tip of the coronoid, the entire sublime tubercle with attachment of the anterior bundle of the medial collateral ligament (subtype 3).

The mechanism is a varus/posteromedial rotation injury with axial loading; for example a fall onto the ulnar side of the hand or forearm with a flexed elbow position. This causes a posteromedial rotatory displacement of the ulna underneath the trochlea with fracture of the anteromedial coronoid. Depending on the subtype, the anterior bundle of the medial collateral ligament may remain sufficient. Associated injuries may include tears of the lateral collateral ligament complex and of the posterior band of the medial collateral ligament, and also of radial head fractures in more severe cases. However, anteromedial coronoid fractures can occur as mainly isolated injuries without other associated fractures.

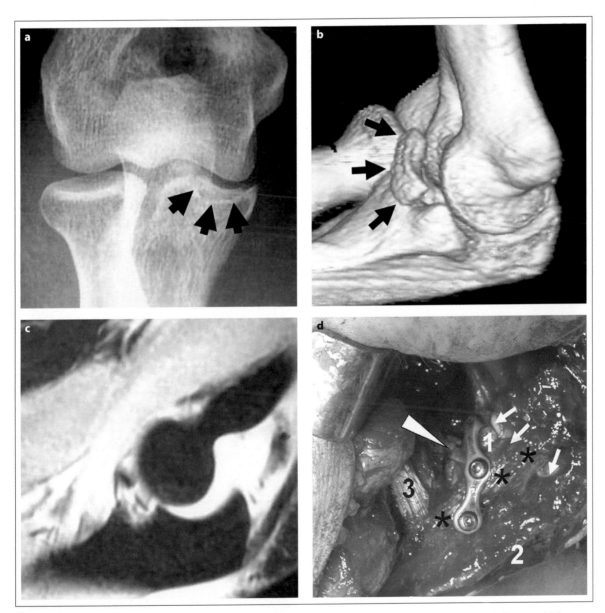

Fig. 4. (a) Anteroposterior radiograph of a 45-year-old woman 7 weeks after subtype 2 anteromedial coronoid fracture (O'Driscoll et al.[6] classification). Double subchondral bone line (marked with arrows) as a sign of displaced coronoid fragment. She presented with severe pain and stiffness. (b) 3D reconstruction of CT scan showing location and size of anteromedial coronoid fragment. (c) MRI indicating instability with posterior subluxation of the ulna. (d) Intra-operative view after medial approach according to Taylor and Scham [16]. (1) Coronoid fragment after osteotomy due to malunion, iliac crest bone graft insertion (*white triangular arrow*), and internal fixation with preshaped plate (Acumed). Asterisks, anterior bundle of medial collateral ligament; white arrows, trochlea. (2) Ulna. (3) Brachialis tendon

Basal Coronoid Fractures

Basal fractures involve at least 50% of the height of the coronoid. These fractures can result in one single fragment, but often they are comminuted.

Subtype 1 basal fractures are usually comminuted. They may have die-punch fragments and fracture lines extending into the proximal radioulnar articulation. The radial head is often fractured, and the ulnohumeral joint is usually unstable (Fig. 5).

Subtype 2 basal fractures consist of coronoid fractures associated with transolecranon fracture dislocation. These fractures sometimes have a single large coronoid fragment.

Diagnosis of Coronoid Fractures

History of a prior elbow dislocation, a radial head fracture, or painful stiffness of an elbow after a "simple" distortion of the elbow or a fall onto the involved extremity are suggestive of a potential coronoid fracture.

Plain anteroposterior and lateral radiographs most often allow an examiner to identify even small coronoid fractures. However, non-displaced coronoid fractures or subtype 1 anteromedial fractures might be difficult to identify on plain radiographs (Fig. 6), or they might even not be recognizable. Additional oblique views might be helpful in such instances.

Certain coronoid fractures show a double subchondral bone line at the medial joint surface on the anteroposterior view (Fig. 4a). An indirect sign of certain anteromedial coronoid fractures is the wedge sign on the varus stress views (Fig. 7b). The cause for the wedge sign or the "simulated" medial joint space narrowing, respectively, is a posteromedial rotatory subluxation of the ulna underneath the trochlea. For optimal identification of

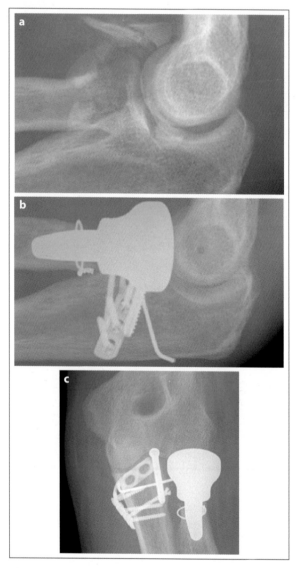

Fig. 5. (**a**) Comminuted basal coronoid fracture subtype 3 (O'Driscoll et al. [6] classification, corresponds to Type III, Regan and Morrey [1] classification) combined with radial head fracture after dislocation of the elbow ("terrible triad" injury). (**b**) One year after internal fixation, radial head replacement and temporary external fixator for 6 weeks. Patient with stable elbow, flexion arc of 10° to 130° and mild pain. (**c**) Anteroposterior view

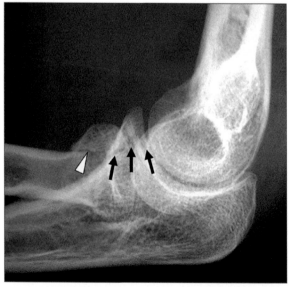

Fig. 6. Lateral radiograph of a 28-year-old patient with a slightly displaced coronoid Type II fracture (Regan and Morrey classification [1]) combined with a radial head fracture (white arrow)

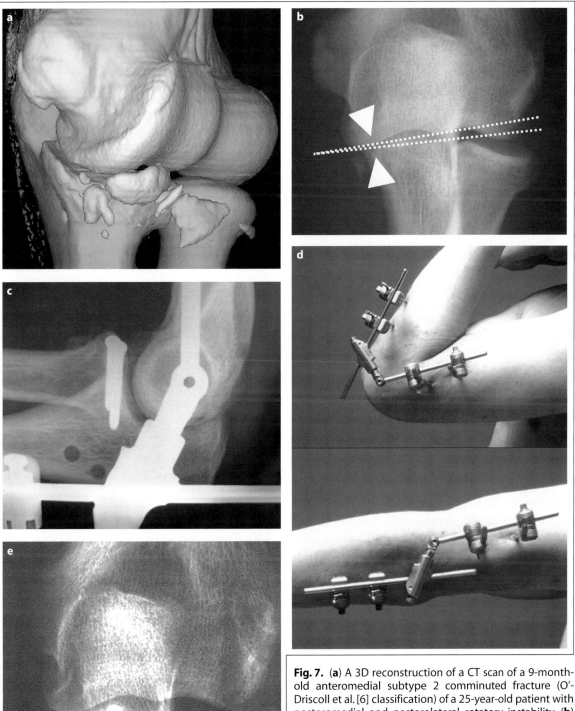

Fig. 7. (**a**) A 3D reconstruction of a CT scan of a 9-month-old anteromedial subtype 2 comminuted fracture (O'-Driscoll et al. [6] classification) of a 25-year-old patient with posteromedial and posterolateral rotatory instability. (**b**) Varus stress view showing wedge sign indicating postero-medial rotatory subluxation of ulna underneath trochlea. (**c**) Postoperative lateral radiograph after internal fixation of main coronoid fragment with 3.5 mm cannulated screws through a lateral Kocher approach, lateral collateral liga-ment reconstruction with palmaris longus autograft and hinged external fixator (Dynamic Joint Distractor 2, DJD 2, Stryker Corp.). (**d**) Hinged external fixator allowing early postoperative mobilization. (**e**) Radiograph 1 year after surgery with stable elbow, full function, and no pain

the size, location, and type of the coronoid fractures, a CT scan with two- and three-dimensional reconstructions gives the best imaging and diagnosis (Figs. 3, 4b, 7a).

Treatment

Type I Coronoid Fractures, Coronoid Tip Fractures

If coronoid Type I fractures or coronoid tip fractures are isolated fractures, they usually are "benign" injuries. They most often do not cause chronic instability, and can be treated like a simple elbow dislocation, with a short-term period of immobilization followed by an early range of motion program [8]. Conservative treatment resulted in good to excellent outcomes in over 90% of the cases in the series of Regan and Morrey [1], and in all cases in the series of Bousselmame et al. [9].

However, if coronoid Type I fractures are associated with radial head fractures, they might be considered severe injuries. These combined fractures have even been called "terrible triad injuries" [7]. In an *in vitro* study we found that an isolated defect of 30% of the height of the coronoid process caused no important instability [5]. In contrast, if a defect of 30% of the height of the coronoid process was associated with a defect of the radial head, the elbows were fully unstable in the laboratory, always resulting in posterolateral rotatory dislocation of the elbow despite of intact collateral ligaments [5]. If these *in vitro* findings were to be applied to patients, terrible triad injuries should be treated with strict preservation of the radial head, i.e. internal fixation of the fractured radial head whenever possible. If preservation of the radial head is not possible, it should not be resected, but replaced to avoid instability. The radial head implant should preferably be of a solid material rather than of Silastic or another soft material, to restore valgus stability [10]. In addition, some bipolar implants may not stabilize the elbow joint in the same manner as rigid devices [5].

With repaired or replaced radial heads, the elbow joints usually turn out to be stable even if small coronoid fragments are not fixed [5]. Small flake fractures (subtype 1 coronoid tip fractures) usually cannot be fixed in a satisfactory manner due to their small size. For subtype 2 coronoid tip fractures that involve about one-third of the height of the coronoid, internal fixation should be attempted in terrible triad injuries. This might be

obtained by direct screw fixation through the same lateral approach as for fixation of the radial head [11]. This is possible with the radial head in place, but significantly facilitated in those cases where the radial head has been resected before replacement. Alternatively, the coronoid fragments can be fixed by indirect screw or Kirschner wire insertion from the posterior ulnar cortex [12].

Stability of the elbow joint is best restored if the coronoid fragments are fixed in an anatomic position. In cases of anatomic but unstable fixation of small or comminuted coronoid fragments, protection by a hinged external fixator for about 6 weeks should be considered [13]. Cast immobilization alone might not be sufficient for protection of the repair, and might result in post-operative stiffness, especially if the immobilization is longer than 3 weeks [1].

The rational for this aggressive treatment of small coronoid fractures in terrible triad injuries is the potential need for later radial head resection due to post-traumatic arthrosis, or removal of radial head prosthesis due to loosening or capitellum erosion. The prognosis might be significantly better in conditions where the coronoid process has been restored compared to those conditions with a deficient coronoid process.

Type II Coronoid Fractures

Isolated Type II fractures represent an intermediate condition. Some of these fractures are stable and result in good outcomes after conservative treatment. In other conditions, these elbows might be unstable and require open reduction and internal fixation. There are no clear guidelines regarding how to determine whether these elbows are stable. A conservative trial might be attempted in all instances. Although a certain instability is always present immediately after an elbow dislocation, after 4 to 5 days of cast immobilization most elbows turn out to be stable, and the lateral plain radiographs show a reduced and centred ulnohumeral joint. However, persisting ulnohumeral subluxation on plain lateral radiographs suggests instability and may require internal fixation of these coronoid fractures.

Type II coronoid fractures combined with radial head fractures are treated like all terrible triad injuries with internal fixation of the coronoid fragments and internal fixation of the radial head whenever possible. If the radial head cannot be fixed, it is replaced. The coronoid fragments are repaired either with direct or indirect screw fixation alone, or using small plates with or without additional screws and K-wires. New pre-shaped plates may be helpful in these rather demanding procedures [6]. Hinged external fixators for about 6 weeks protect unstable coronoid repairs.

Various approaches may be suitable for internal fixation of the coronoid fractures:

- The lateral approaches (according to either Kocher [14] or Kaplan [15]) have the advantage that only one approach is necessary for fixation of the radial head and the coronoid. However, they might be suitable only for non-comminuted coronoid fractures that can be fixed with screws alone.
- The medial approaches (according to either Taylor and Scham [16] or Hotchkiss [17]) are suitable to expose the entire coronoid process including the sublime tubercle with the insertion of the anterior band of the medial collateral ligament (Fig. 4d). These approaches are useful for comminuted and/or for anteromedial coronoid fractures, and allow internal fixation with whatever method necessary. They even allow distal extension of the approach in cases of associated proximal ulnar fractures.
- The anterior approach through the brachialis muscle [18] may allow direct fixation of coronoid fractures, but probably due to the anterior neurovascular structures, this approach has not found wide acceptance.

If lateral and medial approaches are anticipated for fixation of radial head and coronoid fractures, a posterior midline incision is preferable to lateral and medial skin incisions in order to facilitate the approach and to avoid injury to the cutaneous nerves [19, 20]. Using the posterior skin incision it is possible to reach by subcutaneous preparation the lateral and the medial part of the elbow joint, including the possibility of subcutaneous transposition of the ulnar nerve [21].

In the series by Regan and Morrey, 15 of 16 Type II coronoid fractures were treated conservatively. Eight of the 16 cases had a concomitant fracture of the radial head, the medial epicondyle, or the olecranon. Overall, 74% of the 16 fractures had a good or excellent outcome at latest follow-up. In the series by Bousselmame [9] there were 7 Type II fractures. A satisfactory outcome was obtained in 2 of 3 cases with conservative treatment. Of 4 surgical cases, 3 had direct anatomic screw fixation with a satisfactory outcome, and 1 comminuted fracture was fixed using osteosuture alone, resulting in a fair outcome [9].

Type III Coronoid Fractures, Basal Coronoid Fractures

These fractures involve more than 50% of the height of the coronoid. If displaced, they always cause instability [5, 22]. These fractures usually represent more severe injuries, and they are often as-

sociated with other fractures and dislocation of the elbow. Frequently, these fractures are comminuted, and successful internal fixation might not always be achieved. The treatment of choice is open reduction and internal anatomic fixation, usually with plates and eventually with additional screws and K-wires. As for the other coronoid fractures, the threshold to add a hinged external fixator to protect the repair should be minimal, as loss of reduction will result in joint instability, incongruence, and early arthrosis.

Four of 5 Type III fractures had a poor outcome in the series by Regan and Morrey; 3 of them had had a conservative treatment [1].Conversely, there were 2 excellent, 1 good, and 1 fair result in the series by Bousselmame et al. [9]. All 4 latter fractures had been treated by open reduction and internal fixation.

Subtype 2 basal fractures that are associated with a transolecranon fracture dislocation can be repaired in certain instances from posterior through the transolecranon fracture site, especially if the coronoid fragment is of a single large fragment. The transolecranon fractures themselves can afterwards be fixed with 3.5 mm plates.

Anteromedial Coronoid Fractures

These fractures almost always cause posteromedial ulnohumeral joint subluxation and incongruence. Early arthrosis seems to occur in non-operated cases, although long-term data regarding these recently identified fracture patterns are not yet available. Nonetheless, open reduction and plate or screw fixation through a medial approach seems to be the treatment of choice (Fig. 7). In certain subacute or chronic cases, malunited fragments may even require osteotomy to allow anatomic reduction (Fig. 4).

Complications

The most important complication of coronoid fractures is persistent instability of the elbow with posterior, posteromedial, or posterolateral subluxation of the ulnohumeral joint. This complication most often occurs in terrible triad injuries or in isolated Type III, rarely in isolated Type II, and usually not in isolated Type I fractures. The causes are insufficient reduction, nonunion, secondary displacement, and avascular necrosis of coronoid fragments. In these unstable elbow joints, the trochlea rides on the sharp edges of the fractured coronoid

(Fig. 4c). The cartilage wears out rapidly, in certain instances even in months.

Delayed stabilization of coronoid fractures in cases of chronically instable and subluxed ulnohumeral joints often results in persistent ulnohumeral joint subluxation and early arthrosis despite extensive surgical reconstruction of the coronoid and of the collateral ligaments, and despite the use of hinged external fixators. In particular, the duration of the ulnohumeral subluxation and the condition of the cartilage seem to influence the prognosis. If significant cartilage damage of more than 50% of the ulnohumeral joint surface is present, preservation of the joint may no longer be possible.

Although reconstruction of the coronoid fragments with iliac crest autograft or allograft coronoid fragments may be successful in certain instances [23], avascular necrosis and collapse of the fragments often lead to failure and early arthrosis.

Heterotopic bone formation can occur in up to 20% of the Type II coronoid fractures and up to 80% in Type III fractures, often impeding pronation and supination [1]. Prophylaxis using oral nonsteroidal anti-inflammatory medication for 2-3 weeks should therefore be considered in cases of severe coronoid fractures. Salmon calcitonin nasal spray for 2 weeks seems to be even more effective than oral nonsteroidal anti-inflammatory medication [24]. Single-dose radiation therapy may be used in high-risk patients such as those associated with closed-head injury.

Post-operative stiffness depends on the severity of the injury, delay of internal fixation, and on the duration of immobilization, which should be as short as possible, not exceeding 3 weeks [1]. In the series by Regan and Morrey [1], Type II injuries resulted in an average arc of flexion of 12° to 127°, and in an arc of pronation and supination from 83° to 87°. In Type III injuries, the average arc of flexion was 39° to 100°, and the arc of pronation and supination was from 42° to 42°.

Conclusions

The coronoid process is an important stabilizer of the elbow joint. Isolated Type I and most isolated Type II coronoid fractures can be treated conservatively. Coronoid fractures associated with radial head fractures, anteromedial coronoid fractures, and Type III coronoid fractures usually require open reduction and anatomic internal fixation. Repaired but unstable coronoid fractures might be protected with hinged external fixators.

References

1. Regan W, Morrey BF (1989) Fractures of the coronoid process of the ulna. J Bone Joint Surg Am 71:1348-1354
2. O'Driscoll SW, Jupiter JB, King GJW, Hotchkiss RN, Morrey BF (2000) The unstable elbow. J Bone Joint Surg Am 82:724-738
3. Ring D, Jupiter JB, Zilberfarb J (2002) Posterior dislocation of the elbow with fractures of the radial head and coronoid. J Bone Joint Surg Am 84:547-551
4. Terada N, Yamada H, Seki T et al (2000) The importance of reducing small fractures of the coronoid process in the treatment of unstable elbow dislocation. J Shoulder Elbow Surg 9:344-346
5. Schneeberger AG, Sadowski MM, Jacob HA (2004) Coronoid process and radial head as posterolateral rotatory stabilizers of the elbow. J Bone Joint Surg Am 86:975-982
6. O'Driscoll SW, Jupiter JB, Cohen MS et al (2003) Difficult elbow fractures: pearls and pitfalls. Instr Course Lect 52:113-134
7. Hotchkiss RN (1996) Fractures and dislocations of the elbow. In: Rockwood CA Jr, Green DP, Buchholz RW, Heckman JD (eds) Fractures in Adults. Lippincott-Raven, Philadelphia, pp 980-981
8. Cohen MS, Hastings H (1998) Acute elbow dislocation: evaluation and management. J Am Acad Orthop Surg 6:15-23
9. Bousselmame N, Boussouga M, Bouabid S et al (2000) Les fractures de l'apophyse coronoïde. Chir Main 2:286-293
10. King GJ, Zarzour ZD, Rath DA et al (1999) Metallic radial head arthroplasty improves valgus stability of the elbow. Clin Orthop Relat Res 368:114-125
11. Cohen MS (2004) Fractures of the coronoid process. Hand Clin 20:443-453
12. McKee MD, Pugh DM, Wild LM et al (2005) Standard surgical protocol to treat elbow dislocations with radial head and coronoid fractures. Surgical technique. J Bone Joint Surg 87 [Suppl 1]:22-32
13. Cobb TK, Morrey BF (1995) Use of distraction arthroplasty in unstable fracture dislocations of the elbow. Clin Orthop Relat Res 312:201-210
14. Kocher T (1911) Textbook of Operative Surgery. A and C Black, London
15. Kaplan EB (1941) Surgical approaches to the proximal end of the radius and its use in fractures of the head and neck of the radius. J Bone Joint Surg 86
16. Taylor TKF, Scham SM (1969) A posteromedial approach to the proximal end of the ulna for the internal fixation of olecranon fractures. J Trauma 9:594-602
17. Hotchkiss RN (1998) Surgical technique. In: Hotchkiss R (ed) Compass Universal Hinge. Surgical Technique. Smith and Nephew, Memphis, pp 8-12
18. Ameur NE, Rebouh M, Oberlin C (1999) La voie d'abord antérieure transbrachiale de l'apophyse coronoïde. Ann Chir Main 18:220-223
19. Bryan RS, Morrey BF (1982) Extensive posterior exposure of the elbow. A triceps-sparing approach. Clin Orthop Relat Res 166:188-192
20. Dowdy PA, Bain GI, King GJ, Patterson SD (1995) The midline posterior elbow incision. An anatomical appraisal. J Bone Joint Surg Br 77:696-699

21. Morrey BF (2000) Surgical exposures of the elbow. In: Morrey BF (ed) The elbow and its disorders. Sanders Company, pp 116-128

22. Closkey RF, Goode JR, Kirschenbaum D, Cody RP (2000) The role of the coronoid process in elbow stability. A biomechanical analysis of axial loading. J Bone Joint Surg Am 82:1749-1753

23. Kohls-Gatzoulis J, Tsiridis E, Schizas C (2004) Reconstruction of the coronoid process with iliac crest bone graft. J Shoulder Elbow Surg 13:217-220

24. Gunal I, Hazer B, Seber S et al (2001) Prevention of heterotopic ossification after total hip replacement: a prospective comparison of indomethacin and salmon calcitonin in 60 patients. Acta Orthop Scand 72:467-469

CHAPTER 9

Lateral Collateral Ligament Injury

D. STANLEY

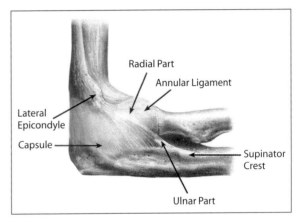

Fig. 1. The anatomy of the lateral aspect of the elbow showing the lateral ligament complex. The radial part, annular ligament and ulnar part (lateral ulnar collateral ligament) are well demonstrated

Introduction

Lateral collateral ligament injuries result from damage to the ulnar part of the lateral ligament complex. They are unlike medial ligament injuries which can be caused by a pure valgus stress since a pure varus stress is uncommonly applied to the elbow joint. These injuries most frequently follow a complete dislocation of the elbow but may also occur as the result of elbow subluxations and fractures. In addition, they are also seen as a result of iatrogenic injury after incorrectly performed tennis elbow surgery and radial head excision.

Pathology

The lateral ligament complex of the elbow comprises the radial collateral ligament, the annular ligament and the lateral ulnar collateral ligament (Fig. 1) [1]. Although any part of this complex may be injured, it is damage to the lateral ulnar collateral ligament that results in posterolateral rotatory instability of the elbow. The ligament takes its origin from the lateral epicondyle of the humerus and attaches to the ulna on the tubercle of the supinator crest. It was first described by Morrey and An in 1985 [2], although earlier in 1958 Martin had noted fibers passing between the supinator crest and humerus. It is most frequently damaged at its humeral origin causing a loss of stability between the lateral aspect of the humerus and the ulna. This allows the entire radio-ulnar joint (radius and ulna) to rotate referable to the humerus and produces the instability symptoms.

Clinical Presentation

Although patients may present at almost any age, the injury is most frequently seen in patients in the second or third decade [3]. The majority are male, and there is usually a history of a first dislocation of the elbow before the age of 15 years, or a nonunion of a lateral epicondyle fracture [4]. On occasion, patients will present with a lateral collateral ligament injury as the result of iatrogenic damage to the ligament caused by a poorly performed radial head excision or tennis elbow surgery [5].

A carefully taken history will often suggest the diagnosis although it is possible to confuse the symptoms – clicking, locking, snapping – with those of a loose body within the joint. The absence of evidence of a loose body on plain radiographs is helpful and should lead the clinician to refocus on the possibility of a ligament injury.

Specific questions that should be asked when this diagnosis is being considered are whether the patient can push themselves out of a chair by locking out the affected elbow in full extension and whether the elbow can be fully extended on performing a "press-up". Both these activities are usually impossible due to apprehension that the elbow will dislocate (Fig. 2).

Clinical examination usually reveals a normal range of movement although the patient may be apprehensive with the elbow fully extended and supinated.

The most sensitive test of this injury is the lateral pivot-shift apprehension test [6]. The patient is asked to lie supine on the examination couch with the shoulder in flexion and the arm above their head. The forearm is supinated and a valgus and axial compression force is applied to the elbow during flexion. As the procedure is performed, the patient senses that the elbow is about to dislocate, becomes apprehensive, and resists the examiner (Fig. 3).

To confirm the instability the patient should be re-examined under general anesthesia with fluoroscopy. The procedure is repeated and as the radius and ulna sublux off the humerus a prominence is produced posterolaterally over the radial head together with a dimple between the radial head and capitellum. As the elbow is flexed to approximately 40° the radius and ulna suddenly reduce with a palpable and visible clunk. Fluoroscopic images taken as the test is performed provide a permanent record of the instability (Fig. 4).

Management

The symptoms associated with lateral collateral ligament injuries frequently affect the patients' ability to perform their work and undertake activities of daily living. As such, since the ligament injury does not heal with time, consideration should be given to surgical repair or reconstruction. In both situations the patient is positioned supine on the operating table with the affected arm across the chest or supported on an arm table. A high tourniquet is applied and the limb exsanguinated.

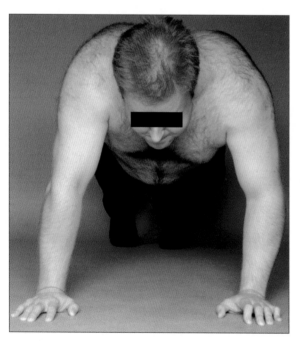

Fig. 2. With a lateral ulnar collateral injury it is impossible to fully extend the elbow when doing a "press-up". The patient is apprehensive that the elbow will dislocate

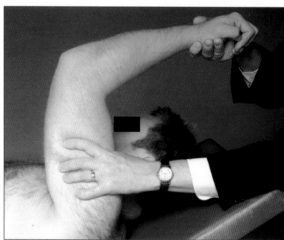

Fig. 3. The lateral pivot-shift apprehension test. The forearm is supinated and a valgus and axial compression forces applied to the elbow during flexion

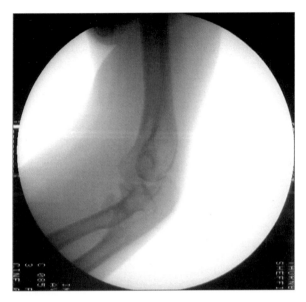

Fig. 4. A fluoroscopic image obtained during the lateral pivot-shift test. The radius and ulna rotate off the distal humerus

Surgical Repair

The lateral aspect of the elbow is exposed through Kochers interval with the triceps and anconeus being reflected posteriorly from the lateral column and the common extensor tendon elevated from the lateral epicondyle so as to allow exposure of the anterolateral aspect of the joint capsule and lateral ligament complex. The damage to the lateral ligament complex is confirmed. This may consist of laxity of the capsuloligamentous complex or avulsion of the ligament from its origin.

If the ligament has been avulsed from the lateral epicondyle, its proximal end is identified and reattachment achieved using non-absorbable sutures inserted into the bone at the anatomical origin of the ligament. Residual laxity is treated by plication of the anterior and posterior capsule.

Surgical Reconstruction

This is usually undertaken for chronic ligament injuries with recurrent instability. A variety of materials have been used to reconstruct the ligament of which palmaris longus is the most common. If this is not available semi-tendinosus, fascia lata, and a toe extensor are acceptable alternatives. My personal preference is to use a strip of triceps tendon

which is easily harvested from the operative field. Whichever material is chosen, however, it is important to have sufficient length to enable an adequate reconstruction. This normally requires a graft of approximately 20 cm in length.

The operative approach to the lateral aspect of the joint is as described for surgical repair of the ligament. The tubercle on the supinator crest is identified by palpation and a drill hole is made in the bone just posteriorly. A second drill hole is placed 1-1.25 cm proximally and the two holes linked using a burr (Fig. 5). A suture is passed through the holes and used to identify the isometric point on the humeral epicondyle (Fig. 6). This is the point at which the suture remains taut in both elbow flexion and extension.

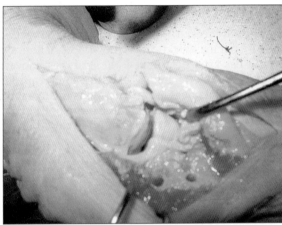

Fig. 5. The first drill hole into the ulna is made just posterior to the supinator crest and the second hole is placed 1–1.25 cm proximally. These are linked using a burr

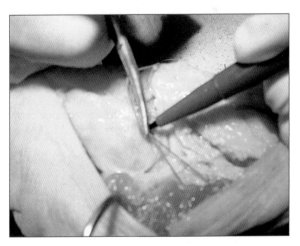

Fig. 6. The isometric point on the humeral epicondyle is identified

Although several methods of ligament reconstruction have been described, all involve passing the graft material with non-absorbable sutures inserted at both ends through the tunnel made in the ulna. The variations in fixation relate to the humeral side of the joint. The technique which I currently use is as follows.

Having identified the isometric point on the humeral lateral epicondyle, a 3.5 mm drill hole is made at that point and directed in the line of the lateral column. Two additional drill holes, sufficient to allow suture passage, are made anterior and posterior to the lateral supracondylar ridge and directed so as to link with the drill hole in the lateral column (Fig. 7). The ends of the graft are then passed into the lateral column with the attached sutures being passed out of the column via the anterior and posterior supracondylar drill holes. The sutures are tensioned to check that the graft does not "bottom out". If this happens the graft must be shortened and the new length checked by repositioning the graft in the lateral column tunnel. Once the appropriate graft length has been determined, the graft is removed from the humeral tunnel and the joint capsule closed. The ligament reconstruction is finally repositioned and the sutures tied over the lateral supracondylar ridge (Fig. 8). The wound is closed using

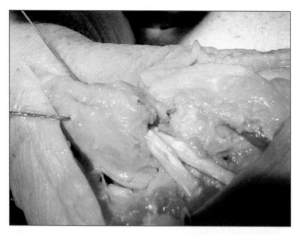

Fig. 8. The joint capsule has been partially closed and the ligament tension checked. The sutures are about to the tied over the supracondylar ridge

absorbable sutures and the arm immobilized with an above-elbow plaster backslab for 2 weeks. This is then removed and progressive flexion and extension permitted using an adjustable brace. The brace is normally removed at 6 weeks. Flexion and extension strengthening exercises should be performed for 6 months after which I allow my patients to undertake any activity as tolerated.

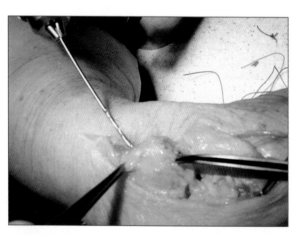

Fig. 7. A 3.5 mm drill hole has been made in the line of the lateral epicondyle (marked with forceps). Drill holes are being made anterior and posterior to the lateral supracondylar ridge to link with the 3.5 mm tunnel

References

1. O'Driscoll SW, Horii E, Morrey BF et al (1992) Anatomy of the ulnar part of the lateral collateral ligament of the elbow. Clin Anat 5:296
2. Morrey BF, An KN (1985) Functional Anatomy of the Ligaments of the Elbow. Clin Orthop Relat Res 201:84-90
3. Morrey BF, O'Driscoll SW (2000) Lateral Collateral Ligament Injury. In: Morey BF, Elbow and its Disorder (Ed.), 3rd Ed W B Saunders Co, Philadelphia Ch, 44:556
4. Malkawi H (1981) Recurrent dislocation of the elbow accompanied by ulnar neuropathy: a case report and review of the literature. Clin Orthop 161:270
5. Morrey BF (1992) Re-operation for failed tennis elbow surgery. J Shoulder Elbow Surg 1:47
6. O'Driscoll SW, Bell DF, Morrey BF (1991) Postero-lateral rotatory instability of the elbow. J Bone Joint Surg Am 73:440

CHAPTER 10

The Complex Dislocations of the Elbow

G.J.W. KING

Introduction

The elbow is the second most frequently dislocated major joint in adults (following the shoulder). Most elbow dislocations do not have an associated fracture and therefore have been termed a simple dislocation [1]. Fortunately, early mobilization following a closed reduction has a low risk of redislocation and generally good long-term results [2, 3]. When an elbow dislocation is associated with a fracture this injury has been termed a complex dislocation [5-7]. These injuries often require surgical treatment to render the elbow stable enough to allow early motion. The presence of intra-articular fractures compromises the intrinsic stability of the elbow and increases the risk of recurrent instability and post-traumatic arthritis. In fact, these injuries historically have had such a poor outcome that when a posterior elbow dislocation is associated with the radial head and coronoid fracture this injury has been referred to as "the terrible triad". In this paper the relevant anatomy, biomechanics, pathophysiology, and treatment approach to these difficult injuries will be reviewed.

Stabilizers of the Elbow

The elbow joint is one of the most intrinsically stable joints of the human body [8, 9]. It consists of the articulation of the trochlea of the distal humerus with the greater sigmoid notch of the proximal ulna as well as the articulation of the capitellum with the radial head. The trochlea and capitellum are tilted anteriorly approximately 30° relative to the long axis of the distal humerus. The tilt of the trochlea functionally increases the prominence of the coronoid process in resisting posterior instability of the elbow. The radial head has a concave dish which articulates with the spherical-shaped capitellum and by virtue of their interacting surfaces also resists subluxation of the elbow. The greater sigmoid notch has a prominent guiding ridge which seats deeply within the trochlear groove of the distal humerus, which further stabilizes the elbow joint.

There are numerous studies that have looked at the stabilizers of the elbow joint [8, 9]. Collectively, these studies demonstrate the primary importance of the ulno-humeral articulation. In the setting of disrupted collateral ligaments, which are routinely injured in patients with an elbow dislocation, the radio-capitellar joint assumes a greater importance in maintaining elbow stability. Dynamic muscle forces are important in maintaining stability in elbows with intact osseous structures, but may contribute to instability in the setting of osseous deficiency. The flexor-pronator origin medially and common extensor origin laterally are important secondary constraints to valgus and varus stability respectively [10, 11]. The brachialis, biceps, and triceps muscles compress the articular surfaces together, thereby stabilizing the elbow. In the setting of osseous deficiencies, these same posteriorly directed muscular forces may contribute to recurrent dislocation of the elbow.

While the elbow capsule has been demonstrated to be an important constraint to varus and valgus stability in the laboratory, the capsule is usually disrupted in patients with elbow dislocations and does not contribute to elbow stability in this setting [12, 13]. The medial collateral ligament has two distinct portions arising from the anterior, inferior aspect of the medial epicondyle [9, 10]. The anterior band is attached to the sublime tubercle on the medial surface of the coronoid and has been shown to be the most important contributor to valgus stability. The posterior band of the medial collateral ligament has a less prominent role in maintaining elbow stability. The medial collateral ligament is routinely disrupted in patients with a dislocation of the elbow; failure usually occurring as an avulsion from the medial epicondyle [12, 14, 15]. The lateral collateral ligament provides an important constraint to varus and posterolateral rotatory stability of the elbow [9, 11-13]. The annular ligament attaches to the anterior and posterior aspects of the radial notch of the ulna, stabilizing the proximal radius to the ulna. The radial collateral ligament originates from the lateral epicondyle and blends with the annular ligament. The lateral ulnar collateral ligament arises from the lateral epicondyle and courses just posterior to the radial collateral ligament blending with the annular ligament to insert on the proximal ulna at the crista supinatoris.

Biomechanical studies have demonstrated that progressive loss of the coronoid process causes a decrease in varus, posteromedial, and posterior elbow stability [16]. The anteromedial facet and sublime tubercle of the coronoid are particularly important in resisting varus and posteromedial rotatory instability. Deficiency of the radial head contributes to a loss of valgus, posterolateral, and posterior stability [17-20]. In the setting of medial collateral lateral ligament insufficiency, repair or replacement of a fractured radial head should be considered. Radial head excision should be avoided due to the gross valgus instability that occurs as a consequence. While ligament repair has not been shown to be advantageous in the majority of simple dislocations, ligament repair is often essential in patients with associated osseous injuries to render the elbow sufficiently stable to allow early range of motion [4, 14, 21, 22].

History

Patients presenting with fracture-dislocations of the elbow fall into two major groups. High-energy injuries are often associated with vehicular accidents or falls from a height, most commonly in younger patients. These injuries typically have more severe osseous and soft tissue damage and may have other associated upper extremity fractures or multisystem trauma. The second group of patients has a low energy fall with less severe osseous and ligamentous injuries such as in elderly patients with osteopenia. While the incidence of associated vascular or neurologic injuries is low, a careful history should be performed to rule these out in all patients with fracture-dislocations of the elbow.

Physical Examination

The diagnosis of an elbow dislocation can usually be made clinically by determining the position of the olecranon process relative to the medial and lateral epicondyles of the elbow. With the elbow in extension these structures are normally on a straight line, while with the elbow flexed to 90° they form an equilateral triangle in the same plane. These anatomical features are also useful in evaluating whether the elbow is reduced following a closed reduction in the emergency department. Prior to reduction, the elbow should be carefully evaluated for the presence of a laceration or puncture wound that would suggest a compound dislocation. Neurological injuries can occur with elbow dislocations, therefore the function of the ulnar, median, and radial nerves should be carefully determined pre- and post-closed reduction. Vascular injuries should be evaluated by determining the presence of distal pulses and capillary refill. Associated upper extremity injuries, such as fractures or dislocations of the wrist, forearm, humerus, and shoulder, should also be sought in patients with complex elbow dislocations. A general physical examination should be carried out as indicated to search for associated traumatic injuries and to determine the patient's suitability for surgical treatment if required.

Imaging

Anterior, posterior and lateral radiographs are obtained in patients with fracture-dislocations of the elbow in the emergency department. Oblique radiographs can be helpful since positioning of the elbow is typically suboptimal in the setting of a dislocation such that multiple views are often necessary to identify the associated osseous injuries. Following a closed reduction, repeat radiographs in a radiolucent splint are helpful as they often identify associated osseous injuries which were not evident on the pre-reduction radiographs. If, following a closed reduction, the associated injuries are not well defined or there is a concern about the presence of a fragment in the joint, the use of computerized tomography should be considered. This provides a better evaluation of the extent and nature of the associated osseous injuries, which may influence operative decision-making. Magnetic resonance imaging has not been routinely employed in clinical practice due to the difficulty in positioning patients with acute elbow injuries for this investigation. Furthermore, since both collateral ligaments are usually disrupted in patients with elbow dislocations it is more appropriate to use computerized tomography to define the osseous injuries since they typically influence decision making for treatment.

Management of Complex Elbow Dislocations

Non-operative Treatment

Complex elbow dislocations can be managed non-operatively if the associated osseous injuries are minor and do not sufficiently destabilize the elbow to prevent the institution of early range of motion. Typical injuries include undisplaced or minimally displaced fractures of the radial head and/or the presence of small fractures of the tip of the coronoid. If the fractures themselves are not sufficiently large or displaced enough to warrant treatment in isolation then it is the presence of residual instability post-reduction which is the primary determinant to non-operative or operative treatment [1]. Patients with larger fractures of the coronoid, involving greater than 10%-20%, typically destabilize the elbow sufficiently such that non-operative treatment is usually unsuccessful [21, 23, 24]. In order to determine whether closed treatment is appropriate, an evaluation of elbow stability should be performed following closed reduction while the patient is under conscious sedation. Following closed reduction of a complex elbow dislocation, the elbow should be placed through an arc of flexion and extension with the forearm maintained in supination, neutral, and pronation while the tracking of the elbow is evaluated fluoroscopically if available.

Biomechanical studies demonstrate that patients who have lateral collateral ligament insufficiency are best rehabilitated with the forearm in pronation while those with residual insufficiency of the medial collateral ligament or coronoid are best rehabilitated with the forearm in supination [10, 11]. Many patients with elbow fracture-dislocations are best rehabilitated in neutral due to the combined injures of both medial and lateral ligaments.

The initial stable arc of motion to prevent recurrent instability and the development of late arthritis is unknown. It is this Author's experience that elbows, which remain stable from full flexion to 40° of extension, can usually be successfully managed non-operatively with early-protected range of motion as long as the associated osseous injuries are minor, as discussed above. If the elbow subluxes or dislocates at greater than 40° of elbow flexion this seems to portend to a high incidence of recurrent instability and a failure of non-operative treatment. A fiberglass splint is optimally employed in patients following a closed reduction of an elbow dislocation, as heavy plaster splints tend to pull the elbow out of joint. It is advisable to keep the elbow splinted at approximately 90° of flexion in the most stable position of forearm rotation for 1 week until the muscular tone of the elbow returns allowing the dynamic stabilizers to assist in maintaining congruity of the elbow. In elderly patients with significant medical comorbidities more unstable elbows can be considered for non-operative treatment by splinting in greater degrees of elbow flexion for longer periods of time; however, this approach should be avoided in younger, more active patients with a greater expectation for function following their injuries. It has been reported that the longer the period of immobilization, the worse the clinical and radiographic outcome of simple elbow dislocations. It is likely that complex dislocations managed with prolonged immobilization would also fair more poorly than those managed with early motion.

Range of motion of stable elbows is initiated with the use of a resting collar and cuff between exercises. Active motion is better than passive motion in maintaining stability of the elbow. More unstable elbows are splinted in a 90° resting splint with the forearm in the appropriate rotation between exercises. As the stability of the elbow improves with the return of muscle tone and soft tissue healing, the resting splint is discarded. Full flexion is permitted but elbow extension is limited to the position of known stability as determined by the post-reduction examination. Elbow extension is gradually increased 10° per week starting from the position of known stability. Pronation and supination are performed with the elbow in the flexed position. An overhead rehabilitation protocol may be beneficial in the setting of more unstable elbows. With the patient supine and the humerus oriented vertically gravity compresses the elbow while it is flexed and extended.

Operative Treatment

Operative management of complex elbow dislocations primarily depends on the extent and degree of associated osseous and ligament injuries requiring treatment to render the elbow sufficiently stable to allow early range of motion.

Fractures of the Radial Head

In patients with displaced radial head fractures involving greater than one-third of the articular surface, open reduction and internal fixation appears appropriate as fixation improves the osseous stability of the elbow and may decrease the incidence of late osteoarthritis [19, 24]. Displaced fragments smaller than one-third of the radial head should be reduced and fixed if it is possible to achieve secure fixation; however, small fragments should be excised if the fixation is tenuous (Fig. 1). Insecure fixation should be avoided, as this will result in a high incidence of early failure due to the stresses across the radial head during the post-operative period. One point five, 2.0, or 2.4 mm screws are generally used for partial ar-

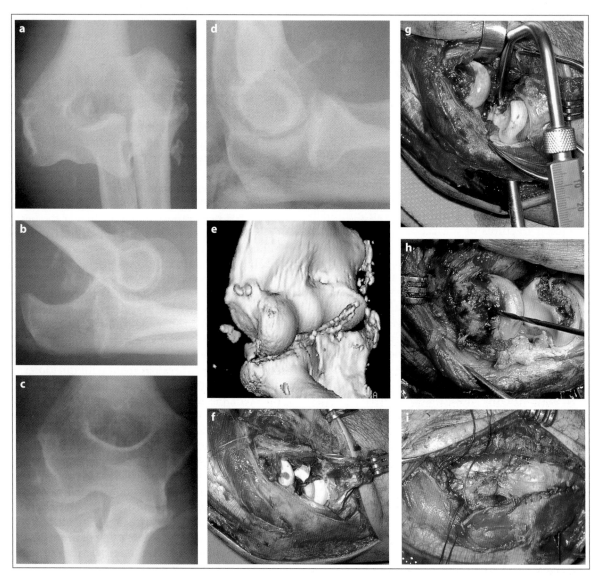

Fig. 1.

Continue →

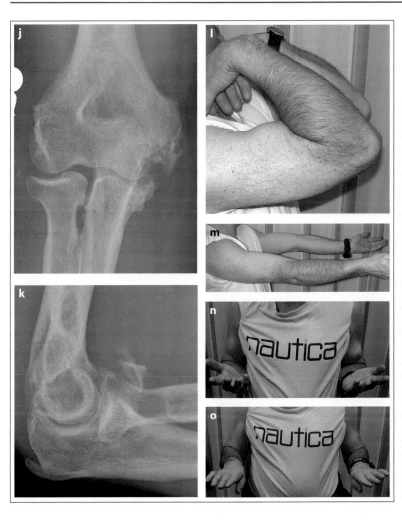

Fig. 1. *Continued* (**a, b**) Anteroposterior and lateral radiographs of a 48-year-old construction worker who fell off a ladder demonstrating a posteromedial dislocation and multiple fracture fragments. (**c, d**) Post-reduction radiographs showing a non-congruous reduction. (**e**) 3D CT scan demonstrates residual subluxation of the elbow with a marginal radial head fracture, a comminuted coronoid fracture and ligament avulsions from the medial and lateral epicondyles. (**f**) Operative photograph demonstrating avulsion of lateral ligaments and common extensor origin from lateral epicondyle. (**g**) Use of targeting guide for placement of drill holes to pass sutures from subcutaneous border of ulna around coronoid and anterior capsule. (**h**) Placement of drill holes for lateral ligament repair. (**i**) Completed repair of extensor origin and lateral ligaments secured to lateral epicondyle.(**j, k**) Anteroposterior and lateral radiographs 1 year following fragment excision of the radial head, suture repair of coronoid and lateral collateral ligament. (**l-o**) Clinical result. The patient had a minimal pain and a stable elbow

ticular fractures (Fig. 2). Noncomminuted neck fractures are fixed with oblique screws placed through the head into the neck [25]. Comminuted head and neck fractures are fixed using locking plate techniques; however, radial head arthroplasty should be considered in selected cases.

In patients with comminuted radial head fractures involving 3 or more fragments, the experience with open reduction and internal fixation has been less favorable [26]. In the setting of an elbow dislocation, the stresses across the radial head/neck fixation are greater, making metallic radial head arthroplasty a more reliable option [27, 28] (Fig. 3). Radial head excision without replacement, while reported in the literature for unreconstructable radial head fractures with an associated dislocation, is not recommended due to a high incidence of residual instability and recurrent dislocation [29].

Fractures of the Coronoid

Regan and Morrey [23] have classified coronoid fractures on the basis of fracture size into Types I, II, and III. Type I consists of a small shear fracture, typically only 2 or 3 mm thick with anterior capsular attachment, Type II up to 50%, and Type III greater than 50%. There is a direct correlation between the size of the coronoid fracture and the loss of stability of the elbow and hence the need for repair. Type I coronoid fractures do not typically require repair in this Author's experience. Our laboratory has recently reported that suture repair of Type I coronoid fractures has a minimal effect of elbow stability in an *in vitro* biomechanical study. Repair or replacement of a fractured radial head and repair of the collateral ligaments has a much greater effect on elbow stability. Placing sutures

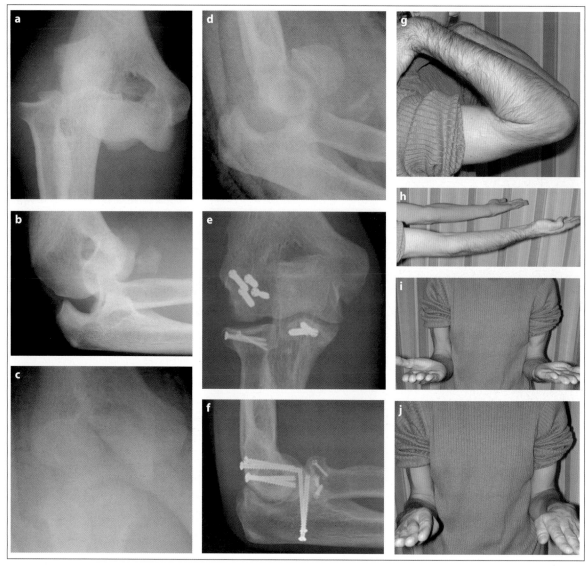

Fig. 2. (**a, b**) Anteroposterior and lateral radiographs of a 24-year-old snowboarder demonstrating a posterolateral dislocation and multiple fractures. (**c, d**) Post-reduction radiographs showing a non-congruous reduction, a fracture of the coronoid, radial head, and capitellum. (**e, f**) Radiographs 1 year following open reduction and internal fixation of the radial head, coronoid, and capitellum. The lateral ligament was also repaired. (**g, j**) Clinical result. The patient had no pain and a stable elbow

around the fragment(s) and anterior capsule and passing these through drill holes in the base of the coronoid fracture onto the subcutaneous border of the ulna can accomplish repair if desired [21]. Larger Type II and III coronoid fractures are fixed with either screws or a buttress plate. Most coronoid fractures can adequately be fixed with screws placed from the subcutaneous border of the ulna. Other Authors prefer fixation placed from the coronoid tip into the ulna from an anterior approach. Large comminuted coronoid fractures

should be fixed with an anteromedial buttress plate. In the setting where a comminuted radial head has been excised in preparation for an implant, access to reduce and fix a coronoid fracture using screws can easily be achieved from a lateral approach. If the radial head is intact, a muscle splitting approach through the common flexor origin can be employed to allow visualization of the coronoid for anatomic reduction and fixation. In order to gain adequate exposure to place an anteromedial buttress plate on a comminuted coro-

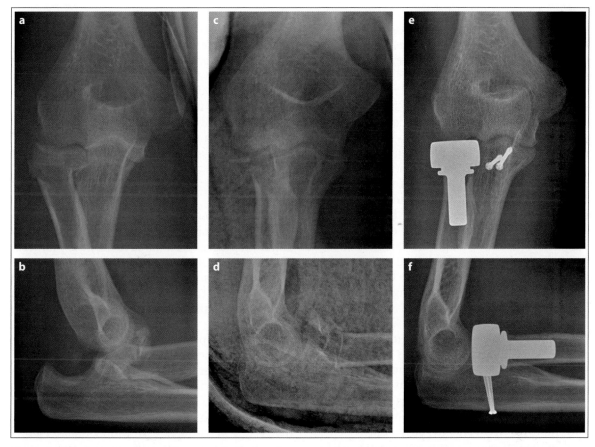

Fig. 3. (**a, b**) Anteroposterior and lateral radiographs of a 28-year-old man involved in a motor vehicle accident demonstrating a posterior dislocation and fractures of the radial head and coronoid. (**c, d**) Post-reduction radiographs showing malalignment of the radial head fracture. (**e, f**) Radiographs 6 months following open reduction of the coronoid and a modular metallic radial head arthroplasty. The patient had minimal discomfort and had a range of flexion from 16° to 135° with full forearm rotation

noid, the humeral head of the flexor carpi ulnaris and flexor pronator mass is elevated anterior to the ulnar nerve.

O'Driscoll [16] has presented a modified classification of coronoid fractures which additionally emphasizes the importance of anteromedial coronoid fractures and their role in posteromedial rotatory and varus instability. Repair of anteromedial coronoid fractures and those involving the sublime tubercle are key to prevent residual instability and post-traumatic arthritis. These injuries should be suspected in patients who have a coronoid fracture without an associated dislocation or radial head fracture. These injuries are often missed due to the subtle nature of their presentation relative to a fracture-dislocation of the elbow, the topic of the current review.

Ligament Repair

Typically the lateral collateral ligament injury is worse than the medial collateral ligament injury in a simple elbow dislocation [12, 13]. In a complex fracture-dislocation the soft tissue injuries may be less severe than in a simple dislocation due to bony failure allowing the elbow to dislocate prior to complete ligament disruption. In the post-operative period, integrity of the lateral collateral ligament is much more important than the medial collateral ligament in maintaining elbow stability. This is due to the fact that the elbow is not typically exposed to valgus stresses in daily life while varus stresses are common, for example, placing the arm across the chest. In view of this, the lateral collateral ligament should always be repaired in operatively treated fracture-dislocations of the elbow. While suture anchors can be employed, ligament repair through drill holes tends to be most efficient. Locking Krackow sutures are placed in the lateral collateral ligament and common extensor origin and drawn through a single drill hole placed at the flexion-extension axis which is located near the lateral epicondyle. By visually converting the articular surface of the capitellum into a circle, the location of the axis position can be estimated as the geometric center of this circle. One drill hole is placed posterior to the lateral column and one anterior to create a large bone bridge for secure repair. The ligament and extensor origin sutures are passed through the axis hole and out through the holes on the lateral supracondylar ridge. This allows the ligaments to be drawn to the bone and tensioned prior to tying over the bone bridge for a tight repair.

Repair of the medial collateral ligament is only performed if the elbow remains unstable following repair of the osseous injuries and the lateral collateral ligament. In the Author's experience medial collateral ligament repair is not commonly required in fracture-dislocations of the elbow. Medial collateral and flexor-pronator origin repair improves elbow stability so should be considered in the setting of a teno-osseous reconstruction. Medial collateral ligament repair is also indicated in the setting of delayed treatment of complex dislocations where the quality of osseous and ligament repair is often less optimal. Finally, medial collateral ligament repair can be helpful in patients who are obese where there is a tendency for the forearm to pull the elbow out of joint simply due to its weight.

External Fixation

Dynamic external fixation is rarely required for the acute management of elbow fracture-dislocations [6, 30]. It is typically used if the elbow remains unstable after all of the osseous and ligamentous structures have been repaired or in the setting where the fixation of any of the aforementioned structures is tenuous. It is particularly useful in the setting of delayed surgical management and in patients with recurrent instability. A number of dynamic external fixators are available for the elbow; each rely on the accurate localization of the flexion-extension axis of the elbow. There are no comparative biomechanical or clinical studies comparing designs. These fixators vary in size and complexity,

all require careful application and aftercare. The incidence of pin tract problems has been high relative to static external fixators used elsewhere.

A static fixator can also be employed if a dynamic fixator is unavailable; however, early removal of a static fixator is desirable to avoid severe stiffness. Trans-articular fixation of the elbow using heavy pins should be avoided due to the risk of pin breakage and an intra-articular infection.

Rehabilitation

As previously outlined in the non-operative management of complex elbow dislocations, the rehabilitation program is tailored to the injury pattern. The goal is to initiate early elbow motion while protecting the soft tissue and osseous repairs and maintaining a congruous reduction. Active motion is better than passive motion in maintaining stability of the elbow due to muscle activation which tends to pull the elbow into joint [9-11]. Active assisted and passive motion initiated by the patient is encouraged after resting muscle tone returns, usually within 1 week of the injury or surgical treatment [1]. Passive mobilization of the elbow by a therapist should be avoided due to the potential risk of heterotopic ossification. Stable elbows are managed with early active motion and a collar and cuff. An overhead rehabilitation protocol, which provides gravity to compress the elbow, may be useful in the setting of residual instability. Flexion and extension of the elbow are performed with the patient supine and the humerus vertical. The medial collateral ligament deficient elbow is rehabilitated in supination, the lateral collateral ligament deficient elbow in pronation [10, 11]. Neutral rotation is used if both ligaments are deficient. If the patient has residual instability, a removable splint at 90° is used in the appropriate position of rotation. An extension block splint or hinged cast-brace can be beneficial for less reliable patients. In patients with severely comminuted fractures and tenuous fixation and/or patients with residual instability following repair a dynamic fixator can be employed [6]. Alternatively, immobilization in a cast, or a static external fixator can be considered until it is safe to initiate motion. A surgical contracture release may be required after fracture and soft tissue healing to achieve a functional range of motion. In general, a congruent stiff elbow has a better prognosis for outcome than an unstable incongruous arthritic articulation. Given the advent of improved techniques and more reliable outcomes for elbow contracture release, this two-stage approach may be considered in special circumstances.

Indomethacin 25 mg three times daily for 3 weeks can be used peri-operatively to prevent heterotopic ossification. Indomethacin should not be used in elderly patients and those with a history of peptic ulcer disease, renal disease, hypertension and those with a history of allergy to anti-inflammatory medication. This medication should be particularly considered in patients who are at high risk such as those with delayed treatment, patients undergoing a second surgical procedure following a failed primary procedure, and patients with an associated head injury. While single dose irradiation can be employed to prevent heterotopic ossification acutely, this author reserves its use for patients undergoing late excision of heterotopic bone for stiffness and for those who are unable to use indomethacin.

Outcome

A functional outcome can be achieved in most acute cases by addressing each of the injured structures and initiating early motion [7, 21]. Pugh and coworkers reported the results of 36 patients with "terrible triad" injuries of the elbow [21]. The authors routinely fixed or replaced the radial head; fixed larger coronoid fractures; and repaired the lateral collateral ligament. The medial collateral ligament was repaired in six patients who had persistent instability. Two patients required hinged external fixation. The functional outcome was good, with 34 patients achieving concentric stability. The flexion extension arc was 112° ± 11° and there were 28 good and excellent results. The outcome of secondary management for recurrent instability is less predictable, stressing the need for adequate primary treatment of complex elbow dislocations.

References

1. Hildebrand KA, Patterson SD, King GJW (1999) Acute elbow dislocations: simple and complex. Orthop Clinics North Am 30:63-79
2. Josefsson PW, Johnell O, Gentz CF (1984) Long-term sequelae of simple dislocation of the elbow. J Bone Joint Surg Am 66:927-930
3. Mehlhoff TL, Noble PC, Bennett JB, Tullos HS (1988) Simple dislocation of the elbow in the adult. Results after closed treatment. J Bone Joint Surg Am 70:244-249
4. Josefsson PO, Gentz CF, Johnell O, Wendeberg B (1989) Dislocations of the elbow and intrarticular fractures. Clin Orthop 246:126-130
5. Broberg MA, Morrey BF (1987) Results of treatment of fracture-dislocations of the elbow. Clin Orthop 216:109-119
6. McKee MD, Bowden SH, King GJ et al (1998) Management of recurrent complex instability of the elbow with a hinged external fixator. J Bone Joint Surg Br 80:1031-1036
7. Ring D, Jupiter JB, Zilberfarb J (2002) Posterior dislocation of the elbow with fractures of the radial head and coronoid. J Bone Joint Surg Am 84:547-551
8. King GJ, Morrey BF, An KN (1993) Stabilizers of the elbow. J Shoulder Elbow Surg 2:165-174
9. Morrey BF, An KN (1983) Articular and ligamentous contributions to the stability of the elbow joint. Am J Sports Med 11:315-319
10. Armstrong AD, Dunning CE, Faber KJ et al (2000) Rehabilitation of the medial collateral ligament-deficient elbow: an in vitro biomechanical study. J Hand Surg Am 25:1051-1057
11. Dunning CE, Zarzour ADS, Patterson SD et al (2001) Muscle forces and pronation stabilize the lateral ligament deficient elbow. Clin Orthop 388:118-124
12. O'Driscoll SW, Morrey BF, Korinek S, An KN (1992) Elbow subluxation and dislocation. A spectrum of instability. Clin Orthop 280:186-197
13. McKee MD, Schemitsch EH, Sala MJ, O'Driscoll SW (2003) The pathoanatomy of lateral ligamentous disruption in complex elbow instability. J Shoulder Elbow Surg 12:391-396
14. Josefsson PO, Gentz CF, Johnell O, Wendeberg B (1987) Surgical versus non-surgical treatment of ligamentous injuries following dislocation of the elbow joint. A prospective randomized study. J Bone Joint Surg Am 69:605-608
15. Ring D, Jupiter JB, Zilberfarb J (2003) Roles of the medial collateral ligament and the coronoid in elbow stability. J Bone Joint Surg Am 85:568-569
16. O'Driscoll SW, Jupiter JB, Cohen MS et al (2003) Difficult elbow fractures: pearls and pitfalls. Instr Course Lect 52:113-136
17. Morrey BF, Tanaka S, An KN (1991) Valgus stability of the elbow. A definition of primary and secondary constraints. Clin Orthop 265:187-195
18. King GJ, Zarzour ZD, Rath DA et al (1999) Metallic radial head arthroplasty improves valgus stability of the elbow. Clin Orthop 368:114-125
19. Beingessner DM, Dunning CE, Beingessner CE et al (2003) The effect of radial head fracture size on radiocapitellar joint stability. Clinical Biomechanics 18:677-681
20. Beingessner DM, Dunning CE, Gordon KD et al (2004) The effect of radial head excision and arthroplasty on elbow kinematics and stability. J Bone Joint Surg Am 86:1730-1739
21. Pugh DMW, Wild LM, Schemitsch EH et al (2004) Standard surgical protocol to treat elbow dislocations with radial head and coronoid fractures. J Bone Joint Surg Am 86:1122-1130
22. O'Driscoll SW, Jupiter JB, King GJ et al (2001) The unstable elbow. Instr Course Lect 50:89-102
23. Regan W, Morrey B (1989) Fractures of the coronoid process of the ulna. J Bone Joint Surg Am 71:1348-354
24. Heim U (1998) Combined fractures of the radius and the ulna at the elbow level in the adults. Analysis of 120 cases after more than 1 year. Rev Chir Orthop 84:142-153

25. Giffin JR, Patterson SD, Johnson JA, King GJW (2004) Internal fixation of radial neck fractures: an in vitro biomechanical analysis. Clinical Biomechanics 19:358-361
26. Ring D, Quintero J, Jupiter JB (2002) Open reduction and internal fixation of fractures of the radial head. J Bone Joint Surg Am 84:1811-1815
27. Harrington IJ, Sekyi-Out A, Barrington TW et al (2001) The functional outcome with metallic radial head implants in the treatment of unstable elbow fractures: a long-term review. J Trauma 50:46-52
28. Moro JK, Werier J, MacDermid JC et al (2001) Arthroplasty with a metal radial head for unreconstructable fractures of the radial head. J Bone Joint Surg Am 83:1201-1211
29. Sanchez-Sotelo J, Romanillos O, Garay EG (2000) Results of acute excision of the radial head in elbow radial head fracture-dislocations. J Orthop Trauma 14:354-358
30. Cobb TK, Morrey BF (1995) Use of distraction arthroplasty in unstable fracture dislocations of the elbow. Clin Orthop 312:201-210

CHAPTER 11

The Fracture-Dislocation of the Forearm (Monteggia and Essex-Lopresti Lesions)

A. CELLI, M.C. MARONGIU, M. FONTANA, L. CELLI

Introduction

The fracture-dislocation of the forearm can be classified into a number of complex forearm lesions.

The most recent literature defines "complex instability of the elbow" as lesions with elbow fractures associated with ruptures of the medial and lateral ligaments [1].

In the same way for the forearm, we define "complex fracture of the forearm" as lesions in which the fracture of one or both bones are associated with dislocation of the distal and proximal radio ulnar joint, or with wrist and elbow dislocation.

In the following discussion we review the anatomy and biomechanics of the forearm functional unit and also the proposal of a new classification of the forearm complex fracture.

In contrast, elbow or wrist dislocation associated with articular fractures are excluded.

The Monteggia and Essex-Lopresti lesions can be classified in this group of complex fractures of the forearm, which are characterized by serious anatomy-pathological damage that modifies the functional unit of the forearm, composed of the radius and ulnar bones, the interosseous membrane (IOM), and the radio-ulnar proximal and distal joints.

The Forearm Joint

The Anatomy and Biomechanics of the Forearm Unit

The forearm can be considered as a single articulating joint where the interdependence of the different functioning units allow forearm rotation and elbow and wrist motion. All of these functions, in particular prono-supination, explain the complex integrated relationships between the bones and soft tissue along the entire length of the forearm.

An understanding of the biomechanics of the forearm is essential for the acute management of complex fractures and also in case of late reconstruction.

The radius and ulna are roughly parallel and joined at each end by a well-constrained joint and in the midportion by the IOM.

The system is relatively tight and it is difficult to injure one of these structures without affecting another part of the system.

Two conditions must be present to allow free and full prono-supination movement:
1. the radius and ulna are of equal length, with normal location and amount of the radial bow;
2. a stable relationship between the radius and ulna at the proximal and distal radio-ulnar joints.

The Shape and Length of the Bones

The ulna is a relatively straight bone, but the radius is much more complex.

Sage [2] pointed out the complexity of the angles and curve in the radial bone. The radius has four small, but consistent curves: two on the frontal plane (about 13° proximally and 6° at the middle shaft) and two in the sagittal plane (about 13° proximally and 9° at the middle shaft). The curves of the radius give it the distinct radial bow necessary to cross over the ulna in pronation while at the same time perpetuating relative tension in the IOM in all positions (Fig. 1).

Schemitsch and Richards [3] confirmed the importance of restoration of the radial bow to forearm function after fracture.

The patient may not be able to achieve full promotion and good grip strength after fractures malunion if the radial curve is not recovered.

These authors [3] described a measurement technique for the amount and location of the maximum radial bow.

Using antero-posterior radiograph with the forearm in neutral rotation, a line is drawn from the bicipital tuberosity to the most ulnar aspect of the radius at the wrist. A perpendicular line (*a*) is then drawn from the point of the maximum radial bow to this line.

We can determine the location of maximum radial bow by dividing the distance from the bicipital

tuberosity to the point of maximum bow (*b*) by the length of the entire bow (*c*) (Fig. 2).

The ulna is essentially fixed by the proximal anatomy (ulno-humeral joint), and the radius at the radiocarpal unit circumscribes a simple cone, with its axis running roughly from the center of the radial head (RH) to the center of the distal part of the ulna (Fig. 3).

The normal range of motion has been described as 71°-75° of pronation and 82°-84° of supination [4].

The Stable Relationship Between the Radius and Ulna

The osseous relationships and the ligaments structure maintain the longitudinal and transverse stability between the radius and the ulna during prono-supination movement. We consider these to be the most important anatomic relationships in the proximal middle and distal forearm that must be taken into consideration in the management of the complex fracture of the forearm.

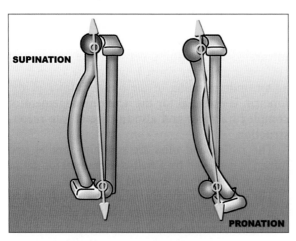

Fig. 1. The radius has a distinct radial bow necessary for crossover the ulna in pronation. The patient may not be able to achieve full pronation and supination if the radial bow is not recovered after fracture

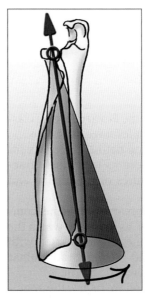

Fig. 3. The rotation of the radius with respect to the ulna describes a simple cone with its axis running roughly from the center of the radial head to the center of the distal part of the ulna. The rotation is guided by the IOM and the triangular fibrocartilage at distal radio-ulnar joint

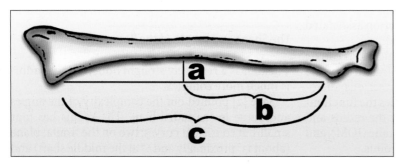

Fig. 2. Technique for measuring the amount and location of the radial bow:
• The amount of the maximum radial bow is determined by measuring in milimeters (*a*).
• The location is determined by dividing the distance from the bicipital tuberosity by the point of maximum bow (*b*) by the length of the entire bow (*c*). The value is expressed as a percentage. Location is b/c × 100

Proximal Forearm

The Proximal Radio Ulnar Joint

The proximal radio ulnar joint (PRUJ) is composed of the RH and the lesser sigmoid fossa of the ulna.

The RH is an elliptic structure where the greatest diameter of the head comes into contact with the lesser sigmoid fossa in full supination.

The stability of the PRUJ is achieved by the surrounding ligaments: the annular, quadrate, and oblique ligaments.

The annular ligament encircling the RH and attached to the anterior and posterior margins of the radial notch of the ulna is the principal structure maintaining the stability of the PRUJ. This ligament is tunnel shaped, with a smaller diameter in the distal aspect than the proximal border. This condition allows approximately 1-5 mm distal migration of the radius and maintains RH stability through the entire range of rotation.

The annular ligament becomes tighter in supination due to the shape of the RH, and has closed relationship with the lateral ulnar collateral ligaments and with the lateral radial collateral ligament. These thickened ligamentous structures prevent RH dislocation and also posterolateral rotator instability (Fig. 4).

The quadrate ligament or ligament of "Denucé" is a thin, fibrous layer between the inferior margin of the annular ligament and the ulna. It consists of a dense anterior border and a thinner posterior border and a thin central fibrous lamina [5] (Fig. 5).

In full supination this anterior border becomes taut around the neck of the radius and draws it against the proximal radio-ulnar notch. In full pronation the posterior fibers become taut and perform a similar function.

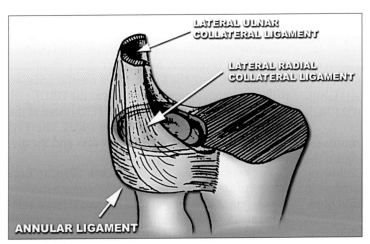

Fig. 4. The lateral collateral ligamentous complex. The lateral ulnar and radial collateral ligament originates from the lateral epicondyle and courses distally to interdigitate with the fibers of the annular ligament. This complex ligamentous structure is the main component in providing stability to the proximal radio-ulnar joint (PRUJ) and to the radio capitellum joint when the elbow is stressed in varus posterolateral rotation

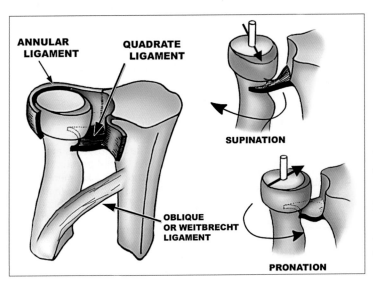

Fig. 5. The proximal radio-ulnar joint can be stabilized by two articular ligaments: the annular ligament and the quadrate ligament. The oblique cord as extrarticular ligament becomes taut in the forearm supination and contribute to avoid RH anterior dislocation. The quadrate ligament increased the joint stability, limiting the radius anterior translation with the anterior fibers during supination and the posterior translation with the posterior fibers during pronation

The oblique ligament or Weitbrecht's ligament extends from the ulna below the radial notch and ends at the radius below the biceps tuberosity (Fig. 5). It becomes taut when the radius is in supination. RH anterior dislocation can occur when the annular ligament, the quadrate ligament, and the oblique ligament are injured, as in the Monteggia's lesion.

The Middle Forearm

The Interosseous Membrane

The interosseous membrane (IOM) runs obliquely between the shafts of the ulna and radius (Fig. 6). Its fibers are separate from the oblique ligament and run in the opposite direction. The central portion of the IOM is thickened and measures about 3.5 cm in width. This is the interosseous ligament (IOL).

The oblique orientation of the IOL allows it to function as both as a restraint to diastasis of the radius and ulna and also provide weight-transfer structure during axial loading. The stout IOL is oriented obliquely, from the stable ulna distally to the mobile radius proximally.

Incision of the IOL reduced longitudinal stability by 71%; however, with the proximal IOM incision, stability decreased by only 11% [6].

The IOL is a constant structure and accounts for most of the longitudinal support of the radius if the RH is resected. The proximal migration following RH resection occurs when the IOL is injured as in the Essex-Lopresti lesion, resulting in painful ulno-carpal impingement.

When the forearm is compressed, the IOL may be loaded when transferring tension load from the radius to the ulna [7]; about 60% of the force applied was transmitted through the radius.

The Distal Forearm

The Distal Radio-Ulnar Joint

The distal end, or head, of the ulna consists of a rounded, conical expansion covered over almost three quarters with articular cartilage.

The articular surface of the radius is flatter than that of the ulna. This implies that rotation in the distal radio-ulnar joint (DRUJ) must include translation as well as rotation with less than 10% of surface at extremes of rotation. The joint-surface contact is optimal when the forearm is in the neutral position. In full pronation we have dorsal minimal joint surface contact (posterior translation of the ulnar head), otherwise in full supination the minimal joint surface contact is volar (the ulna translates anteriorly).

The DRUJ should be a critical focus in the treatment of distal radius fractures.

In these cases the fractures reduction should be performed with the forearm in a neutral position using the stable ulna head as a support and guiding tool for the fragment. Also, the fracture should be immobilized with the forearm in a neutral position with maximum articular contacts at the DRUJ.

The triangular fibro cartilage (TFC) is one of the most important stabilizers of the DRUJ. The TFC has two components: the articular disk and the distal radio-ulnar ligament.

The articular disk is a biconcave fibrocartilage structure interposed between the ulnar aspect of the carpus and the distal ulnar dome. It has a variable thickness depending upon the relative length of the ulna (ulnar variance).

The organized, longitudinally oriented fibers emerge as a bundle from the volar and dorsal peripheral fibers of the articular disk.

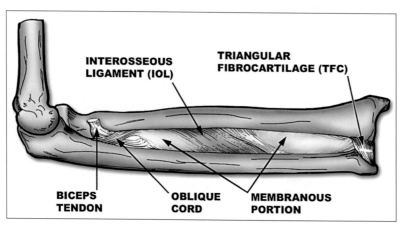

Fig. 6. The interosseous membrane (IOM). The central portion is thicker and functions as a ligament (IOL) to prevent axial translation. In the proximal part of the IOL the oblique cord improves the radio-ulnar stability, avoiding anterior and lateral radius dissociation. In both the proximal and distal parts of the IOM the tissue is more membranous

These bundles are called dorsal and volar distal radio-ulnar ligaments.

The TFC is able to convert the compressive force transmitted axially through the carpus into a tensile force that is borne by the triangular fibrocartilage.

Moore et al. [8] have shown in cadaver studies that 5 mm of radial shortening can occur before disruption of the ligaments complex (TFC of the DRUJ) and when the shortening is greater than 10 mm the disruption involves the IOL.

During the forearm rotation the radioulnar joint is controlled by components of the TFC. When the forearm is pronated, the dorsal-radio-ulnar ligament becomes taut and seats the ulnar head against the dorsal rim of the sigmoid notch.

In supination, the volar radio-ulnar ligament displaces the ulnar head against the volar radial rim.

Classification

We have developed a simple system to characterize and approach the complex fractures of the forearm. This new classification brings into focus the traumatic lesions that modify the functional unit of the forearm, and correlates joint instability (PRUJ, DRUJ, elbow, and wrist) with the associated ulna and radius fractures.

We believe that this system can guide the surgeon in clinical assessment and operative approach as well as targeting the parameters (instability and fractures) to follow the postoperative evaluation.

The necessity to classify these lesions arises because the literature is not sufficiently clear as to how to frame these types of damage involving the forearm joint.

Differently in the AO group principles [9] for the treatment of the fractures, complex fractures of the forearm are characterized only by bone comminu-

tion or bone loss in which anatomical reduction can be difficult to obtain.

Any references in the AO classification were reported to be elbow- and wrist-associated lesions.

Our classification of complex fractures of the forearm (Table 1) is based on the more current principles accepted for the treatment of elbow lesions, where the fractures are correlated to elbow instability. In the same way forearm fractures become complex when they are associated with forearm joint instability or elbow and wrist instability.

The treatment of the forearm complex fracture poses a unique challenge: the open reduction and internal fixation (ORIF) of the forearm fractures.

This is a necessity for restoration of proximal or distal joint stability to recover forearm rotation.

The ORIF goals are anatomic restoration and maintenance of the length and shape of the forearm bones and also axial and rotational alignment, which are useful to recover elbow or wrist stability.

In the following discussion we review the management of the principal and more frequent forearm complex fractures that involve the elbow joint and are more critical in maintaining upper extremity function: the Monteggia lesions and the Essex-Lopresti lesion.

Monteggia's Lesions

Clinical Assessments and Treatment Options

In 1814 Monteggia described [10] the fractures of the ulna at the proximal third associated with an anterior dislocation of the RH, which is recognized today as the most common type of these groups of lesions.

Table 1. Classification of complex fractures of the forearm

One bone involved	Instability	Complex fracture of the forearm
Fracture of the ulnar diaphysis	PRUJ	Monteggia's lesion Bado I, II, III
Fracture of the radius diaphysis	DRUJ	Galeazzi's lesion
Fracture of the radius distal metaphysis	DRUJ	Wrist complex fracture
Fracture of the RH	DRUJ + IOL	Essex-Lopresti's lesion
Two bones involved	**Instability**	**Complex fracture of the forearm**
Fracture of the radius and ulna	PRUJ dislocation	Monteggia's lesion Bado IV
Fracture of the radius and ulna	Elbow dislocation	Elbow complex fracture
Fracture of the radius and ulna	PRUJ + DRUJ dislocation	Floating radius
Fracture of the radius and ulna	Wrist dislocation	Wrist complex fracture

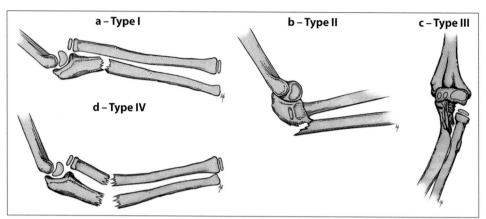

Fig. 7. Monteggia's lesions. Bado's classification

Watson-Jones in 1943 [11] introduced a first classification where the location of the RH dislocation is related to mechanism of injury:

- fractures that occur with extension mechanism are related to anterior dislocation of the RH;
- fractures that occur with flexion mechanism are related to posterior dislocation of the RH;
- fractures with lateral mechanism are related to lateral dislocation of the RH.

In 1967 Bado [12] coined the term "Monteggia's lesion" to define this type of fracture; he also recognized four different types of Monteggia's lesion; these classifications described the full spectrum of those injuries and it became universally accepted.

Monteggia's lesions described by Bado are classified by the fracture of the ulna and the position of the RH dislocation (Fig. 7):

- type I (55%-78%) (Fig. 7a): anterior dislocation of the RH with anteriorly angulated fracture of the ulnar shaft (most common in children);
- type II (10%-15%) (Fig. 7b): posterior dislocation of the RH with posteriorly angulated fracture of the ulnar shaft (most common in adults);
- Type III (7%-20%) (Fig. 7c): antero-lateral or lateral dislocation of the RH with fracture of the ulnar metaphysis (most common in children);
- Type IV (5%) (Fig. 7d): fractures of the ulna and radius with anterior dislocation of the RH (most rare).

Monteggia's lesions are complex fractures of the forearm; in types I-III of Bado's classification, the fractures of the ulna are associated with the dislocation of the proximal radio ulnar joint; in contrast, in type IV, the radio ulnar joint dislocation is associated with the fracture of the proximal third of the radius and a fracture of the ulna at the same level.

Bado and some other authors have defined numerous equivalent types of these lesions that cannot be included in Bado's classification [13-16].

Jupiter [17] defines four different subgroups of the posterior Monteggia lesion (Type II Bado classification) based on the location of the ulnar fracture:

- type IIA: the fracture involves olecranon and coronoid process;
- type IIB: the fracture involves the metaphyseal and diaphyseal ulnar juncture;
- type IIC: the fracture is diaphyseal;
- type IID: the fracture is located in the proximal third of the ulnar shaft.

Monteggia's lesion does not occur as a high percentage; it is present in 7% of ulna fractures and in 0.7% of elbow lesions. There can be some difficulty in the diagnosis and treatment and this may justify the high percentage of unsatisfactory outcomes.

Mechanism of Injury

The mechanism of injury of type I has been debated; a direct blow to the posterior aspect of the ulna seems to be the injury that produces this lesion [18].

Evans [19] postulated in cadaver experiments that type I is usually secondary to a fall in which the hand is fixed while the forearm is forced in full pronation. The oblique fracture of the ulna occurs that lead the radius anteriorly through the annular ligament disruption.

The annular ligament, the ligament of Denucé, and the Weitbrecht ligament become tighter in supination depending on the elliptic shape of the RH.

A mechanism of injury with the forearm forced in ipersupination is similar to that of a posterolateral elbow dislocation and could explain the type II lesion.

Penrose [20] in cadaver experiments has confirmed that these injures are caused by a direct and rotational force in supination.

The type III mechanism of injury almost always occurs in children and is presumed to be due to a fall on the outstretched arm, with adduction force leading to varus angulation of the ulna and lateral dislocation of the radius.

A particular aspect of the pathology is the lesion of the annular ligament; it may be transected with pieces interposed between ulna and radius. In the child with ligamentous laxity the annular ligament may be intact but displaced up and over the RH. In these situations, the intact annular ligament may prevent complete reduction of the RH.

Clinical Assessment

The presenting signs and symptoms vary according to the type, degree, and time (acute or chronic lesions) of injuries.

In general Monteggia's lesion is characterized by acute pain and marked tenderness and functional incapacity to move the elbow. In particular in type I and IV lesions, the forearm and the hand are fixed in pronation. During clinical evaluation of these two types, shortening of the forearm can be observed and also the RH can be palpated in the ante-cubital fossa.

Otherwise, the RH can easily be palpated posteriorly in type II; usually this lesion is characterized by a more proximal ulnar fracture angulated posteriorly.

In type III, the forearm is often in midrotation; the ulnar fracture is angulated laterally and the RH can easily be palpated.

A careful neurologic examination is mandatory with this injury because it is more frequently associated with acute lesion of the posterior interosseous nerve (PIN). Most nerve injuries have been associated with the Bado type II lesion where the PIN can be compromised by traction, impingement, or entrapment in the arcade of Frohse.

Radiological Findings

Adequate radiological evaluation is necessary to obtain a correct diagnosis. Usually two X-ray evaluations are performed; one in antero-posterior view and the second in lateral view.

Most of the time the ulnar fracture is easily diagnosed, but RH dislocation can be missed. Morrey [21] summarized the difficulty of diagnosing Monteggia's lesion with different observations:
1. the dislocation of the RH can be missed because of the poor quality of the X-ray;
2. the RH can be minimally displaced and this can be difficult to visualize;

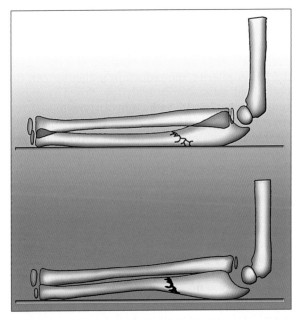

Fig. 8. The ulnar bow sign. In the lateral view the posterior border of the ulna is represented by a straight line. In the treatment of the ulnar shaft fracture in Monteggia's lesion type I, Bado's classification, when the straight line is lost, with anterior bowing of the posterior border the radial head dislocation is often unreduced. In case of isolated RH dislocation, the ulnar bow sign is considered a sign of the occult ulnar shaft fracture (variant of type I Monteggia injuries)

3. sometimes the RH dislocation can be reduced during the maneuvers involved in performing the X-ray evaluation.

Lincoln and Mubarak [22] described the ulnar bow sign in isolated cases of anterior RH dislocation. This radiological sign presents when the midshaft of the ulna is bowed anteriorly in type I Monteggia lesions when the anatomical ulnar straight line along the postural border of the ulna is lost or not recovered, and bows anteriorly, and the RH is dislocated or subluxated anteriorly (Fig. 8).

In the literature the incidence of missed Monteggia's lesions ranges from 16% to 52% [18, 23, 24].

Radiological evaluation can help to reduce this percentage, but the X-ray must be performed in the correct position and the evaluation done with particular attention, not only to the ulnar fracture, but also to the relationship between the radius and the capitellum joint.

Treatment

Monteggia's lesion can be treated with open or closed methods; the choice depends on the type of fracture, the time of the reduction and on the patient's age. The first aim is to obtain the reduction of the ulna, recovering the length, and to correct all angular deformity of the ulnar shaft. This permits reducing RH dislocation. If the patient is a child and the RH is anterior, the reduction maneuver can be performed satisfactorily with the closed method. Under anesthesia ulna reduction can be achieved, recovering the correct length and normal angulations.

This permits reducing the RH dislocation; reduction of the RH can be facilitated by flexion of the elbow over 90° and pushing the RH posteriorly. The flexion of the elbow around 110°-120° helps to maintain the reduced RH. It is necessary to check the correct reduction of the RH and to perform an X-ray evaluation at the end of this maneuver. The elbow is placed in a cast for 4-5 weeks in midrotation to reduce the traction by the bicipital tendon. Surgical treatment in children is indicated in type I after a failure of the closed reduction. In contrast, in type IV and in comminuted fractures of the ulna, the primary treatment for children is open reduction and stable fixation.

In adults, Monteggia's lesion requires an open treatment to obtain the best outcome. The surgical treatment must provide for:
1. patient's position: we prefer the lateral decubitus but it can also be performed in a supine position; a tourniquet is useful (Fig. 9a, b);
2. surgical approach: posterior mid-line or postero-lateral can be used. All these incisions allow to expose the ulna, the olecranon, and the RH, and if necessary to show the coronoid process (Fig. 10a, b). We are able to expose the lateral collateral ligament (LCL) and the annular ligament and to perform an anterior capsulotomy if it is interposed between the capitellum and the RH, preventing its reduction;
3. stable reduction of the ulna fracture: generally after this time the RH can easily be reduced (Fig. 11);
4. if a reduction of the RH after stable fixation of the ulna is not obtained, it must be checked (Fig. 12). It is advised to check the RH reduction before performing stable fixation of the ulna fracture, and this can be done using clinical evaluation and intraoperative X-ray. If we find an instability of the RH it is necessary to open the space between the anconeus and flexor carpis ulnaris, exposing the LCL complex, and after detaching the extensor carpi ulnaris from the ulna, the radio ulnar joint, and the annular ligament can be exposed. If it is necessary to expose the radial neck to reconstruct the annular ligament, the supinator muscle must be detached by 2 cm from its ulnar insertion (Fig. 13);
5. post-operative treatment: early motion is indicated, protected with brace for 4-6 weeks, in par-

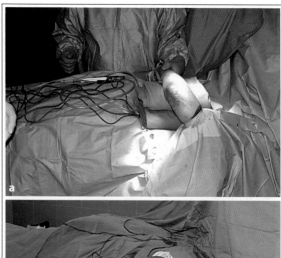
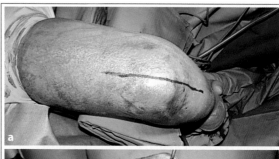

Fig. 9 a, b. The patient can be placed in a supine or lateral decubitus

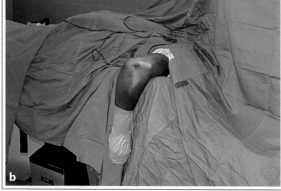
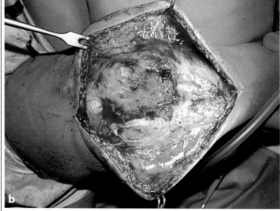

Fig. 10 a, b. The posterior midline skin incision is performed; the medial and lateral cutaneous flaps are elevated

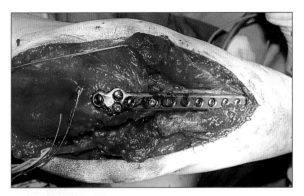

Fig. 11. The anatomical and stable fixation of the ulna fracture must be obtained

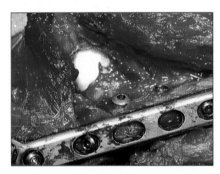

Fig. 12. The RH reduction must be checked after ulna reduction and stable fixation

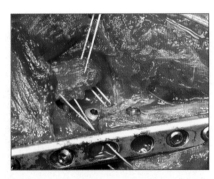

Fig. 13. The annular ligament is repaired or reinforced, detaching the extensor carpi ulnaris from the ulna

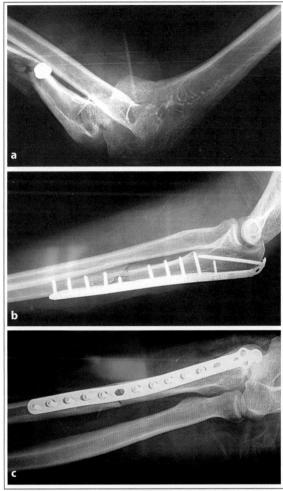

Fig. 14 a-c. Type I Monteggia's fracture: preoperative and post-operative X-ray evaluations. The anatomical and stable fixation of the ulna allows the reduction of the RH

To improve the outcomes we suggest a decision-making algorithm for the treatment of a Monteggia fracture in children and in adults that includes a summary of our preferred method of treatment (Table 2) (Figs. 14, 15).

Essex-Lopresti's Lesion

Clinical Assessments and Treatment Options

In 1951, Essex-Lopresti [27] described the proximal migration of the radius following the surgical excision of comminuted radial-head fracture. In 1992, Trousdale [28] described 20 cases defining this lesion as a longitudinal radio-ulna dissociation

ticular in case of reconstruction of the ligaments.

The results reported in the literature are excellent in children [14, 25] when the lesion is recognized and treated early. However, outcomes reported for adults have been less successful [26].

The poor results have been related principally to ulnar fracture malalignment or nonunion that allow RH subluxation or when the ORIF is not reliable enough to allow early motion.

The type II and type IV lesions generally have poorer results than does a type I lesion [12].

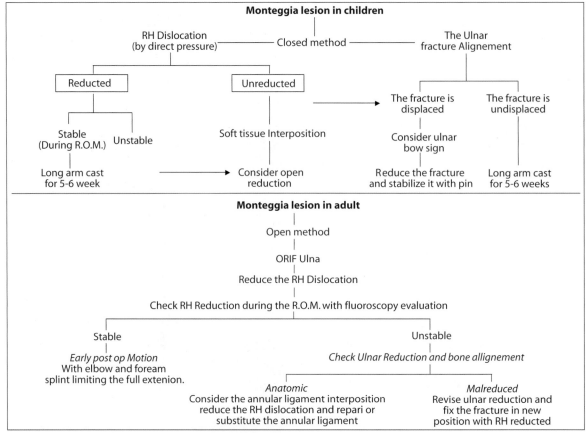

Monteggia lesion in children

RH Dislocation
(by direct pressure) ———— Closed method ———— The Ulnar
fracture Alignement

| Reduced | | Unreducted |

Stable
(During R.O.M.)   Unstable

Soft tissue Interposition

The fracture is
displaced

The fracture is
undisplaced

Consider ulnar
bow sign

Long arm cast
for 5-6 week

Consider open
reduction

Reduce the fracture
and stabilize it with pin

Long arm cast
for 5-6 weeks

Monteggia lesion in adult

Open method

ORIF Ulna

Reduce the RH Dislocation

Check RH Reduction during the R.O.M. with fluoroscopy evaluation

Stable

Unstable

Early post op Motion
With elbow and foream
splint limiting the full extenion.

Check Ulnar Reduction and bone allignement

Anatomic
Consider the annular ligament interposition
reduce the RH dislocation and repari or
substitute the annular ligament

Malreduced
Revise ulnar reduction and
fix the fracture in new
position with RH reduced

Table 2. Decision-making algorithm for the treatment of a Monteggia fracture in children and in adults

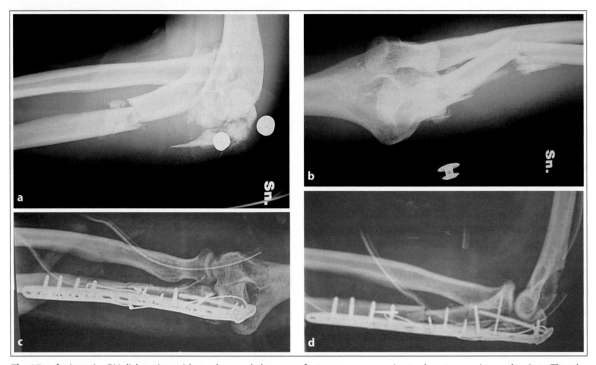

Fig. 15 a-d. Anterior RH dislocation with an ulnar and olecranon fracture: pre-operative and postoperative evaluations. The olecranon and ulnar fracture is stabilized using a long contour plate to recover the anatomical length and angulation of the ulna

(LRUD). The Essex-Lopresti lesion compromises the stability of the entire forearm axis: where the lack of the RH is associated with IOM lesion it can be stretched or attenuate acutely or with time.

Appropriate treatment of the Essex-Lopresti injury requires an understanding of the biomechanics of forearm stability and an early diagnosis in the acute lesion. When the patient presents a RH comminuted fracture, the possibility of acute or chronic development of the Essex-Lopresti lesion must be considered.

Numerous studies have shown the ability of the IOM and trangular fibro cartilage complex (TFCC) at DRUJ to maintain axial forearm stability. After RH excision, the IOM provides stability for 71% and TFCC for 8% [29, 30]. Only if both the IOM and TFCC are disrupted, does significant proximal migration of the radius occur [31].

Clinical Assessment

Proximal translation of the radius of about 2 mm in most patients occurs after RH excision [32] without clinical symptoms. Otherwise, once the radius has translated to a proximal position of more than 10 mm, functional impairment occurs (Fig. 16).

Forearm rotation decreases because the distal ulna loses its position in the sigmoid notch of the radius and becomes subluxed in more dorsal and distal position; in addition, the wrist extension is blocked because the distal ulna abuts against the dorsal carpus. In this way the common symptoms reported by patients with primary resection of the RH and secondary forearm longitudinal instability are:
- pain in the posterior aspect of the wrist (increased with forearm supination) and in the elbow when the proximal stumps of the radius abut against the capitellum;
- loss of range of motion in the forearm supination and in the wrist extension (Fig. 17);
- evidence of posterior prominence of the distal ulna at the wrist (fixed subluxation) (Fig. 18);
- associated elbow valgus instability (Fig. 19).

The Longitudinal Instability Manœuvers

- Axial stress test [33]. Manual compression was applied through the hand and wrist. A proximal radial migration of 5 mm has to be considered indicative of instability.
- Radius pull test [34]. With the patient in the supine position; the shoulder is abducted at 90° and internally rotated, the elbow is bended to 90° and the forearm is held in neutral rotation.

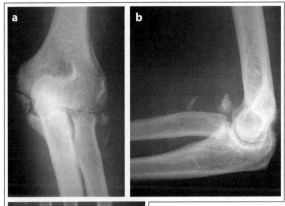
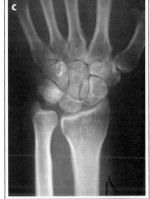

Fig. 16 a-c. After RH resection, if the IOM and the triangular fibrocartilage at the wrist are damaged, the entity of the proximal migration of the radius can be evaluated with X-rays

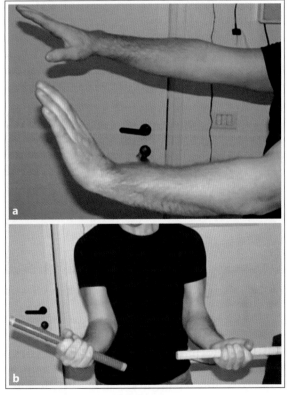

Fig. 17 a, b. The loss of the wrist extension and forearm supination

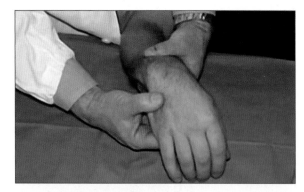

Fig. 18. The posterior prominence of the distal ulna at the wrist

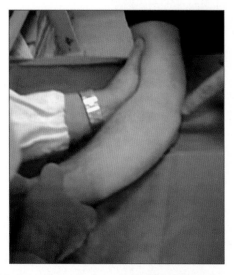

Fig. 19. Sometimes the Essex-Lopresti lesion can be associated with valgus instability with pain on the medial side

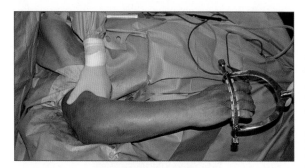

Fig. 20. The radius pull test: the positive test is with more than 3 mm of proximal radial migration

The positive pull test is with ≥3 mm of proximal radial migration; the migration of 6 mm or more is observed in gross instability of the forearm with injuries of the IOM and of the triangular fibro-cartilage complex (TFCC) (Fig. 20).

These maneuvers are highly sensitive for acute lesions and they provide useful information in chronic lesions regarding the possibility of correcting forearm longitudinal instability with RH replacement.

Imaging Studies Are Helpful to Define

1. With X-ray view or TC:
   - distal radius joint subluxation;
   - proximal migration of the radius;
   - positive ulnar variance;
2. With dynamic fluoroscopic evaluation, which demonstrates the possibility of correcting forearm longitudinal instability with axial traction (Fig. 21) [34];
3. With MRI to assess the anatomic status of the IOM and to depict tears (Fig. 22).

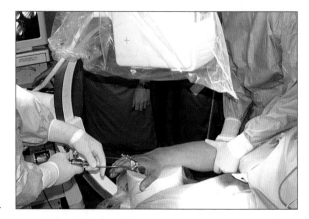

Fig. 21. The dynamic fluoroscopic evaluation demonstrates the possibility of correcting the forearm longitudinal instability with axial traction

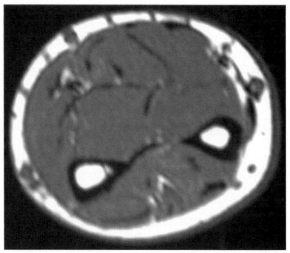

Fig. 22. The MRI can be used to evaluate the status of the IOM

Surgical Options

The advantage of surgical treatments is that they restore the DRUJ relationship (Fig. 23) by:

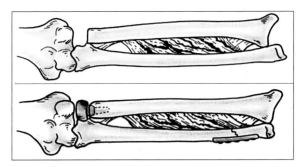

Fig. 23. The surgical treatment must restore the anatomical relationship between the radius and the ulna

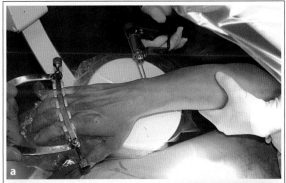

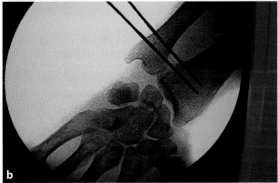

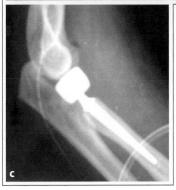

Fig. 24 a-c. Axial traction reduces the ulnar variance; DRUJ reduction in full supination is maintained with transient transarticular pins. The RH replacement is performed, recovering the correct length of the radius

- lengthening the radius;
- shortening the ulna.

The choice of the surgical option depends on the reducibility from positive to neutral the ulnar variance at the wrist:

1. The forearm axial traction reduces ulnar variance. We perform RH replacement and afterwards DRUJ reduction with forearm in full supination maintained with a transient transarticular pin (about 3-5 weeks) (Fig. 24).
2. The forearm axial traction does not reduce the ulnar variance (fixed subluxation).
   The options are radial replacement with:
- distal ulna-shortening osteotomy;
- Darrach resection [35];
- Sauvé Kapandji reconstruction [36].

Conclusions

The fractures-dislocations of the forearm must be classified as complex fractures because they damage the functional unit of the forearm.

We proposed a new classification of complex fractures of the forearm to describe the lesions characterized by bone fractures and the instability of the proximal and distal joints.

The Monteggia and Essex-Lopresti lesions must be included in this classification because the fractures of one or both forearm bones are associated with the dislocation of proximal and distal articulation. The treatment of choice for these lesions must recover the correct anatomy of the ulna and radius and the congruence of the proximal and distal joints.

Correct clinical evaluation and early treatment are critical for successful treatment of these lesions; late treatment is often correlated to poor outcomes.

We would like to conclude by quoting Putnam: "Most adverse outcomes in forearm fractures are related to a failure to recognize injury to the proximal or distal radio-ulnar joints or a failure to a appreciate the loss of reduction after it has begun".

Acknowledgements

The Authors would like to thank Mrs. Marongiu Betti for her contribution in creating the schematic drawings to support the forearm anatomic descriptions.

References

1. Morrey BF (1997) Complex instability of the elbow. J Bone Joint Surg Am 79:460
2. Sage FP (1959) Medullary fixation of fractures of the forearm: a study of the medullary canal of the radius and a report of fifty fractures of the radius treated with a present triangular nail. J Bone Joint Surg Am 41:1489-1516
3. Schemitsch EH, Richards RR (1992) The effect of malunion on functional outcome after plate fixation of fractures of both bones of the forearm in adults. J Bone Joint Surg Am 74:1068-1078
4. Boone DC, Azen SP (1979) Normal range of motion subjects. J Bone Joint Surg Am 61:756-759
5. Spinner M, Koplan EB (1970) The quadrate ligament of the elbow-wrist relationship to the stability of the proximal radio-ulnar joint. Acta Orthop Scand 41:632-647
6. Hotchkiss RN, Kai-nan A, Sowa DT et al (1989) An anatomic and mechanical study of the interosseous membrane of the forearm: pathomechanics of proximal migration of the radius. J Hand Surg Am 14:256-261
7. Halls AA, Travil A (1960) Transmission of pressures across the elbow joint. Anat Rec 150:243-248
8. Moore TM, Lester DK, Sormiento A (1985) The stabilizing effect of soft tissue constraints in artificial Galeazzi fractures. Clin Orthop 194:189-194
9. Monteggia GB (1814) Instituzioni Chirurgiche, vol 5. Maspero, Milan
10. Muller ME, Allower M, Schneider R, Willenegger H (1979) Manual of internal fixation: techniques recommended by AO Group, 2nd ed. Springer-Verlag, Heidelberg Berlin New York
11. Watson-Jones R (1943) Fractures and joint injures, 3rd edn. Livingston, Edinburgh
12. Bado JL (1967) The Monteggia lesions. Clin Orthop 50-71
13. Willey JJ, Galey JP (1985) Monteggia injures in children. J Bone Joint Surg Br 67:728-731
14. Letts M, Locht R (1985) Monteggia fractures-dislocation in children. J Bone Joint Surg Br 67:724-731
15. Darmans JP, Rang M (1990) The problem of Monteggia fracture dislocations in children. Orthop Clin North Am 21:251-256
16. Stanley EA, Dela Sarza JF (2001) Monteggia fracture dislocation in children. Rockwood and Greens fractures in children. Lippincott, New York 5:529-562
17. Jupiter JB, Leihovic SJ, Ribbons W, Wilk RM (1991) The posterior Monteggia lesion. J Orthop Trauma 5:395-402
18. Speed JS, Boyd HB (1940) Treatment of fractures of the ulna with dislocation of head of radius (Monteggia fracture). JAMA 115:1699-1703
19. Evans EM (1949) Pronation injures of the forearm with special reference to the anterior Monteggia fracture. J Bone Joint Surg Br 31:578
20. Penrose JH (1951) The Monteggia fractures with posterior dislocation of the radial head. J Bone Joint Surg Br 33:65
21. Morrey BF (1992) Fractures and dislocation of the elbow. In: Gustilo RB (ed) Fractures and dislocation. Chicago Year Book, Medical Publishers
22. Lincoln TL, Mubarak SJ (1994) Isolated traumatic radial head dislocation. J Pediatr Orthop 14:454-457
23. Boyd HB, Bools JC (1969) The Monteggia lesion: A reviw of 159 cases. Clin Orthop 66:94
24. Reckling FW, Codell LD (1968) Unstable fracture-dislocation of the forearm: The Monteggia and Galeazzi lesions. Arch Surg 996-999
25. Kalamachi A (1986) Monteggia fracture-dislocation in children. J Bone Joint Surg Am 68:615-619
26. Reckling FW (1982) Unstable fracture-dislocation of the forearm (Monteggia and Galeazzi lesions). J Bone Joint Surg Am 64:857-863
27. Essex-Lopresti P (1951) Fractures of the radial head with distal radio-ulnar dislocation. J Bone Joint Surg Br 33:244-247
28. Troudale RT, Amadio PC, Cooney WP, Morrey BF (1992) Radio ulnar dissociation a review of 20 cases. J Bone Joint Surg Am 74:1486-1497
29. Hotchkiss RN (1998) Fractures of the radial head and related unstability and contracture of the forearm. Instr Course Lect 47:173-177
30. Hotchkiss RN (1994) Injuries to the interosseus ligament of the forearm. Hand Clin 10:391-398
31. Robinowitz RS, Light TR, Havey RM, Gourinemi P, Patwardhan AG, Vrbos L (1994) The role of the interosseous membrane and triangular fibrocartilage complex in forearm stability. J Hand Surg Am 19:385-393
32. Morrey BF, Chao EY, Huy FC (1979) Biomechanical study of the elbow following excision of the radial head. J Bone Joint Surg Am 61:63-68
33. Davidson PA, Moseley JB, Tullos HS (1993) Radial head fracture. A potentially complex injury. Clin Orthop 297:224-230
34. Smith AM, Urhonosky LR, Castle JA, Rushing JT, Ruch DS (2002) Radius pull test: Predictor of longitudinal forearm unstability. J Bone Joint Surg Am 84:1970-1976
35. Darrach W (1913) Partial excision of the lower shaft of the ulna for deformity following Cole's fracture. Ann Surg 57:764
36. Sauvè L, Kapandy M (1936) Nouvelle technique de traitment chirurgical des luxations recidivantes isolèe de l'extremitè inferieure du cubitus. J Chirurgie 47:589-594

CHAPTER 12

The Instability after Radial Head Excision

S.L. JENSEN

Introduction

The most common clinical scenario leading to consideration of radial head excision is a comminuted radial head fracture in which rigid internal fixation is not feasible. Other indications for radial head excision may be painful mal- or non-union after conservatively or operatively treated fracture [1-3], failed internal fixation [3-5], as a supplement to a synovectomy in inflammatory arthritis [6], and various developmental deformities including congenital/chronic dislocation of the radial head [7].

It is convenient to look upon the radial head as part of two joint systems: (1) the elbow, consisting of the articulation between the humerus and the forearm as an entity, and (2) the forearm, consisting of the articulations between the radius and the ulna. Excision of the radial head may affect each of these joint systems by leading to an acute increase in joint laxity. If severe enough, such excess laxity may cause symptomatic clinical instability. The radial head also plays an important role in force transmission, and excision may change the way forces are distributed from the hand through the forearm and to the elbow. While this does not necessarily cause symptoms immediately, load changes in ligaments and joints may lead to pathological changes with time.

Fractures of the radial head are frequently associated with other injuries to the elbow or forearm, the presence of which may unfavorably moderate the destabilizing effect of radial head excision. Injury to the medial collateral ligament of the elbow is common with varying degrees of valgus instability as a result [8]. Radial head fractures may also complicate elbow joint dislocations, during which the lateral and usually also the medial collateral ligament is torn [9, 10]. The lateral collateral ligament is particularly important, since insufficiency of the lateral collateral ligament may predispose to re-dislocation or lead to recurrent elbow instability in the form of posterolateral rotatory instability [11, 12]. Other fractures may impair the stability normally provided by the congruous joint surfaces of the elbow, including fractures of the coronoid process, the olecranon, and humeral epicondyles/condyles [8, 13-15]. The combination elbow joint dislocation and fractures of the radial head and coronoid has been recognized as a particularly unfavorable condition [16].

In the forearm, an axial trauma may result in a radial head fracture associated with dislocation of the distal radio-ulnar joint, a combination referred to as the Essex-Lopresti lesion [17, 18]. This uncommon condition is characterized by acute proximal dislocation of the radius due to disruption of the structures stabilizing the forearm joints including the interosseous membrane [19]. The injury may not be entirely ligamentous, as fractures in the forearm may be included [20, 21]. Combined Essex-Lopresti lesion and elbow joint dislocation have also been reported [20-23].

Radial head fractures are traditionally classified into three types according to Mason [24]: undisplaced, displaced segmental, and comminuted. Radial neck fractures have been included in this classification [25]. Johnston [26] added a fourth type, which was any fracture associated with elbow dislocation. Morrey [27] divided fractures into simple and complex irrespective of morphology, depending on whether the fracture is complicated by other fractures or ligamentous injuries.

In this chapter, the current experimental and clinical documentation for instability after radial head excision will be discussed. The documentation for the use of radial head replacement will also be reviewed and discussed, as will other techniques for restoring stability.

Experimental Studies

Elbow Joint Laxity

Morrey et al. [28] investigated valgus laxity in cadaver elbows with a constant valgus moment generated by the effect of gravity on the forearm, and they found that excision of the radial head in the otherwise intact elbow joint induced no or very little increase in valgus laxity. This finding was later confirmed by other investigators using a similar model where the valgus moment was defined to 0.75 Nm [29]. If, however, radial excision is done secondary to division of the medial collateral ligament, more laxity is added to the increased laxity already present due to medial collateral ligament insufficiency [28, 30-32]. Hence, Morrey et al. [28] defined the medial collateral ligament as a primary and the radial head as a secondary valgus stabilizer (Fig. 1). It has been shown that the radial head also increases internal rotatory laxity, but again only if done secondary to division of the medial collateral ligament [32].

Jensen et al. [29] showed that radial head excision in the otherwise intact joint increases varus and external (posterolateral) rotatory laxities of the elbow; similar to, but in a lesser degree than the increased laxities seen after division of the lateral collateral ligament (Fig. 2) [33]. It was hypothesized that the lateral collateral ligament, which normally is distended in its course around the radial head, becomes slack after excision and thereby relatively insufficient. The findings that a repair of the ligament after radial head excision with recreation of tension could almost restore normal laxity confirms this hypothesis [34]. Division of the lateral collateral ligament and radial had excision has an additive effect on varus and external rotatory laxities (Fig. 2) [34].

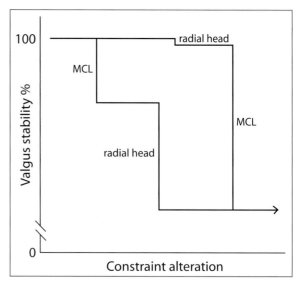

Fig. 1. Schematic representation of the primary role of the medial collateral ligament (anterior portion) and secondary role of the radial head as valgus constraints of the elbow. (Modified from [28])

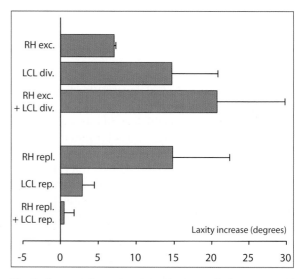

Fig. 2. Increase in posterolateral rotatory laxity compared with the intact elbow after various alterations in radial head and lateral collateral ligament constraint (*LCL div.*: lateral collateral ligament division; *LCL rep.*: lateral collateral ligament repair; *RH exc.*: radial head excision; *RH repl.*: radial head replacement)

In earlier studies of valgus stability, experimental protocols with determination of load-placement relationships were employed. Pribyl et al. [35] as well as Hotchkiss and Weiland [36] showed that the valgus stiffness of the elbow calculated as the slope of the load-displacement curve is reduced to about 70% of normal after radial head excision (Fig. 3). A medial shift of the pivoting point was provided as an explanation for this finding. The resulting smaller valgus moment arm after radial head excision increases the tension experienced by the medial collateral ligament for the same external load applied to the forearm (Fig. 4) [36]. It was

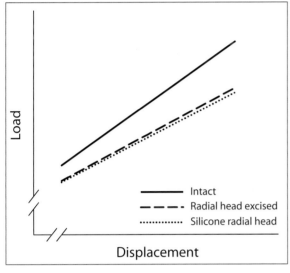

Fig. 3. Valgus load-displacement relationship for the intact elbow, after radial head excision, and replacement with a silicone prosthesis. (Modified from [6])

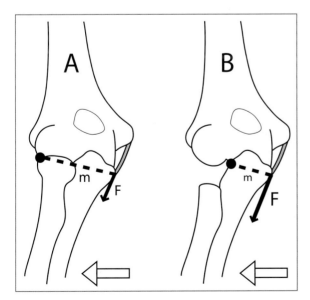

Fig. 4. Moment arm (m) and force (F) in the medial collateral ligament before (A) and after (B) radial head excision during application of identical valgus load. (Modified from [6])

also shown that silicone radial head replacement does not improve valgus stiffness after radial head, whereas an implant made of a stiffer material provides some improvement [35, 36].

King et al. [30] and Pomianowski et al. [31] investigated the ability of radial head replacement to improve valgus laxity after radial head excision in cases of medial collateral ligament disruption. A silicone implant did not reduce laxity, whereas three different metallic implants reduced laxity almost to the level before radial head excision [30, 31]. Jensen et al. [32] investigated laxity in more directions and found that with a metallic prosthesis, valgus laxity was restored completely to the level before radial head excision, whereas internal rotatory laxity was not completely restored. As for radial head excision in cases of lateral collateral ligament disruption, metallic radial head arthroplasty experimentally provides the same constraint as the native radial head (Fig. 2) [34].

Radial head replacement in case of disruption of either collateral ligament may at best substitute for the native radial head. It has been shown that combining arthroplasty with ligament repair restores laxity completely [32, 34]. The radial head, however, is a valgus stabilizer only secondary to the medial collateral ligament, and it appears that an isolated repair of the medial collateral ligament stabilizes valgus stability almost as well as the combined procedures [32]. In addition, after radial head excision in elbows with experimental disruption of the lateral collateral ligament, isolated repair of the ligament restores laxity almost as efficiently as combined ligament repair and radial head replacement (Fig. 2) [34].

The combination of radial head and coronoid fractures has been studied in experimental models simulating posterolateral elbow dislocation. Deutch et al. [37] showed that with the lateral collateral ligament intact, radial head and coronoid excision each increased posterolateral (external) rotatory laxity. The combined excisions lead to subluxation, which was prevented by metallic prosthetic replacement of the radial head [37]. In a similar investigation, Schneeberger et al. [38] showed that excision of the radial head increased posterolateral rotatory laxity, whereas the additional removal of 30% of the coronoid resulted in complete dislocation. Both a rigid and a floating (bipolar) radial head prosthesis reduced laxity, but the rigid implant performed better. With 50% or more of the coronoid removed, reconstruction of the coronoid in addition to radial head prosthetic replacement was necessary to restore laxity.

Forearm Load Distribution and Laxity

Several experimental studies, most using forearm models with load cells, have provided information regarding how forces are transferred from the wrist to the elbow during axial load. In the intact forearm, nearly all wrist force is picked up in the distal radius [39, 40]. The oblique fibers of the interosseous membrane transmit a part of this force to the ulna [39, 40]. The result is a more equal distribution of forces between the radius and ulna at the elbow, but still with relatively more force in the radio-capitellar joint [39-43]. A central thick band within the interosseous membrane is the functional structure regarding load transfer [43-45]. Markolf et al. [46, 47] showed that substantially more force is transferred through the interosseous membrane during varus alignment of the forearm compared to valgus alignment when the radial head is in contact to the humerus. Forearm rotation also affects load sharing with most force transmitted over the radio-capitellar in pronation [40, 48].

After radial head excision, the loss of radio-capitellar support allows the radius to slide more proximally, increasing the tension in interosseous membrane and also in the distal radio-ulnar joint [49]. The fraction of applied wrist force that normally would be directed through the radio-humeral joint is now shifted to the ulna mainly through the interosseous membrane and to a lesser extend through the distal radio-ulnar joint (Fig. 5) [49]. The central band of the interosseous membrane becomes the main restraint to proximal displacement of the radius, providing as much as 71% of the resistance against proximal displacement, whereas the distal radio-ulnar joint provides only 8% [45, 50].

With a 9.1 kg load, Rabinowitz et al. [43] found that up to 7 mm proximal migration of the radius was possible with the soft tissue structures intact. In contrast, Smith et al. [51] observed that proximal displacement was only 0.5 mm average after isolated radial head excision when pulling the proximal radius with 9.1 kg. After additional transection of either the distal radio-ulnar joint or the interosseous membrane, displacement was 1.3 mm and 3.5 mm respectively, but if both soft tissue structures were divided, displacement reached 9.5 mm. Based on their results, the investigators proposed the radius "pull test" highly indicative for disruption of the interosseous membrane if translation of the radius was greater than 3 mm.

A silicone replacement does not offer the same stiffness in the radio-capitellar joint as metallic replacement or the native radial head, and is about five times less stiff than the central band of the in-

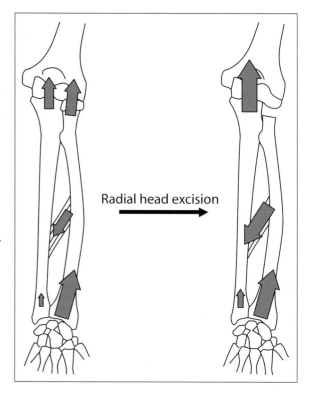

Fig. 5. Graphic illustration of load distribution in the forearm before and after radial head excision. Size of arrows approximates the relative forces based on results from several studies

terosseous membrane [45, 52, 53]. In case the interosseous membrane is disrupted, titanium but not silicone radial head replacement, provides nearly the same resistance to proximal migration as the intact membrane [50]. Neither is it possible to restore normal load sharing between the proximal radius and ulna with a silicone implant [42]. With metallic prostheses of anatomical length, it is possible to normalize load transfer to the distal ulna, also if the interosseous membrane has been divided [54]. Still, if no load is transmitted through the membrane, the radio-humeral joint load will remain increased.

Graft reconstructing the interosseous membrane has been proposed as an alternative to radial head arthroplasty in order to prevent proximal migration of the radius. Sellman et al. [50] demonstrated that a polyester cord reconstruction may provide 94% of the stiffness of the intact interosseous membrane. Others have investigated various autologous grafting materials, and showed that bone-patellar tendon-bone graft is superior to both single-stranded flexor carpi radialis and palmaris longus tendon in preventing migration, but neither is as efficient as the native interosseous membrane [55, 56]. Tomaino et al. [57] found that load sharing in the forearm could not be reproduced with an Achilles tendon graft, but later the same research group tested a flexor carpi radialis graft, which could restore forearm load transfer if the graft was double-stranded [58].

Clinicals Studies

Early Instability After Radial Head Excision

Early instability after radial head excision has been reported only for complex fractures associated with other injuries to the elbow or more rarely the forearm. In a series of elbow joint fracture-dislocations, Wheeler and Linscheid [13] observed that among elbow dislocations with no other associated fractures but the radial head, two out of nine patients who had their radial head excised sustained re-dislocation of the elbow. One patient who also had a coronoid process fracture, experienced re-dislocation although the elbow was immobilized in a cast. Josefsson et al. [14] reported a series of elbow joint fracture-dislocations treated with radial head excision and found that re-dislocation occurred in four elbows in all of which a simultaneous coronoid fracture was present. Hotchkiss [59] termed this unfavourable combination (elbow joint dislocation, radial head fracture, coronoid process fracture) the "terrible triad" of the elbow. Ring et al. [15] published a series of 11 patients with this injury. All four patients, who had their radial head excised, re-dislocated in the post-operative splint.

The short term results after radial head arthroplasty in complex radial head fractures has been reported in several papers. Generally stability was accomplished, but radial head replacement was used on a routine basis (usually with fixation of associated fractures), and it is not reported whether a prothesis was actually necessary to achieve stability [2, 52, 60-62]. Harrington and Tountas [63] gave details for selected cases, noting that radial head excision lead to instability in patients with an associated medial collateral ligament injury, with fracture of the coronoid, and with a fracture of the proximal ulna; all of which became stable after prosthetic replacement. In that series repair of the collateral ligaments was not performed [63]. In a later follow-up by Harrington et al. [8] the decision for replacement of the radial head was based on peri-operative findings of valgus-varus instability, but neverthless

those authors took the approach of never repairing associated collateral ligament injury.

Pugh et al. [64] reported 36 "terrible triad" lesions, among which the radial head was fixed or replaced (n=20) depending on fracture configuration. Coronoid fractures and the lateral collateral ligament were always repaired. Because of residual subluxation, additional repair of the medial collateral ligament was necessary in six and hinged external fixation in two cases. In a series of radial head fracture-dislocations and no other major fractures, Frankle et al. [65] used the same strategy and described that additional medial collateral repair and/or external fixation was required in three of eight radial head replacements. Moro et al. [66] reviewed 25 fracture-dislocations; eight elbows were still unstable after radial head replacement and additional repair of the medial collateral ligament was performed. Sanchez-Sotelo et al. [67] reported of 10 patients who were treated for an elbow fracture dislocation in which the only associated fracture was a comminuted radial head fracture treated by excision without replacement. Although the lateral collateral ligament was repaired, two patients still showed gross posterolateral instability and the elbows were temporarily transfixed.

In 1951 Essex-Lopresti [18] described a case of radial head excision which lead to immediate proximal dislocation of the radius. Curr and Coe [17] had reported a similar injury a few years earlier. It was suggested that disruption of the interosseous membrane and distal radio-ulnar joint had occurred along with the radial head fractures as a result of a longitudinal compression force on the radius [18]. McDougall and White [68] found that proximal displacement of the radius was more common than previously appreciated, but distinguished between rare cases of acute displacement and more common cases of late displacement occurring years after radial head excision. Edwards and Jupiter [19] reported seven cases of radial head fractures with an acute proximal displacement of 5-10 mm. Sowa et al. [23] found acute displacement of 15 mm in one patient, but also seven cases where proximal migration of 3-11 mm was detected with a delay of days to months.

There are only a few reports on the treatment of Essex-Lopresti injuries, probably reflecting their rarity. Essex-Lopresti [18] originally suggested prosthetic replacement of the radial head if the fracture could not be repaired. Edwards and Jupiter [19] reported that radial length could be restored with a silicone radial head prosthesis, but additional temporary fixation of the distal radio-ulnar joint was used and recommended. Trousdale et al. [21]

reported a patient in whom silicone replacement yielded a fair result, but resection of the distal ulna was performed six moths later. Sowa et al. [23] reported that proximal migration recurred after removal of radio-ulnar transfixation, although the radial head had been replaced with a silicone implant. A few cases of Essex-Lopresti injuries were included in series of metallic radial head replacements [62, 66]. Details were not provided regarding the achievement of normal radial length, but no symptoms were reported, that could be attributed to radio-ulnar longitudinal instability.

Late Consequences

Several follow-up studies exist, but the effect of radial head excision can be difficult to evaluate, because the studies often include a mixture of simple and complicated fractures. In the best studies, the follow-up period is more than 10 years and a clear distinction is made between simple fractures and those complicated by other injuries [1, 69-74].

An increase in elbow valgus angle of 5°-10° is consistently reported after radial head excision in otherwise intact upper extremities [69-72]. Herbertsson et al. [1] reported a 3° increase in a large series of 61 patients followed for 18 years, comprising both simple and complex fractures. Ikeda and Oka [73] reported 8° after 10 years, but failed to mention associated injuries. Coleman et al. [71] found that valgus angulation was positively correlated with follow-up time and the degree of fracture comminution (Mason classification). Janssen and Vegter [72] could not demonstrate valgus laxity with stress radiographs, although seven of 21 patients in their series had an increased valgus angulation of 5°-10°.

Most patients have degenerative arthritic changes in the ulno-humeral joint, but this is usually graded as mild [1, 69-73]. There appears to be no correlation between valgus angulation and degeneration in the elbow, but degeneration is more severe in Mason Type III fractures [71]. Except for the study by Ikeda and Oka [73], only a few patients are reported to have elbow pain, and usually only mild. [1, 69, 72] Herbertsson et al. [1] showed chronic pain to be more common in fracture-dislocations. Some investigators found association between elbow degeneration and pain [72, 74], while others did not [70, 71].

Most studies report proximal migration of the radius with an average ulna plus deformity of about 2 mm [69-74]. In the series of Coleman et al. [71] patients with migration of 2 mm or more were all male laborers and had longer follow-up times.

Degenerative changes in the wrist are uncommon and always mild [71-74]. Only a small number of patients have wrist pain and there appears to be no correlation with ulna plus deformity [69-71, 74]. Reduced grip strength has been reported in some cases [71-73], but in a large series of 61 patients, no such could be demonstrated [1].

There is only one study documenting the long-term results after radial head prosthetic replacement. Harrington et al. [8] reviewed 20 patients an average of 12 years after metallic replacement of a radial head fracture complicated with a mixture of injuries, including 15 elbow dislocations. Nine had radiographic osteoarthritis at the elbow, but all were restricted to the ulno-humeral joint. Six patients had no pain at all. Some loss of extension and supination was present. Strength was somewhat reduced compared with the uninjured limb, including grip strength by 13%. There was no sign of proximal migration of the radius and no patient had wrist pain. Four prostheses were removed because of pain, but the elbows remained stable after this.

Harrington's [8] series of radial head replacement can not be compared with series of radial head excision in which all or most fractures are simple. Josefsson et al. [14] however reported the results of 19 elbow joint fracture-dislocations after an average of 14 years: 15 patients had their radial head excised; 11 of these had radiographic signs of osteoarthritis in the elbow, and 6 complained of elbow pain. The average increase in carrying angle was 9° [14]. Broberg and Morrey [75] reported five patients with fracture-dislocations who all had the radial head removed primarily. All patients had mild or moderate arthritis in the elbow, all but one had mild pain, and some extension deficit (always less than 20°) was present [75].

Discussion

With the advances in surgical techniques and implants, most radial head fractures are amenable to internal fixation. Still, reconstruction of a comminuted fracture is technically difficult and not without complications. Less satisfactory results have been reported for comminuted (Mason Type III) and for complex fractures, and secondary excision of the radial head may often be necessary due to technically failure or nonunion [3-5]. It is therefore recommendable that internal fixation is reserved for relatively straightforward fracture patterns in which a stable anatomic reduction can be achieved, whereas comminuted fractures are better treated by excision with or without radial head replacement [3, 5].

Experimental as well as clinical studies support the motion that the biomechanical consequences of radial head excision strongly depend on the existence of associated injuries. There is a correlation between the comminution of the radial head fracture and the existence/extent of complicating lesions [13,15,76]. A comminuted radial head fracture should therefore alert the surgeon that other potentially destabilizing injuries may exist. Fluoroscopic stress testing of the elbow or forearm is a useful intra-operative tool if there is any doubt as to the state of the collateral ligaments or interosseous membrane [51, 62]. Soft tissue injuries may also be detected preoperatively with ultrasonography or MRI scanning [77, 78]. In fracture-dislocations, pre-operative CT scanning with 3-D reconstruction should be used liberally. For instance, a fracture of the coronoid may be mistaken for a fragment from the radial head on plain radiographs, with potential detrimental consequences for stability and result of treatment [15].

Experimental data indicate that in otherwise intact elbows, excision of the radial head increases varus and posterolateral laxities, probably by introducing slackness in the lateral collateral ligament. Theoretically, posterolateral rotatory instability may develop, but it has never been documented following excision of simple radial head fractures, although O'Driscoll et al. [11] briefly mentioned that they had seen such a case. It may be speculated that subtle posterolateral rotatory instability contributes to functional elbow pain after radial head excision, but it has not been looked for in follow-up studies. At our institution, when performing surgery on the radial head, we approach it by a partial or total transection of the lateral collateral ligament complex at its insertion on the supinator crest of the ulna. We do this primarily because it gives a good access to the radial head, but in cases where in the radial head is excised, it also has the advantage that tension in the ligament can be restored during reinsertion.

As documented by several biomechanical investigations, the radial head plays a central role in the transmission of forces from the hand to the elbow. After isolated radial head excision, there is no increase in valgus laxity, but experimental studies suggest that the medial collateral ligament is put under increased tension during activities involving valgus stress. In the forearm, longitudinal laxity increases only slightly, but load is redistributed with substantially more force acting on the interosseous membrane during axial stress. These changes in the elbow and forearm may attenuate the ligaments over time and explain the invariable findings of cubitus valgus and proximal radial migration in long-term clinical follow-up studies. The late clinical results after excision of simple radial head fractures are favorable, with only a few patients complaining of elbow or wrist pain, and there appears to be no correlation with these symptoms and the occurrence of valgus angulation and ulna plus deformity. After radial head excision, all elbow joint load is shifted to the ulno-humeral joint, suggesting why mild degenerative changes in the elbow are common findings. Ulno-humeral osteoarthritic changes, however, have been reported with comparable frequencies after arthroplasty, suggesting that they may be related to the initial traumatic event rather than the radial head excision itself [8].

After radial head excision, the central band of interosseous membrane is the most important constraint to proximal migration of the radius. If disrupted, and particularly if also the distal radio-ulnar joint is damaged, severe acute longitudinal radio-ulnar laxity develops. Clinically, the onset of proximal migration is sometimes more insidious perhaps representing cases where the distal radio-ulnar joint is initially intact or only part of the membrane is torn [23]. Radio-ulnar instability is often overlooked, and proximal migration sometimes becomes apparent only after excision of the radial head, leading to poor results which are difficult to redress [21]. Initial restoration of radial length with reconstruction or replacement of the radial head and distal radio-ulnar pinning have yielded satisfactory results, but with silicone implants proximal migration can recur after removal of radio-ulnar transfixation [19, 21, 45]. Experimentally, metallic radial head replacement as well as reconstruction of the functional important central band of the interosseous membrane is a more promising option and may make temporary transfixation unnecessary, but clinical experience with this is limited [79].

Excision of the radial head in the presence of elbow joint collateral ligament injuries such as occurring during an elbow dislocation or during severe valgus trauma results in severe instability both experimentally and clinically. If an elbow joint dislocation is also associated with a fracture of the coronoid process ("terrible triad"), the risk of frank re-dislocation is high, even within a retaining splint. Experimentally, prosthetic replacement of the radial head reduces laxity, but it is not always sufficient to maintain adequate stability as to prevent dislocation in clinical settings. Based on clinical experience, it is recommended that fractures of the coronoid process be fixed, and with additional repair of ligament injuries (at least the lateral collateral ligament), stability sufficient to allow early post-operative mobilization can nearly always be obtained. Experimental studies support that with this approach immediate stability can be achieved, but also suggest that with proper repair of the ligaments replacing the radial head may not be necessary. Most clinical studies have primarily aimed at a replacement of the radial head, and other strategies need further investigation.

There is much evidence that silicone radial head implants are biomechanically insufficient. In addition, complications such as mechanical failure and arthritis have frequently been reported [80, 81]. Metallic implants are better, and they experimentally approximate the constraint provided by the native radial head. Capitellar wear, however, is a major concern with the use of metallic prostheses, although there was no radiographic evidence of such in the long-term follow-up by Harrington et al. [8] Selecting the correct height of the prosthesis is important not only to re-establish normal kinematics of the elbow and load-sharing in the forearm, but also to avoid increased radio-capitellar pressure [82]. The radio-capitellar contact area is reduced with metallic implants which may further increase the risk of abnormal wear [83]. Capitellar erosion has been reported after metallic radial head replacement, and not infrequently prostheses are removed because of pain [8, 52, 84]. In such cases stability seems to persist, and the prosthesis may have served its purpose well by protecting soft tissue during healing [8].

Conclusions

Radial head excision can be performed in other wise intact upper extremities without risk of symptoms related to early or late instability. Radial head excision performed alone results in severe instability and is contraindicated if a radial head fracture is complicated by other injuries to the elbow or radio-ulnar joints. Metallic prosthetic replacement is an adjunct to gain immediate stability, but sufficient stability requires soft tissue repair and fixation of associated fractures.

References

1. Herbertsson P, Josefsson PO, Hasserius R et al (2004) Fractures of the radial head and neck treated with radial head excision. J Bone Joint Surg Am 86:1925-1930
2. Smets S, Govaers K, Jansen N et al (2000) The floating radial head prosthesis for comminuted radial head fractures: a multicentric study. Acta Orthop Belg 66:353-358
3. Ring D, Quintero J, Jupiter JB (2002) Open reduction and internal fixation of fractures of the radial head. J Bone Joint Surg Am 84:1811-1815
4. Esser RD, Davis S, Taavao T (1995) Fractures of the radial head treated by internal fixation: late results in 26 cases. J Orthop Trauma 9:318-323
5. King GJ, Evans DC, Kellam JF (1991) Open reduction and internal fixation of radial head fractures. J Orthop Trauma 5:21-28
6. Woods DA, Williams JR, Gendi NS et al (1999) Surgery for rheumatoid arthritis of the elbow: a comparison of radial-head excision and synovectomy with total elbow replacement. J Shoulder Elbow Surg 8:291-295
7. Hresko MT, Rosenberg BN, Pappas AM (1999) Excision of the radial head in patients younger than 18 years. J Pediatr Orthop 19:106-113
8. Harrington IJ, Sekyi-Otu A, Barrington TW et al (2001) The functional outcome with metallic radial head implants in the treatment of unstable elbow fractures: a long-term review. J Trauma 50:46-52
9. Josefsson PO, Gentz CF, Johnell O, Wendeberg B (1987) Surgical versus non-surgical treatment of ligamentous injuries following dislocation of the elbow joint. A prospective randomized study. J Bone Joint Surg Am 69:605-608
10. McKee MD, Schemitsch EH, Sala MJ, O'Driscoll SW (2003) The pathoanatomy of lateral ligamentous disruption in complex elbow instability. J Shoulder Elbow Surg 12:391-396
11. O'Driscoll SW, Bell DF, Morrey BF (1991) Posterolateral rotatory instability of the elbow. J Bone Joint Surg Am 73:440-446
12. Olsen BS, Sojbjerg JO (2003) The treatment of recurrent posterolateral instability of the elbow. J Bone Joint Surg Br 85:342-346
13. Wheeler DK, Linscheid RL (1967) Fracture-dislocations of the elbow. Clin Orthop 50:95-106
14. Josefsson PO, Gentz CF, Johnell O, Wendeberg B (1989) Dislocations of the elbow and intraarticular fractures. Clin Orthop 246:126-130
15. Ring D, Jupiter JB, Zilberfarb J (2002) Posterior dislocation of the elbow with fractures of the radial head and coronoid. J Bone Joint Surg Am 84:547-551
16. Hotchkiss RN (1996) Fractures and dislocations of the elbow. In: Rockwood CA, Green DP, Bucholz RW, Heckman JD (eds) Fractures in adults, 4 edn. Lippincott-Raven Publishers, pp 929-1024
17. Curr JF, Coe WA (1946) Dislocation of the inferior radio-ulnar joint. Br J Surg 34:74-77
18. Essex-Lopresti P (1951) Fractures of the radial head with distal radio-ulnar dislocation. Report of two cases. J Bone Joint Surg Br 33:244-247
19. Edwards GS Jr, Jupiter JB (1988) Radial head fractures with acute distal radioulnar dislocation. Essex-Lopresti revisited. Clin Orthop 234:61-69
20. Kazuki K, Miyamoto T, Ohzono K (2005) A case of traumatic divergent fracture-dislocation of the elbow combined with Essex-Lopresti lesion in an adult. J Shoulder Elbow Surg 14:224-226
21. Trousdale RT, Amadio PC, Cooney WP, Morrey BF (1992) Radio-ulnar dissociation. A review of twenty cases. J Bone Joint Surg Am 74:1486-1497
22. Malik AK, Pettit P, Compson J (2005) Distal radioulnar joint dislocation in association with elbow injuries. Injury 36:324-329
23. Sowa DT, Hotchkiss RN, Weiland AJ (1995) Symptomatic proximal translation of the radius following radial head resection. Clin Orthop 317:106-113

24. Mason ML (1954) Some observations on fractures of the head of the radius with a review of one hundred cases. Br J Surg 42:123-132

25. Johansson O (1962) Capsular and ligament injuries of the elbow joint. A clinical and orthrographic study. Acta Chir Scand 287:1-159

26. Johnston GW (1962) A follow-up of one hundred cases of fracture of the head of the radius with a review of the liiterature. Ulster Med J 31:51-63

27. Morrey BF (2000) Radial head fractures. In: Morrey BF (ed) The elbow and its disorders. 3 edn. W.B. Saunders Co, Philadelphia, pp 341-364

28. Morrey BF, Tanaka S, An KN (1991) Valgus stability of the elbow. A definition of primary and secondary constraints. Clin Orthop 265:187-195

29. Jensen SL, Olsen BS, Sojbjerg JO (1999) Elbow joint kinematics after excision of the radial head. J Shoulder Elbow Surg 8:238-241

30. King GJ, Zarzour ZD, Rath DA et al (1999) Metallic radial head arthroplasty improves valgus stability of the elbow. Clin Orthop 368:114-125

31. Pomianowski S, Morrey BF, Neale PG et al (2001) Contribution of monoblock and bipolar radial head prostheses to valgus stability of the elbow. J Bone Joint Surg Am 83:1829-1834

32. Jensen SL, Deutch SR, Olsen BS et al (2003) Laxity of the elbow after experimental excision of the radial head and division of the medial collateral ligament. Efficacy of ligament repair and radial head prosthetic replacement: a cadaver study. J Bone Joint Surg Br 85:1006-1010

33. Olsen BS, Vaesel MT, Sojbjerg JO et al (1996) Lateral collateral ligament of the elbow joint: anatomy and kinematics. J Shoulder Elbow Surg 5:103-112

34. Jensen SL, Olsen BS, Tyrdal S et al (2005) Elbow joint laxity after experimental radial head excision and lateral collateral ligament rupture: efficacy of prosthetic replacement and ligament repair. J Shoulder Elbow Surg 14:78-84

35. Pribyl CR, Kester MA, Cook SD et al (1986) The effect of the radial head and prosthetic radial head replacement on resisting valgus stress at the elbow. Orthopedics 9:723-726

36. Hotchkiss RN, Weiland AJ (1987) Valgus stability of the elbow. J Orthop Res 5:372-377

37. Deutch SR, Jensen SL, Tyrdal S et al (2003) Elbow joint stability following experimental osteoligamentous injury and reconstruction. J Shoulder Elbow Surg 12:466-471

38. Schneeberger AG, Sadowski MM, Jacob HA (2004) Coronoid process and radial head as posterolateral rotatory stabilizers of the elbow. J Bone Joint Surg Am 86:975-982

39. Birkbeck DP, Failla JM, Hoshaw SJ et al (1997) The interosseous membrane affects load distribution in the forearm. J Hand Surg Am 22:975-980

40. Pfaeffle HJ, Fischer KJ, Manson TT et al (2000) Role of the forearm interosseous ligament: is it more than just longitudinal load transfer? J Hand Surg Am 25:683-688

41. Halls AA, Travill A (1964) Transmission of pressures across the elbow joint. Anat Rec 150:243-248

42. Gupta GG, Lucas G, Hahn DL (1997) Biomechanical and computer analysis of radial head prostheses. J Shoulder Elbow Surg 6:37-48

43. Rabinowitz RS, Light TR, Havey RM et al (1994) The role of the interosseous membrane and triangular fibrocartilage complex in forearm stability. J Hand Surg Am 19:385-393

44. Shepard MF, Markolf KL, Dunbar AM (2001) The effects of partial and total interosseous membrane transection on load sharing in the cadaver forearm. J Orthop Res 19:587-592

45. Hotchkiss RN, An KN, Sowa DT et al (1989) An anatomic and mechanical study of the interosseous membrane of the forearm: pathomechanics of proximal migration of the radius. J Hand Surg Am 14:256-261

46. Markolf KL, Lamey D, Yang S et al (1998) Radioulnar load-sharing in the forearm. A study in cadavera. J Bone Joint Surg Am 80:879-888

47. Markolf KL, Dunbar AM, Hannani K (2000) Mechanisms of load transfer in the cadaver forearm: role of the interosseous membrane. J Hand Surg Am 25:674-682

48. Morrey BF, An KN, Stormont TJ (1988) Force transmission through the radial head. J Bone Joint Surg Am 70:250-256

49. Shepard MF, Markolf KL, Dunbar AM (2001) Effects of radial head excision and distal radial shortening on load-sharing in cadaver forearms. J Bone Joint Surg Am 83:92-100

50. Sellman DC, Seitz WH Jr, Postak PD, Greenwald AS (1995) Reconstructive strategies for radioulnar dissociation: a biomechanical study. J Orthop Trauma 9:516-522

51. Smith AM, Urbanosky LR, Castle JA et al (2002) Radius pull test: predictor of longitudinal forearm instability. J Bone Joint Surg Am 84:1970-1976

52. Knight DJ, Rymaszewski LA, Amis AA, Miller JH (1993) Primary replacement of the fractured radial head with a metal prosthesis. J Bone Joint Surg [Br] 75:572-576

53. Carn RM, Medige J, Curtain D, Koenig A (1986) Silicone rubber replacement of the severely fractured radial head. Clin Orthop 209:259-269

54. Markolf KL, Tejwani SG, O'Neil G, Benhaim P (2004) Load-sharing at the wrist following radial head replacement with a metal implant. A cadaveric study. J Bone Joint Surg Am 86:1023-1030

55. Tejwani SG, Markolf KL, Benhaim P (2005) Reconstruction of the interosseous membrane of the forearm with a graft substitute: a cadaveric study. J Hand Surg Am 30:326-334

56. Skahen JR, III, Palmer AK, Werner FW, Fortino MD (1997) Reconstruction of the interosseous membrane of the forearm in cadavers. J Hand Surg Am 22:986-994

57. Tomaino MM, Pfaeffle J, Stabile K, Li ZM (2003) Reconstruction of the interosseous ligament of the forearm reduces load on the radial head in cadavers. J Hand Surg Br 28:267-270

58. Pfaeffle HJ, Stabile KJ, Li ZM, Tomaino MM (2005) Reconstruction of the interosseous ligament restores normal forearm compressive load transfer in cadavers. J Hand Surg Am 30:319-325

59. Hotchkiss RN (1996) Dislocations of the elbow and intraarticular fractures. In: Rockwood CA, Green DP, Bucholz RW, Heckman JD (eds) Rockwood and Green's fractures in adults. 4 edn. Lippincott-Raven, Philadelphia, pp 929-1024

60. Judet T, Garreau de Loubresse C, Piriou P, Charnley G (1996) A floating prosthesis for radial-head fractures. J Bone Joint Surg Br 78:244-249

61. Popovic N, Gillet P, Rodriguez A, Lemaire R (2000) Fracture of the radial head with associated elbow dislocation: results of treatment using a floating radial head prosthesis. J Orthop Trauma 14:171-177

62. Ashwood N, Bain GI, Unni R (2004) Management of Mason type-III radial head fractures with a titanium prosthesis, ligament repair, and early mobilization. J Bone Joint Surg Am 86:274-280

63. Harrington IJ, Tountas AA (1981) Replacement of the radial head in the treatment of unstable elbow fractures. Injury 12:405-412

64. Pugh DM, Wild LM, Schemitsch EH et al (2004) Standard surgical protocol to treat elbow dislocations with radial head and coronoid fractures. J Bone Joint Surg Am 86:1122-1130

65. Frankle MA, Koval KJ, Sanders RW, Zuckerman JD (1999) Radial head fractures associated with elbow dislocations treated by immediate stabilization and early motion. J Shoulder Elbow Surg 8:355-360

66. Moro JK, Werier J, MacDermid JC et al (2001) Arthroplasty with a metal radial head for unreconstructible fractures of the radial head. J Bone Joint Surg Am 83:1201-1211

67. Sanchez-Sotelo J, Romanillos O, Garay EG (2000) Results of acute excision of the radial head in elbow radial head fracture-dislocations. J Orthop Trauma 14:354-358

68. McDougall A, White J (1957) Subluxation of the inferior radio-ulnar joint complicating fracture of the radial head. J Bone Joint Surg Br 39:278-287

69. Stephen IB (1981) Excision of the radial head for closed fracture. Acta Orthop Scand 52:409-412

70. Goldberg I, Peylan J, Yosipovitch Z (1986) Late results of excision of the radial head for an isolated closed fracture. J Bone Joint Surg Am 68:675-679

71. Coleman DA, Blair WF, Shurr D (1987) Resection of the radial head for fracture of the radial head. Long-term follow-up of seventeen cases. J Bone Joint Surg Am 69:385-392

72. Janssen RP, Vegter J (1998) Resection of the radial head after Mason type-III fractures of the elbow: follow-up at 16 to 30 years. J Bone Joint Surg Br 80:231-233

73. Ikeda M, Oka Y (2000) Function after early radial head resection for fracture: a retrospective evaluation of 15 patients followed for 3-18 years. Acta Orthop Scand 71:191-194

74. Morrey BF, Chao EY, Hui FC (1979) Biomechanical study of the elbow following excision of the radial head. J Bone Joint Surg Am 61:63-68

75. Broberg MA, Morrey BF (1987) Results of treatment of fracture-dislocations of the elbow. Clin Orthop 216:109-119

76. Davidson PA, Moseley JB Jr, Tullos HS (1993) Radial head fracture. A potentially complex injury. Clin Orthop 297:224-230

77. Wallace AL, Haber M, Sesel K, Sonnabend DH (1999) Ultrasonic diagnosis of interosseous ligament failure in radioulnar dissociation. Injury 30:59-63

78. Starch DW, Dabezies EJ (2001) Magnetic resonance imaging of the interosseous membrane of the forearm. J Bone Joint Surg Am 83:235-238

79. Ruch DS, Chang DS, Koman LA (1999) Reconstruction of longitudinal stability of the forearm after disruption of interosseous ligament and radial head excision (Essex-Lopresti lesion). J South Orthop Assoc 8:47-52

80. Worsing RA, Engber WD, Lange TA (1982) Reactive synovitis from particulate silastic. J Bone Joint Surg Am 64:581-585

81. Stoffelen DV, Holdsworth BJ (1994) Excision or Silastic replacement for comminuted radial head fractures. A long-term follow-up. Acta Orthop Belg 60:402-407

82. Van Glabbeek F., Van Riet RP, Baumfeld JA et al (2004) Detrimental effects of overstuffing or understuffing with a radial head replacement in the medial collateral-ligament deficient elbow. J Bone Joint Surg Am 86:2629-2635

83. Liew VS, Cooper IC, Ferreira LM et al (2003) The effect of metallic radial head arthroplasty on radiocapitellar joint contact area. Clin Biomech 18:115-118

84. Van Riet RP, Van GF, Verborgt O, Gielen J (2004) Capitellar erosion caused by a metal radial head prosthesis. A case report. J Bone Joint Surg Am 86:1061-1064

CHAPTER 13

The Radial Head Prosthesis: Historical Perspective

C. ROVESTA, C. MINERVINI, G. BONANNO, L. CELLI

Introduction

In case of an irreducible comminuted radial head fracture, a simple resection is possible to allow a precocious mobilization of the elbow. But to avoid the valgus deviation and the riding up of the radius that can happen after the resection. The medical literature reported the substitution of the radial head with a prosthesis for the first time 64 years ago.

This prosthesis has had a continuous evolution in the attempt to resolve the principal problems related to its implant:

1. to replace a bony structure that seems anatomically simple but that is really complex and varying from individual to individual;
2. to guarantee a stability and consolidation between the prosthesis and the radius;
3. to allow a precocious and complete movement of the elbow in flexion-extension and pronation-supination without pain;
4. to avoid over time the wear (and tear) of the humeral cartilage.

To solve these problems, the research has developed a better prosthesis design, has worked on the components modularity, and on the materials' proprieties.

Regarding the materials, the research has developed materials that have the proprieties of biocompatibility and long-term stability.

Over time the materials have been improved by trying to obtain the nearest coefficient of elasticity to the bone's coefficient, to reduce a precocious wear (and tear) in the contact with the humeral condyle, and avoiding, however, prohibitively expensive material.

Biomechanical solutions have been introduced that favor the adaptation of the prosthesis to the humerus, reducing the stresses of it (the components' articulations).

To improve and to make more stable over time the union between the radius and the prosthetic stem, the cementation between the stem of a different shape and the coating, which allows a better osteointegration, has been avoided.

Models have been built already assembled before the surgery, to make the implant easier and to minimize the damage to the periarticular soft tissue of the elbow.

After 65 years of history and study about the prosthesis of radial head we have not yet reached an ideal prosthesis.

Historical Revision

The first author that published an article regarding the use of prosthesis for the head of the radius was Speed [1].

After numerous experimentations and design changes, they installed a bearing (ferrule caps) in Vitallium on three patients with a comminuted fracture of the radial head (Fig. 1a).

They concluded that such a method is satisfactory since it "...can bring to a complete resumption

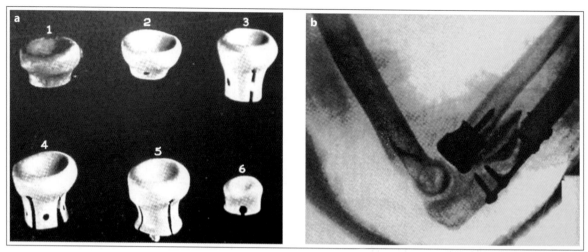

Fig. 1. (**a**) Ferrule caps for the head of the radius: different sizes used by Speed-Kellog [1]. (**b**) X-ray implant: no shortening of the radius and complete ROM

of the elbow articulation functionality, preventing also the shortening of the radius..." (Fig. 1b).

Ten years later Creyssel and De Morgues [2] used a model of a prosthesis in nylon, which is a more elastic material compared to Vitallium, to reduce the stress on the humeral condyle.

Also, Cherry [3] made use of an acrylic prosthesis to treat the fractures of the radial head.

In addition, in Italy we have the first example of the use of a metallic endo-prosthesis over 60 years ago (Fig. 2a). In 1952, Albonico [4] published research regarding the implant in two patients of "...endo prosthesis in Vitallium in substitution of the radial head removed because of the fracture..." (Fig. 2b). The first patient, a 20-year-old carpenter, presented with absence of pain, normal mobility

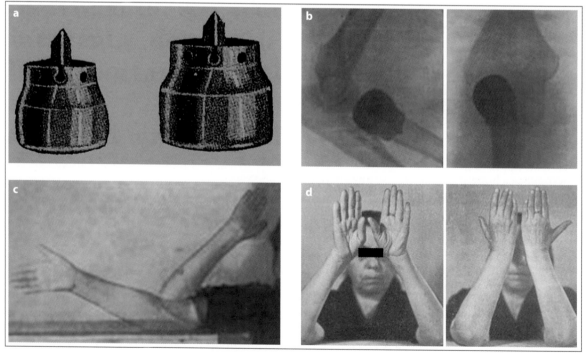

Fig. 2. (**a**) Metallic endo-prosthesis used by Albonico [4]. (**b**) X-ray implant in a 60-year old woman. (**c**) Limitation of 20° of extension and complete flexion. (**d**) Absence of pain and good function in prono-supination

and trophism after one year. The second patient, a 60-year-old woman, presented with absence of pain, limitation of 20° of extension, and good function after 10 months (Figs. 2c, d) [4].

Beginning in 1968, Swanson [5] began to use a prosthesis made of silicone. He published the good results he experienced with his prosthesis and proposed a diffusion of the use of it "since introduces facility of implant, it was well tolerated and it was a prosthesis with low costs" (Fig. 3).

Swanson developed the concept of using a pros-

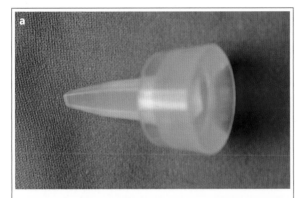
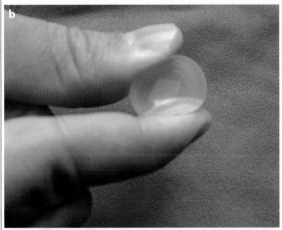
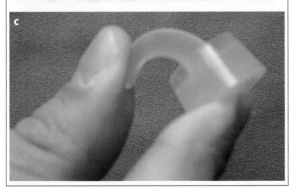

Fig. 3. (**a**) Prosthesis of silastic "Swanson". (**b**) High deformability of the head. (**c**) High flexibility of the stem

thesis in silastic as a spacing that replaces the inevitable traumatic loss of the radial head. In 18 patients checked in 1973 and 1981 "...the silicone implant is a profit, sure and reliable alternative in the treatment of the fractures comminuted of the radial head and in the failures of resection of the radial head..." [5].

When the diffusion of this implant began in the early 1980's, some criticism arose about its use because of the frequent break-ups of the prosthesis that caused a deviation in valgus, or production of fragments that were often the cause of a secondary synovitis [6].

These Authors emphasized, in addition to the frequent complications, the bad mechanical proprieties of silastic, which is easily deformed and which does not provide resistance to the axial load.

For these reasons, beginning in the early 1990's, the materials used for the prosthesis changed to more rigid materialssuch as ceramic, cobalt-chrome, or titanium.

Polyethylene, with its high molecular weight (UHMWPE), seems a good material because it better transmits the load on the humerus in comparison to silicone, and in a more physiological way in comparison to the metals and to ceramic [7].

More recently, prostheses made of pyrocarbon have been used because pyrocarbon introduces mechanical proprieties more similar to the bone.

Such similarity reduces the possibility of wear (and tear) on the humeral condyle. For the same reason, to reduce the stresses of the prosthesis thereby providing a greater adaptability to the humerus, which allows articular movements between stem and cephalic component, the one-piece prosthesis has been replaced with the bipolar prosthesis. The bipolar prosthesis simply has a rotator movement between the head and stem and introduces a mobility on all planes with an articulation "ball in socket" as in Judet's prosthesis or in the radial head prosthesis (KPS) [8, 9].

A cause of failure of this prosthesis can be the mobilization due to the lack of correspondence between the stem and the endomedullar canal. For this to improve, the congruence of the stem beside the cementation, modeled stems, grooves on the neck, or a stem of greater length were used (as in Judet's prosthesis).

In recent years, a prosthesis has been proposed without cement with a stem that introduces a system with expansion life and prosthesis with anatomical form.

Over time the modularity of the prosthesis is strengthened with subsequentl stems of different dimensions that can be assembled with heads of different heights and diameters, in order to promote a greater possibility of adaptation to the anatomical variations.

Currently on the market there are a series of a monoblock prostheses (KNITS, SOLAR, ASCENSION) or bipolar prostheses (BIPOLAR, GUEPAR, KPS), other models that introduce a greater modularity (AVANTA, EVOLVE, MOPYC), and a "custom made" prosthesis (BIOCLONE), which is made of different material with or without cement.

Discussion

The ideal radius prosthesis should have the same anatomical shape and dimension as the radius of the patient. It should be made of a material with the same coefficient of elasticity as the bone, creating a stable and lasting contact between the stem and the radial diaphysis that resists repeated micro trauma, without causing damage to the humeral cartilage. It should also be easy to install.

Anatomical Form and Prosthetic Design

Generically, the radial head of a man is wider than a woman's. Differences based on race, side, or age do not exist; the radial head diameter is proportional to the bodily dimension.

Anatomical studies by Skalki et al. [10], Goupta et al. [7], Van Riet et al. [11] and Mahaisavarlya et al. [12] directly conducted on a dead body or on a dead body with TC integrated with CAD, has underlined that:
1. the radial head has an irregular form (middle diameter 20.5 mm);
2. the central point of the head is close to the central point of the concavity but not coincident;
3. there is no direct correlation between the dimension of the head and that of the medullary canal of the radius that is tightened and irregular (7.4 mm ± 1,4);
4. the angle of the neck is different in comparison to the dialysis (16° ± 5.5°).

These factors can explain why it is difficult to realize a prosthetic model that corresponds to the different anatomical proprieties of the patient.

Beredjiklian et al. [13] define a "mismatch" of the relationship between the prosthetic components of the radial head and the morphology of the proximal radius.

Using MRI they have measured the anatomical dimensions of the head and of the radial neck and

is currently comparing them with the prostheses available on the market.

In 39% of the cases, the neck sizes of the prosthesis were overvalued compared with medullary canal.

The prosthesis stabilization towards the extreme proximal of the radius is submitted to the contact of the head base with the proximal extremity of the radius, but above all to the congruence of the stem with the neck medullary canal and superior part of the diaphysis.

For this reason the prosthesis shape has been changed from a cylindrical shape to a truncated cone, with inclination that matches the neck obliquity (AVANTA) (Fig. 4) ; in other models an expansion stem is used (MOPYC) (Fig. 5).

The stem surface in contact with the bone has to form good osteo-integration. To facilitate the stem stability as regards the radius, many prosthetic models use cementation; with this one it is possible to use thinner and longer stems (Judet) (Fig. 6).

The modularity therefore is essential for better suiting the prosthesis to the anatomical variables and eventually to compensate for technical errors.

For this reason we can have prosthesis heads of different diameters (18-24 mm), different heights (standard or long), with a modular neck of different dimensions (5-10 mm), with short or long stem, or an expansion stem that can be rectilinear or tilted, cemented or not cemented; the result is a notable number of possible assemblages, raising the costs in comparison to the monoblock prostheses, however.

Despite the ample modularity, any implant tested with all the various types of prostheses is able to restore stability in valgus as the original radial

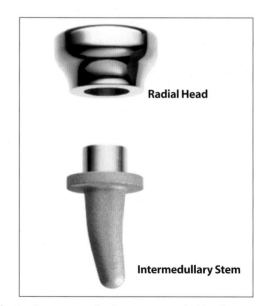

Radial Head

Intermedullary Stem

Fig. 4. Avanta prosthesis: uncementeded implant

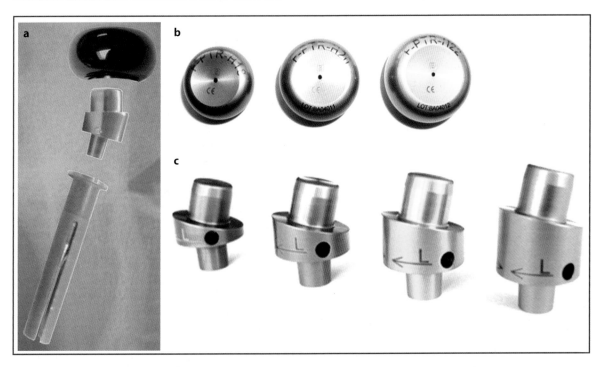

Fig. 5. (**a**) Mopyc prosthesis: hight modularity. (**b**) Different sizes of the head. (**c**) Different sizes of the neck

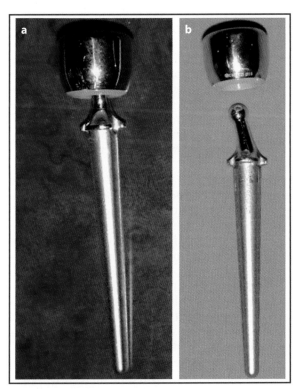

Fig. 6. (**a**) Judet prosthesis: modularity components. (**b**) Long stem cemented

head; this is probably due to the incapability of repeating the physiological shape and size of the original radial head.

For this, using X-ray in anterioposterior and laterals of both the elbows with a standardized marker, a sketch of the prosthesis is created "custom made" that can be assembled with the head and stem in stainless steel (BIOCLONE).

Prosthetic Components Mobility

In 1996, Judet et al. [8] began using a "floating" prosthesis radial head, which is in two articulated parts semiconstrained with a spherical extremity of the stem, with an angle of 15°, contained in the cephalic component as a "ball in socket", which allows a free rotation and an arc of 35° in monoplanar movement in every direction [8].

A more recent model prosthesis (KPS) is biarticulated with a straight, short stem that allows an arc of angular movement of 30°.

The 3° of freedom of movement of this articulation "ball in socket" model permits an automatic positioning of the prosthesis head towards the humeral condyle and the concave radial notch of the ulna; it also compensates for small anatomical differences of the prosthesis in comparison to the original head.

Therefore, the stress is reduced on the stem (less loosening) and the distribution of the loads is improved on the humeral condyle, and the movement between the head and the humeral cartilage is reduced (less stress on the cartilage).

The mobility of the bipolar implant raises issues for discussion regarding how much it can contribute to the stability of the elbow.

Can a bipolar implant be as efficient as a monoblock prosthesis to give back stability of the elbow in valgus, after medial collateral ligament (MCL) lesion?

Pomianowski et al. [14] have appraised on a dead body the stability of the elbow after substitution of the radial head with a Knits-type monoblock prosthesis, a prosthesis made of Vitallium and polyethylene, and a bipolar Judet Vitallium-polyethylene-Vitallium prosthesis, quantifying the instability with an electromagnetic tracing lens.

The average of laxity in valgus with a MCL lesion and prosthetic implant was greater in comparison to that with an intact radial head before the resection.

The implants appeared similar as to stabilization unless in neutral position of the forearm, in which the elbow laxity was greater with the implant of Judet in comparison to the monoblock and to the KPS (perhaps due to the angular design of the neck).

Prosthetic Material

The first prostheses of radial head were made out of stainless steel, which was then replaced with a less rigid acrylic material [3].

Subsequently, Swanson et al. [5] used, from 1968, a silicone prosthesis (SILASTIC) that introduces a high deformability with transmission of 50% of the strength on the humeral condyle, without preventing deviation in valgus under high loads with possibility of fragmentation of the prosthesis [6].

Pribyl et al. [15] introduced an acrylic implant which better resisted the deviation in valgus in comparison to the silicone model, which is more easily deformed.

Due to the low resistance of the silicone, Harrington recommended the use titanium in transplantations when stability was at its lowest point after excision of the head [16].

Due to direct experience with the radial head prostheses and information obtained by the studies performed, above all on hip and knee replacement, there was an inducement to seek new materials for the radial head prostheses.

In fact, the ideal prosthesis should be made of material which has good biocompatibility, is not deformable (whatever stress that transfers to the humeral condyle should avoid deviation in valgus), but which distributes the load on the cartilage in a homogeneous way so as to not cause any damage; therefore, with a coefficient of elasticity similar to that of the bone (= 17).

The metallic (titanium, cobalt-chrome, Vitallium) and ceramic implants have a high coefficient of elasticity, from 7 to 15 times more than the coefficient of the bone, and therefore they can resist more without deformation; however, conversely, they cause a usury of the condyle cartilage [7], since being too rigid they don't distribute the load in a homogeneous way.

Polyethylene, which has a high molecular weight (UHMWPE), is a rigid enough polymer (less elasticity) to mostly transmit the load on the humerus in comparison to silicone and in more physiological way in comparison to the metals.

This polyethylene is characterized by the best mechanical and physiological proprieties in comparison to the polymers previously used in prostheses of hip and knee, which had given unsatisfactory results regarding contact with the cartilage.

Biomechanical analysis has, however, shown that an intramedullary stem polymeric would not have enough resistance to absorb the stresses of articular movements under effort.

To address this issue recent prostheses have been constructed from the union of various materials.

The Judet's "floating" consisting of an high density polyethylene radial head contained in a cobalt-chrome capsule, that articulates with the spherical extremity of a long stem in cobalt-chrome that is cemented in the medullary canal.

The KPS prosthesis is constituted of a head made of polyethylene with high molecular weight (UHMWPE), which directly articulates with the humerus and with the spherical extremity of a short stem of cobalt-chrome-molybdenum (Vitallium).

The choice of Vitallium or chrome-cobalt rather than titanium made by many authors (Skalski, Knight, Judet) is because when the polyethylene articulates with Vitallium it creates a smaller number of deposits in the spherical articulation (ball in socket) in comparison to titanium.

In recent years prostheses have been built with the head made of pyrocarbon, which introduces a coefficient of elasticity similar to that of the bone (= 20); therefore with good transmission of the force and stress on the humeral condyle with a low coefficient of friction. The stem is not cemented in expansion titanium.

Conclusions

We have been searching for the ideal radial head prosthesis ever since it was first developed 65 years ago. The biomechanical and materials studies have resulted in the introduction of various prostheses to the market, including monoblock (KNITS, SOLAR), assembled (ASCENSION), or with intrinsic particularity (JUDET, GUEPAR, KPS), with extreme modularity (AVANTA; EVOLVE, MOPYC), "custom made" prostheses (BIOCLONE), and stem not cemented rectilinear, with angle or to expansion or cemented, smooth or irregular. The prostheses are built with different materials, sometimes assembled to resist to deformation with a coefficient of elasticity closer to the bone coefficient.

The prosthesis design and the modularity also make it easier to implant with a technique as least invasive as possible.

Despite these factors, any prosthesis model, currently usable and applied with the correct technique, is able to work as well as the original radial head. For this, as suggested by Pomianowski et al. [14] the open reduction with internal fixation is preferable to the replacement to recreate the anatomy of the proximal limb of the radius.

References

1. Speed K (1941) Ferrule caps for the head of the radius. Surg Gyn Obst 73:845-850
2. Creyssel J, de Morgues G (1951) Résection de la tete radiale avec endhoprothèse en nylon. Lyon Chir 46:508
3. Cherry JC (1953) Use of acrylic prosthesis in the treatment of fracture of the head of the radium. J Bone Joint Surg Br 35:70-71
4. Albonico P (1952) Endoprotesi in Vitallium in sostituzione del capitello radiale asportato per frattura. Chir Org Mov XXXVII:134-143
5. Swanson AB, Jaeger SH, La Rochelle D (1981) Comminuted fractures of the radial head. J Bone Joint Surg Am 63:1039-1049
6. Vanderwilde RS, Morrey BF, Welberg MW, Vinh TN (1994) Inflammatory arthritis after failure of silicone rubber replacement of the radial head. J Bone Joint Surg Br 76:78-81
7. Goupta GG, Lucas G, Hanh DL (1997) Biomechanical and computer analysis of radial head prostheses. J Shoulder Elbow Surg 6:37-48
8. Judet T, Garreau de Loubresse C, Piriou P, Charnley G (1996) A floating prosthesis for radial head fractures. J Bone Joint Surg Br 78:244-249
9. Knight DJ, Rymaszewski LA, Amis AA, Miller JH (1993) Primary replacement of the fractured radial head with a metal prosthesis. J Bone Joint Surg Br 75:672-576
10. Skalski K, Swieszkowski W, Pomianowski S et al (2004) Radial head prosthesis with a mobile head. J Shoulder Elbow Surg 13:78-85
11. Van Riet R, Van Glabbeek F, Verstreken J (2001) Current concepts in the treatment in the radial head fractures in the adult. A clinical and biomechanical approach. Acta Orthop Belg 67:430-441
12. Mahaisavariya B, Saekee B, Vander Sloten J (2004) Morphology of the radial head: a reverse engineering based evaluation using three-dimensional anatomical data of radial bone. Proc Inst Mech Eng 218:79-84
13. Beredjiklian PK, Nalbantoglu U, Potter HG, Hotchkiss RN (1999) Prosthetic radial head components and proximal radial morphology: a mismatch. J Shoulder Elbow Surg 8:471-475
14. Pomianowski S, Morrey BF, O'Driscoll SW (2001) Contribution of monoblock and bipolar radial head prostheses to valgus stability of the elbow. J Bone Joint Surg Am 83:1829-1834
15. Pribyl CR, Kester MA, Brunet ME (1986) The effect of the radial head and prosthetic radial head replacement on resisting valgus stress at the elbow. Orthopedics 9:723-726
16. Harrington IJ, Toutas AA (1981) Replacement of the radial head in the treatment of unstable elbow fractures. Injury 12:405-412

CHAPTER 14

The Swanson Radial Head Prosthesis

B. MARTINELLI

In fractures where osteosynthesis was not feasible, prosthetic replacement for the radial head has been resorted to, using Silastic implants (Fig. 1) [1, 2]. Prosthetic replacement is the intervention of choice to avoid the possible complications of resection: e.g. loss of radio-humeral contact, elbow instability, worsening of cubitus valgus (the radial head [3] is, in fact, a secondary stabilizer in opposing valgus stress and it plays a primary role whenever there is a simultaneous impairment of the medial collateral ligament), radial shortening, distal radio-ulnar subdislocation (the interosseous membrane and the triangular fibrocartilage are involved) [4-6]; ossification starting from the resection surface, reduction of elbow movement width, reduction in supinatory excursion, wrist pain, and delayed functional recovery.

Ten to 30 years [7] after surgery, we had the opportunity to carry out follow-up examinations on 60 patients (between 25 and 75 years of age, with a 2 to 1 prevalence of female patients), 50 cases with isolated fractures and 10 with fractures associated with elbow dislocation, and this is what we observed:
- the clinical results are more than satisfactory, with total recovery of the elbow function, and they remain unchanged over time;
- the best clinical results are obtained in recent, isolated fractures;
- clinical results are less satisfactory in the presence of associated lesions (elbow dislocation), thus requiring a delay of movement recovery;
- follow-up radiographic patterns overlap those of the immediate post-operative period until 4 years after surgery on average;

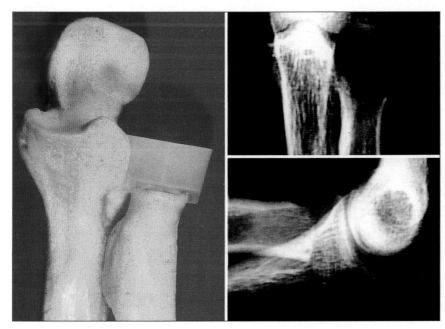

Fig. 1. A Silastic prosthesis on a model and *in vivo*

Fig. 2. Radiographic patterns of the regressive changes that are likely to affect a prosthetic implant: reduction in height, fissuring, detachment from the stem, stem mobilization, fragmentation

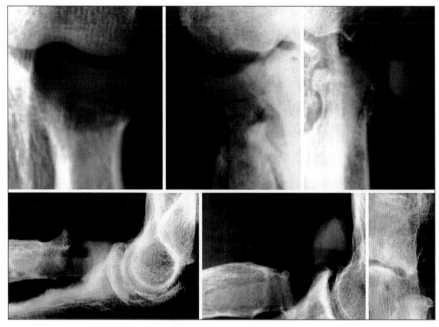

– after 4 years, the prosthesis only shows its limited duration in time at radiography, which shows a reduction in height, fissuring in the prosthetic head, detachment from the stem, and a complete or partial fragmentation of the prosthesis.

In order to explain the observations made in our case study, we focused our attention on the biomechanics of the radial head and the properties of the prosthesis material, in search for any factors explaining the deterioration and reactions induced by the implant.

The maximum force (compression) on the radial head was demonstrated [8] to occur in the extension position, while it decreases (to turn into traction force) as the elbow flexion increases; the extent of the force varies according to the force exerted by the biceps and depending on the forearm position (maximum in pronation and minimal in supination).

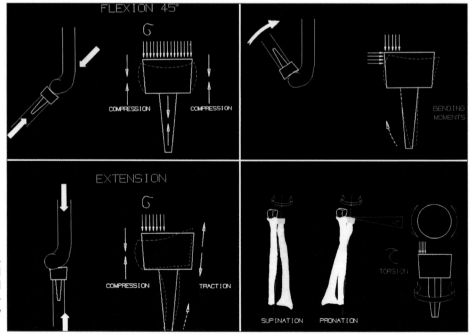

Fig. 3. Compression, traction, flexion, and torsion forces exerted on the prosthetic implant during the elbow joint movements

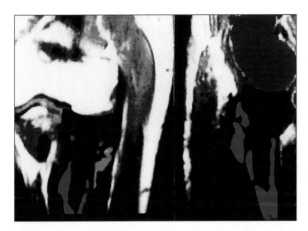

Fig. 4. NMR highlighting the bone-prosthesis interface tissue

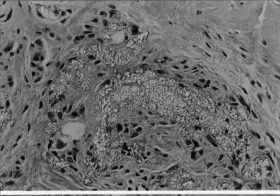

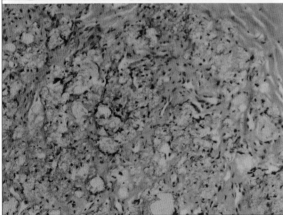

Fig. 5. Infiltration of silicon particles in the intra- and periarticular tissues surrounded by foreign-body giant cells; there are no signs of infection

In everyday activity, the radial head undergoes a series of stresses with compression, shear, and torsion forces which obviously involve the prosthetic implant. This always remains in a lifted position and, therefore, is forced to work under pre-compression. Owing to the flexibility of its material,

the implant is more subjected to the traction, shear, and torsion forces. The prosthesis is made of a silicon rubber, which is liable to change in composition over time due to the attack by blood fluids, with the tendency of silicon to harden and lead, in turn, to a rupture-load reduction, as well as to a reduction in the resistance to fatigue, until it disaggregates with the release of particles and fragments.

Thanks to the Silastic texture, the implant, once placed, can maintain a certain degree of mobility leading to the formation of a bone-prosthesis interface tissue; moreover, mobility induces a wearing process of the prosthesis with the release of silicon particles [9, 10] which give rise to foreign-body reactions in the interface tissue, the synovial membrane, and the capsular wall.

Considering the statements made about biomechanics and the characteristics of the implant material, the mobilization of the Silastic implant for the radial head is to be regarded as an unavoidable and growing consequence, although it appears after some years (at least 4, according to our study).

In conclusion, in the light of our experience with 60 patients treated with Silastic prostheses for the radial head, we may state that:

- none of the disorders that may be correlated to simple resection were ever complained about;
- satisfactory clinical results were always obtained, with excellent and good evaluations by the Mayo Clinic Functional Score;
- only two patients had to be re-entered to remove the multifragmented prostheses which caused occasional articular blocks;
- the foreign-body tissue reactions caused by the degradation of the material never had any clinical repercussions due to the total absence of intolerance to Silastic and the maintenance of articular functionality, even after implant degradation.

This notwithstanding, if we are convinced, as we are, that prosthetic replacement of the radial head is to be preferred to simple resection, one should also recognize that the material of the prosthesis should be selected among other, less wearable components, which are to be resistant enough not to trigger off all the above-mentioned processes: today, despite the more than satisfactory results obtained, the use of a Silastic prosthesis is no longer recommendable, as there are other available materials providing resistance to biomechanical stress and not inducing foreign-body reactions, with osteoinductive and osteoconductive properties which are a prerequisite for implant stability.

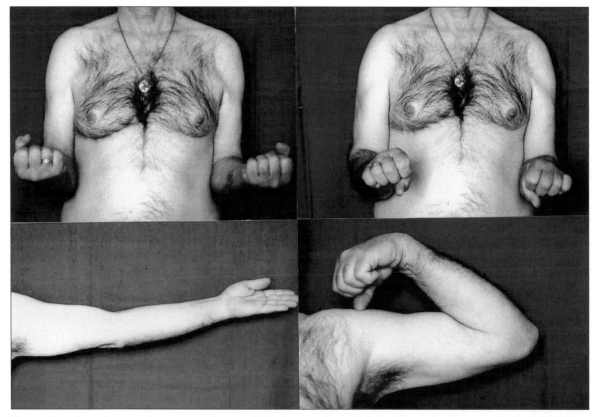

Fig. 6. Elbow joint functionality 30 years after radial head replacement with a Silastic prosthesis

References

1. Swanson AB, Jaeger SH, La Rochelle D (1981) Comminuted fractures of the radial head. J Bone Joint Surg Am 63:1039-1049
2. Morrey BF, Askew L, Chao Y (1981) Silastic prosthetic replacement for the radial head. J Bone Joint Surg Am 63:454-458
3. Morrey BF (1997) Complex instability of the elbow. J Bone Joint Surg Am 79:460-469
4. Taylor TKF, O'Connor BT (1964) The effect upon the inferior radio-ulnar joint excision of the head of the radius in adults. J Bone Joint Surg 46:83-88
5. Hotchkiss RN, An KN, Sowa DT (1989) An anatomic and mechanical study of the interosseous membrane of the forearm: pathomechanics of proximal migration of the radius. J Hand Surg Am 14:256-261
6. Rabinowitz RS, Light TR, Havey RM (1994) The role of interosseous membrane and triangular fibrocartilage complex in forearm stability. J Hand Surg Am 19:385-393
7. Martinelli B (1975) Fractures of the radial head treated by substitution with silastic prosthesis. Bull Hosp Joint Dis 36:61-65
8. Morrey BF, An KN, Stormont TJ (1988) Force transmission through the radial head. J Bone Joint Surg Am 70:250-256
9. Gordon M, Bullough PG (1982) Synovial and osseous inflammation in failed silicone-rubber prosthesis. J Bone Joint Surg Am 64:574-580
10. Worsing RA, Engber WD, Lange TA (1982) Reactive synovitis from particulate silastic. J Bone Joint Surg Am 64:581-585

CHAPTER 15

Bipolar Radial Head Prosthesis

A. CELLI

Introduction

Bipolar implant is one type of radial head prosthesis available for the treatment of comminuted fractures of the radial head associated with joint instability.

However, the anatomical variability of the radial head makes it difficult to recover perfect skeletal anatomy using an implant, even with the modular components now available.

Recent studies [1-4] have attempted to define the main parameters of the proximal radius anatomy in order to recover joint congruity and conformity with the prosthesis. In particular, the diameter and shape of the articular surfaces, the length of the neck and the neck-shaft angle have been measured [1].

Similarly, the anatomical characteristics and the relationship of the radial head with the lesser sigmoid cavity and the capitellum have been considered [1].

The need to replace the radial head with a prosthesis is based on the biomechanical role that it plays in the elbow, in stabilizing the joint on both an axial and a frontal plane, and in transmitting force from the hand to the shoulder, thus contributing to the longitudinal stability of the forearm.

Sixty percent of the forces that cross the elbow are transmitted through the radial head, during the simple movement of flexion-extension and these reach approximately three times body weight [5, 6].

The resection of the radial head for the treatments of acute comminutive fracture or of post-traumatic elbow stiffness, modifies the elbow biomechanics, thus causing an overload on the medial collateral ligament and on the medial portion of the ulno-humeral joint and in particular on the coronoid process that can reach the values of nine times body weight [5, 7].

The interpretation of this medial overload (ligamentous and skeletal) of the elbow joint, can be understood if one considers the important function played by the radial head in stabilizing the elbow in valgus stress, thus assisting the function of the medial collateral ligament [6]. Its absence entails an increase in the strain on the medial collateral ligament with possible precocious osteoarthritic evolution of the ulno-humeral joint [8, 9].

These considerations demonstrate that when reconstruction is not possible the replacement of the radial head becomes essential for recovering osteoarticular stability, and for avoiding precocious osteoarthritic evolution in the ulno-humeral joint [5, 10, 11].

In the designing of the different models of radial head prosthesis, authors have attempted to resolve the anatomical variability with a range of solutions, devising prosthetic implants with great modularity of both the stem and the radial cup, and in some models it is also possible to modify the height of the neck and to improve the adaptation of the prosthesis head to the articular surface using a joint between the stem and the cup that enables varying degrees of freedom [4].

However, all the Authors agree on one point; the radial head prostheses must be made of metal to withstand strain during the compression and rotation it is subject to, and this is not possible with silastic prostheses [10, 12-14].

Metal prostheses are also able to withstand longitudinal strain in the event of injury to the interosseous membrane, as in the case of Essex-Lopresti injuries [13].

On the basis of these considerations, in the early 1990's, T. Judet designed a bipolar radial head prosthesis (Fig. 1). This kind of prosthesis is characterized by the presence of a floating cup joined to a cemented stem, thus allowing a complete mobility of the cup around the stem of 180° and 35° on each plane (Fig. 2).

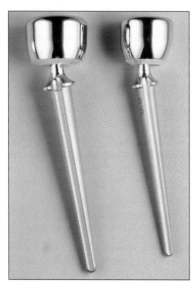

Fig. 1. The bipolar radial head prosthesis: two stems with two different necks (short, long) and two cups

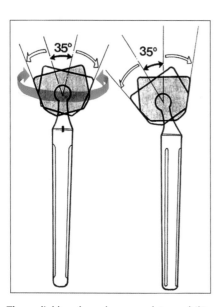

Fig. 2. The radial head cup has complete mobility around the stem of 180° and 35° on each plane

This dual mobility between stem and cup makes it possible to improve the congruity of the implant with both the capitulum and the lesser sigmoid cavity during flexion-extension and pronation-supination [15, 16].

Indication and Contraindication of Prosthetic Implants

Various factors influence the decision of radial head replacement.

In acute pathology, imaging studies make it possible to define the type of radial head fracture, and to decide if the reduction and synthesis of the fracture is possible; further factors to be considered are the other possible associated injuries, such as the ligamentous lesions or the fracture of the coronoid process.

The presence of coronoid fractures, even of type I of the Regan-Morrey classification, is an indication of capsulo-ligamentous damage that must be considered in the surgical choice of the radial head [5, 1-22]. In comminuted fractures of the radial head it is also useful to perform an X-ray of the wrist, in order to exclude distal radioulnar dissociation as a consequence of an Essex-Lopresti injury.

Good results after resection of the radial head in the case of comminuted fractures not associated with ligamentous lesions are reported by numerous authors with long follow-ups [23-30].

However, numerous authors also report complications arising after radial head resection, such as the proximal migration of the radius [26, 28, 30, 31], the reduction in strength, cubitus valgus [26, 31], pain and functional limitation of the wrist [22, 26, 32], ulnar neuropathy [31], and degeneration of the ulno-humeral joint [26, 28, 30, 31].

In a recent study performed in our Institute of 40 patients between 1977 to 2003, treated with resection of the radial head with an average follow-up of 121.4 months (range from 12 to 469 months), the osteoarthritic alterations of the ulno-humeral joint were observed in 30% of cases and the majority were absolutely asymptomatic; a further observation highlighted during this study was the presence in 50% of an ossification on the medial compartment not present at the time of trauma, which only appeared years later.

Several Authors recommend fragment synthesis for radial head fractures, when possible, whereas resection is to be performed when the radial head is irreparable, with an absence of associated ligamentous injuries and preferably in patients over 65 years of age, and prosthesis implants are to be used in irreparable fractures associated to ligamentous injuries above all in young patients [5, 10, 11, 17, 33].

Recently the implant of radial head prosthesis was introduced also in posttraumatic conditions, for inappropriate management of acute radial head fracture or during the treatment of post-traumatic stiff elbow, with simultaneous resection of the radial head in case of malunion.

A further indication is in misidentified Essex-Lopresti injuries in which a limitation in the movement of both elbow and wrist with pain arises after excision of the radial head.

The contraindications of prosthetic implant occur in radial head fractures with skin exposure, in which case it is preferable to perform resection later, once the exposure has healed, in intrarticular infections or for the capitulum humeri erosion.

Bipolar Prosthetic Implants

The bipolar or floating prosthesis (Fig. 1) (Tournier SA, Sanino-Ismier, France) designed by T. Judet in the early 1990's is composed of two components: the stem and the cup. The core of the cup is made of high-density polyethylene coated with chrome cobalt that forms the articular surface of the radial head. The stem is also made of chrome-cobalt and has a neck with a spherical end which articulates in a semiconstrained manner with the cup (Fig. 3).

The prosthetic neck has an angle to the stem of 15°, which reproduces the normal curve of the radius and that is defined as supination curvature

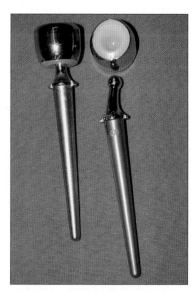

Fig. 3. The bipolar radial head cup is made of high polyethylene coated with chrome cobalt; the stem is also is chromo-cobalt

and the spherical end allows the radial cup free movement in uniplanar rotation through 180° and 35° in any direction.

The 15° of the supination curvature reproduces the normal offset of the radial head and its correct position is essential for avoiding incorrect alignment of the stem with the mobile cup that leads to undesirable tilting of the mobile cup with reduction in valgus stability.

This semiconstrained joint makes it possible to give the maximum contact between the joint surface of the radial head and the capitulum and the lesser sigmoid cavity during movements.

The modularity of this implant is constituted by two sizes of the cup: 19 mm and 22 mm, with an identical height of 14 mm and with two stem diameters of 8 mm with a length of 60 mm and a second of 6.5 mm and length of 55 mm. Recently, two different neck lengths were introduced, one short and one regular for each of the two stem components.

All bipolar prosthesis components are interchangeable to permit a greater adaptability to anatomical variants.

Surgical Technique

Under regional or general anesthesia and with a tourniquet in position, the patient is placed in a supine position.

The skin incision can be lateral if just one surgical time is performed on the lateral compartment of the elbow, whereas in cases in which the ulnohumeral joint or the ligamentous reconstructions of the two compartments can be associated it should be made posteriorly, on the midline.

Both incisions allow, either directly with lateral access or by detaching the lateral skin flap with posterior access, to identify the Kocker interval, as a thin strip of fat between the anconeus and the ulnar extensor muscles (Fig. 4).

Having identified the interval, one proceeds by detaching the two muscles coagulating the vessels inside, attempting to respect the lateral ligamentous complex that lies immediately underneath and presents an interdigitation with the tendon fibers (Fig. 5).

The forearm is placed in full pronation in order to move the posterior interosseous nerve away from the radial neck. The annular ligament, if intact, is exposed together with the lateral collateral ligament in both its anterior and posterior bands (Figs. 6, 7).

If the annular ligament is not damaged, the incision is made, respecting the posterior band of the lateral collateral ligament.

Often the incision of the annular ligament alone does not allow a clear view of the radial neck espe-

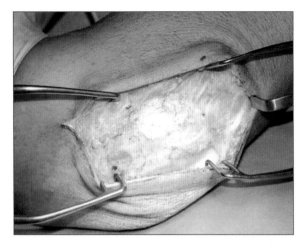

Fig. 4. The kocher is identified as a thin strip of fat between the anconeus and the extensor carpis ulnaris muscles

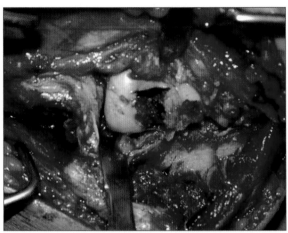

Fig. 7. The radial head is exposed

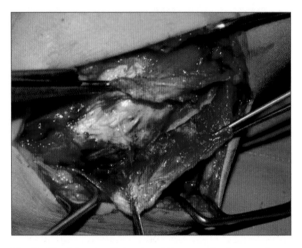

Fig. 5. The lateral collateral and the annular ligaments are exposed under the two muscles

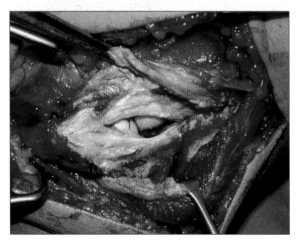

Fig. 6. The incision of the ligament is made respecting the posterior band

cially in chronic cases where the scar tissue or presence of ossification necessitate wider exposure.

In such cases, again keeping the forearm prone, it is possible to detach the two ends of the supinator muscle from the ulna for a few centimeters, in order to obtain better exposure of the radial neck for removing the radial head fragments and more wide debridment.

This makes it possible to expose the lesser sigmoid cavity, which represents an important reference point for deciding the correct degree and level of radius osteotomy.

Using a special instrument (cutting guide), it is possible to view the height of the osteotomy, again checking the correct congruence with the lesser sigmoid cavity and deciding whether to use an implant with a short or regular neck (Fig. 8).

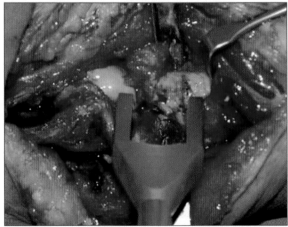

Fig. 8. The height of the osteotomy is decided with the cutting guide

Having performed the cut, one proceeds with the preparation of the intramedular canal with the two brushes depending on the size of the stem.

One prepares the trial stem with the 19-mm or 22-mm cup, depending on the size of the resected radial head or by checking which of these two cups best fits with the lesser sigmoid cavity (Fig. 9).

The evaluations to be made with the trial implant are related to its correct positioning with congruence to the capitulum and with the lesser sigmoid cavity and the height of the radial head implant. This is an important parameter as positioning a prosthesis too high in relation to the articular plane of the ulno-humeral produces an overstaffing effect with reduction in movements, especially in the extreme degrees, with pain and erosion of the capitulum; whereas, on the other hand, the positioning of an implant with too distal resection entails valgus instability.

From our point of view, it becomes essential for the success of the operation to pay great attention to this stage and in addition to use a cutting guide. Regarding the visual assessment of the relationship that exists between the radial cup and the ulno-humeral joint, it is useful to perform a fluoroscopic exam with the trial components in place in order to observe their correct positioning and height.

The correct height can be shown using the fluoroscope by focusing attention on the space between the radio-humeral and radio-ulnar joints, which must have the same level (Fig. 10). This can be shown with an antero-posterior view with the elbow fully extended and supine or with the elbow flexed; however, in this case, the medial margin of the ulno-humeral joint must be considered, as an implant positioned too high produces a decrease in this space.

In the lateral view, the prosthesis cup must be level with the articular surface of the coronoid process.

The subsequent stage entails the cementing of the stem using cement containing antibiotics and a small needle, which is introduced inside the radial canal while it still has a low viscosity in order to allow better distribution.

Keeping the forearm fully pronated, one positions the definitive stem, attempting to obtain parallelism between the thumb and the 15° angle of the radial neck (Fig. 11).

The correct position of the 15° supination curvature is essential for obtaining a correct alignment between the mobile radial head and the radial shaft, in order to obtain good stability of the implant even in postero-lateral rotation.

Once the stem has been positioned, the radial cup must be fitted onto the spherical joint of the neck.

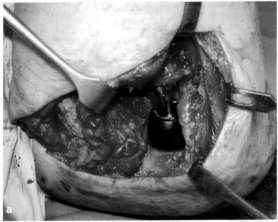
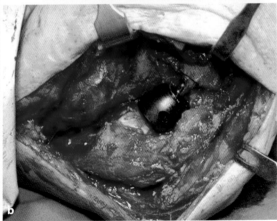

Fig. 9 a, b. The trail implant is seated and the flexion-extension and prono-supination movements are tested

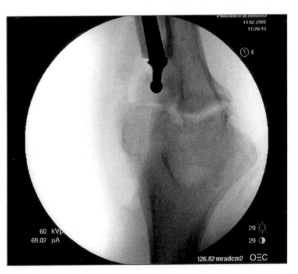

Fig. 10. The trial implant allows all the evaluations also using the fluoroscopy

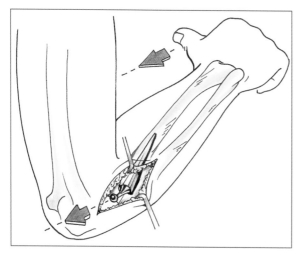

Fig. 11. The definitive stem is cemented keeping the forearm in full pronation and with the 15° angle of neck parallel to the thumb

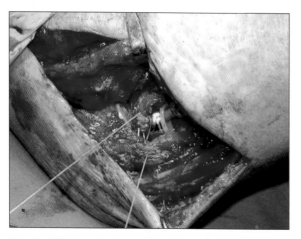

Fig. 12. The lateral collateral ligament and the annular ligament are repaired

The procedure continues with the evaluation of pronation-supination and flexion-extension movements and with a check on valgus stress stability using a fluoroscope if necessary.

The annular ligament is repaired (Fig. 12) and if necessary one performs the retensioning or reconstruction of the lateral collateral ligament. In cases in which damage of the medial compartment is associated (fracture of the coronoid process or damage of the medial collateral ligament), one proceeds with the medial surgical time using the same posterior surgical access by detaching the medial skin, which makes it possible to see the medial compartment.

Postsurgical treatment consists of early motion in flexion-extension and pronation-supination, using an elbow articular brace for the first 3 weeks.

Our Experience

In our experience, we have been using the bipolar implant since 2000 on 45 patients.

We have performed a retrospective study on the prostheses implanted prior to 2004. There were 23 cases, 10 of which were acute injuries; 8 for Mason type 3 fractures, with the association of ulno-humeral dislocation and fracture of the coronoid process, and 2 cases with Mason type 3 fractures of the radial head and lateral collateral ligament damage.

The other 13 implants were used in chronic cases, specifically, 3 for severe valgus instability and the remaining 10 for chronic dislocation and subluxation of the ulno-humeral joint.

The group of implants performed on acute lesions was composed of 3 men and 7 women, with an average age of 61 years (41-71 years); 5 cases involved the right side and 5 the left side.

We checked all patients clinically and radiographically with an average follow-up of 28 months (13-41 months); the data obtained from clinical assessments was analyzed using the Broberg-Morrey Score.

According to this score, we obtained the following results: satisfactory results in 9 cases and in 1 case an unsatisfactory result due to the limited recovery of elbow movements associated with the presence of pain during manual activities.

The average recovery of movement in this group was in flexion-extension of 123.5° and in pronation-supination of 166.4°. Pain was absent in 9 patients and moderate pain was experienced by 1 patient after lengthy manual activity.

With regard to radiographic evaluations, sclerosis of the capitulum humeri was visible in 2 cases and periprosthetic ossifications were present in one case.

Evaluations on stability with the aid of the fluoroscope by means of valgus stress tests and with the manoeuver described by O'Driscoll [39] for the posterior-lateral rotational instability demonstrated complete stability in all patients without opening of the medial articular border or posterior-lateral dislocation of the prosthesis.

The group of implants performed on chronic lesions consisted of 13 patients, 8 males and 5 females, with an average age of 41 (29-58 years old); in 8 cases the right side was involved and in 5 cases the left side.

The group was checked both clinically and radiographically, with an average follow-up of 16 months (3-34 months); the data obtained from clinical assessment was analyzed using the Broberg-Morrey Score.

Using this score we obtained satisfactory results in 11 patients, whereas in the other two there was no recovery of the arc of functional movement, which was associated in one case to pain in the wrist and Broober-Morrey score results were unsatisfactory.

The average recovery of movement in this group was 100.6° in flexion-extension and 157.6° in pronation-supination; pain was absent in 9 patients, and 4 patients experienced moderate pain.

The radiographical evaluations did not show signs of prosthetic loosening; however, in one case periprosthetic ossifications were observed and in another a distal dissociation of the radius of less than 1 mm.

The stability evaluations performed using the fluoroscope were conditioned by limited range of motion in flexion-extension of some of these patients.

We decided to evaluate the correct position of the prosthetic implant by checking the articular level between the radio-humeral and the ulna-humeral and this was at the same level in 10 patients, whereas the remaining three had a slight asymmetry in both articular planes.

Valgus stability was preserved in all patients, whereas one patient presented postero-lateral rotational instability with a lateral dislocation of the cup shown using the fluoroscope.

Discussion

Various reports have been published using bipolar prostheses in the treatment of acute damage.

In 1996 Judet et al. [16] reported their experience using this type of prosthesis on 5 patients with an average follow-up of 49 months, evaluated using the Broberg and Morrey score. They obtained two excellent results and in the remaining three cases they reported good results. The prosthesis was implanted for Mason type III fractures and a single patient had an associated coronoid process fracture.

In 1998, Judet 35 reported his study updated to 22 cases evaluated using the Broober-Morrey score at an average follow-up of 12 months. Twenty-one satisfactory results and 1 unsatisfactory result were obtained.

In 2000, Smets et al. [22] reported their experience using the bipolar prosthesis on 13 cases with a follow-up of 25.2 months and evaluated using the Mayo elbow performance score: 7 proved to be excellent, 2 good, 1 sufficient, and the remaining 3 unsatisfactory. In one of these cases, the prosthesis had to be removed. The cause of the unsatisfactory results in the 3 cases was pain with limited range of motion.

In 2000, Popovic [17] reported the use of bipolar prostheses in acute pathology on 11 patients with Mason type 3 fractures of the radial head associat-

ed with elbow dislocation, the data were analyzed using the Booberg-Morrey score, obtaining satisfactory results in 8 patients; the remaining 3 patients presented an unsatisfactory result due to the presence of limited range of motion and pain during daily living activities.

In 2002, Holmenschlager et al. [36] published their experience in acute cases using this type of prosthesis on 16 patients, evaluated at an average follow-up of 18 months using the Booberg-Morrey score: 14 patients obtained a satisfactory result and two an unsatisfactory one; these were patients with associated radius or coronoid process fractures.

In 2003, Frosch et al. [37] reported their experience with this type of implant on 10 patients with 11 implants. At an average follow-up of 5 years, 9 patients (10 implants – one patient died due to causes not connected to the elbow injury) were assessed using the Broberg-Morrey score.

Satisfactory results were obtained in 7 patients (8 implants) and the remaining 2 were unsatisfactory.

Fewer studies are available in literature regarding bipolar radial head implants used to treat chronic posttraumatic conditions.

In 1996, Charnley et al. [38] described a case report on the use of a bipolar prosthesis in a posttraumatic ankylosis with a follow-up of 3 years and an excellent result regarding movement recovery and no complication on the prosthesis.

In 1996, Judet [16] published his results on the use of the bipolar prosthesis in 7 cases implanted during treatment of the trauma outcome, checked at an average follow-up of 43 months using the Broberg-Morrey score, which obtained 5 satisfactory and 2 unsatisfactory results, the latter connected to nonrecovery of movement.

Once again in 1998, Judet [35] reported the use of the bipolar prosthesis on 30 patients checked at an average follow-up of 12 months using the Broberg-Morrey score: 24 obtained satisfactory results, the remaining 6 unsatisfactory results.

In 2004, Van Riet et al. [39] published a case report on a bipolar prosthesis implants approximately 16 months after radial head resection that developed an erosion of the capitulum with a reduction in range of motion and pain, which, when evaluated with the Mayo elbow performance score, gave an unsatisfactory result.

We intended to evaluate the various results obtained in literature and in our experience in order to show the potential success percentages for this type of prosthetic implant in both acute pathology and in the treatment of posttraumatic conditions. Of a total of 84 Judet bipolar prostheses, implanted by the various authors as reported in literature on acute injury pathology, satisfactory results were obtained with an average of 85%, with an average follow-up of 34.2 months.

In the treatment of post-traumatic conditions, the bipolar prosthesis was used in 50 cases and satisfactory results were obtained in an average of 78% cases, with an average follow-up of 28.3 months.

We believe that the majority of complications arise not from an incorrect design of the prosthesis, which the various biomechanical studies also show to be adequate and comparable to other non-bipolar models [1, 11, 40] but rather due to the implant surgical technique [40].

In general, radial head prostheses are not simple to implant. If properly positioned in length and in the supination curvature of 15°, the Judet's mobile cup prostheses make it possible to obtain excellent results in a high percentage of cases in both acute and posttraumatic patients with a relatively long follow-up (Fig. 13).

The most frequent complications that influenced results in most studies were reduction in range of motion, pain, and the potential persistence of valgus and of postero-lateral rotatory instability.

We believe that many such complications can be reduced with the correct positioning of the implant: prostheses positioned too high exert compression on the capitulum with a limitation of the extreme degrees of the flexion-extension movement, erosion of the capitulum, and pain; on the other hand, prostheses positioned too low do not provide a sufficient

barrier against instability. One advantage that we observed in our study of the use of this type of implant in chronic pathology lies in the capacity to allow pronation-supination movement even when the cup is blocked and this is shown by the analysis of the mean values of recovery of pronation-supination between chronic and acute pathology data.

Conclusions

When properly positioned, the bipolar radial head implants allow good recovery of the pronation-supination and flexion-extension movements.

The mobile cup's ability to adapt to the surface of both the capitulum and the lesser sigmoid cavity is a considerable advantage in chronic patients where these relationships are altered.

We must consider that no prosthetic implant currently on the market has the ability to recover the normal anatomical variability of the radial head; however, they do make it possible to reduce the stress on the ulno-humeral joint and to contribute to the stability of the elbow, thus assisting the action of the ligaments and the coronoid process [1-4, 41].

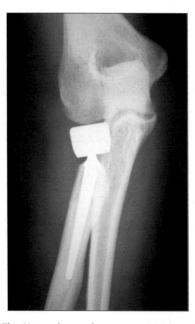

Fig. 13. The X-ray shows the correct position of the implant with the articular space between the capitellum and the radial head cup and the correct position from the ulno-humeral joint

References

1. Van Riet RP, Van Glabbeek F, Neale PG et al (2004) Anatomical considerations of the radius. Clin Anat 17:564-569
2. Johnson JA, Beingessner DM, Gordon KD et al (2005) Kinematics and stability of the fractured and implant-reconstructed radial head. J Shoulder Elbow Surg 14[Suppl S]: 195S-201S
3. Van Riet RP, Glabbeek F, Baumfeld JA et al (2004) The effect of the orientation of the noncircular radial head on elbow kinematics. Clin Biomech 19:595-599
4. King GJW, Zanzour ZDS, Patterson SD, Johnson JA (2001) An anthropometric study of the radial head: implications in the design of a prosthesis. J Arthroplasty 16:112-116
5. King GJW (2004) Management of comminuted radial head fractures with replacement arthroplasty. Hand Clinics 20:429-441
6. Morrey BF, An KN (2005) Stability of the elbow: osseous constraints. J Shoulder Elbow Surg 14[Suppl S]:174S-178S
7. Amis AA, Miller JH, Dowson D, Wright V (1981) Biomechanical aspects of the elbow: joint forces related to prosthesis design. Eng Med 10:65-68
8. Jensen SL, Olsen BS, Sojbjerg JO (1999) Elbow joint kinematics after excision of the radial head. J Shoulder Elbow Surg 8:238-241
9. King GJW, Beingessner DM, Gordon KD et al (2002) The influence of radial head excision and replacement on the kinematics and laxity of the elbow with and without ligamentous injury. American Shoulder and Elbow Surgeons 19th Annual Meeting. Pebble Beach, California, Oct 30-Nov 2

10. King GJK, Zanzour ZDS, Rath DA et al (1999) Metallic radial head arthroplasty improves valgus stability of the elbow. Clin Orthop 368:114-125

11. Pomianowski S, Morrey BF, Neale PG et al (2001) Contribution of monoblock and bipolar radial head prostheses to valgus stability of the elbow. J Bone Joint Surg Am 83:1829-1834

12. Hotchkiss RN, Weiland AJ (1987) Valgus stability of the elbow. J Orthop Res 5:372-377

13. Sellman DC, Seitz WH Jr, Postak PD, Greenwald AS (1995) Reconstructive strategies for radioulnar dissociation: a biomechanical study. J Orthop Trauma 9:516-522

14. Pribyl CR, Kester MA, Cook SD et al (1986) The effect of the radial head excision and prosthetic radial head replacement on resisting valgus stress at the elbow. Orthopedics 9:723-726

15. Judet T, Massin P, Bayeh PJ (1994) Radial head prosthesis with mobile cup: preliminary results in recent and secondary elbow traumatology. Revue de Chirurgie Orthopédique 80:123-130

16. Judet T, Garreau de Loubresse C, Piriou P, Charnley GA (1996) A floating prosthesis for radial-head fractures. J Bone Joint Surg Br 78:244-249

17. Popovic N, Gillet P, Rodriguez A, Lemaire R (2000) Fracture of the radial head with associated elbow dislocation: results of treatment using a floating radial head prosthesis. J Orthop Trauma 14:171-177

18. Harrington IJ, Sekyi-Otu A, Barrington TW et al (2001) The functional outcome with metallic radial head implants in the treatment of unstable elbow fractures: a long-term review. J Trauma 50:46-52

19. Harrington IJ, Tountas AA (1981) Replacement of the radial head in the treatment of unstable elbow fractures. Injury 12:405-412

20. Knight DJ, Rymaszewski LA, Amis AA, Miller JH (1993) Primary replacement of the fractured radial head with a metal prosthesis. J Bone Joint Surg Br 5:572-576

21. Moro JK, Werier J, MacDermid JC et al (2001) Arthroplasty with a metal radial head for unreconstructable fractures of the radial head. J Bone Joint Surg Am 3:1201-1211

22. Smets S, Govaers K, Jansen N et al (2000) The floating radial head prosthesis for comminuted radial head fractures: a multicentric study. Acta Orthop Belg 66:353-358

23. Coleman DA, Blair WF, Shurr D (1987) Resection of the radial head for fracture of the radial head. Long-term follow-up of seventeen cases. J Bone Joint Surg Am 9:385-392

24. Hergenroeder PT, Gelberman R (1982) Distal radioulnar joint subluxation secondary to excision of the radial head. Orthopedics 3:649-650

25. King B (1939) Resection of the radial head and neck: an end-result study of thirteen cases. J Bone Joint Surg Br 1:839-857

26. Mikic ZD, Vukadinovic SM (1983) Late results in fractures of the radial head treated by excision. Clin Orthop 181:220-228

27. Broberg MA, Morrey BF (1986) Results of delayed excision of the radial head after fracture. J Bone Joint Surg Am 8:669-674

28. Janssen RP, Vegter J (1998) Resection of the radial head after Mason type-III fractures of the elbow: follow-up at 16 to 30 years. J Bone Joint Surg Br 80:231-233

29. Leppilahti J, Jalovaara P (2000) Early excision of the radial head for fracture. Int Orthop 24:160-162

30. Ikeda M, Oka Y (2000) Function after early radial head resection for fracture: a retrospective evaluation of 15 patients followed for 3-18 years. Acta Orthop Scand 71:191-194

31. Swanson AB, Jaeger SH, La Rochelle D (1981) Comminuted fractures of the radial head. The role of silicone-implant replacement arthroplasty. J Bone Joint Surg Am 3:1039-1049

32. Stephen IB (1981) Excision of the radial head for closed fracture. Acta Orthop Scand 2: 409-412

33. Rymaszewski LA, Sharma S (2002) Radial head replacement. Curr Orthopaedics 16:331-340

34. O'Driscoll SW, Bell DF, Morrey BF (1991) Postero-lateral rotatory instability of the elbow. J Bone Joint Surg Am 73:440-446

35. Judet T, Piriou P, Garreau de Loubrese C (2001) Prothese de tete radiale a cupule flottante. In: Allieu Y, Masmejean E (eds) Cahiers d'enseignement de la SOFCOT, Protheses du coude. Elsevier, pp 257-263

36. Holmenschlager F, Halm JP, Winckler S (2002) Fresh fractures of the radial head: results with the judet prosthesis. Rev Chir Orthop Reparatrice 88:387-397

37. Frosh KH, Knopp W, Dresing K et al (2003) A bipolar radial head prosthesis after comminuted radial head fractures: indications, treatment and outcome after 5 years. Unfallchirurg 106:367-373

38. Charnley G, Judet T, De Loubresse C et al (1996) Case report: articulated radial head replacement and elbow release for post head-injury heterotopic ossification. J Orthop Trauma 10:68-71

39. Van Riet RP, Van Glabbeek F, Verborgt O, Gielen J (2004) Capitellar erosion by a metal radial head prosthesis. A case report. J Bone Joint Surg Am 86:1061-1064

40. Judet T, Morrey BF, Pomianowski S et al (2002) The importance of rotational seating of radial head prostheses in achieving valgus stability of the elbow. J Bone Joint Surg Am 84:2102

41. Van Glabbeek F, Van Riet RP, Baumfeld JA et al (2005) The kinematic importance of radial neck length in radial head replacement. Med Eng Physics 27:336-342

CHAPTER 16

Evolve™ Modular Metallic Radial Head Arthroplasty

G.J.W. KING

Introduction

Radial head fractures are the most common fracture of the elbow [1]. Undisplaced fractures or small (< 33% of radial head) minimally displaced fractures (< 2 mm) can be treated with early motion with an excellent outcome in the majority of patients [2, 3]. Small displaced fractures which cause painful crepitus or limited motion are managed with fragment excision if they are too small or osteopenic to be treated with open reduction and internal fixation (ORIF) [4-6]. Larger displaced fractures are typically managed with ORIF with good outcomes in most patients [7-11]. However, comminuted fractures that have three or more parts have faired poorly with ORIF [10]. These comminuted radial head fractures are generally treated with radial head excision, with or without radial head replacement. In the setting of an associated injury to the medial collateral, lateral collateral, or interosseous ligaments, radial head excision is contraindicated due to its important role as a valgus, varus and axial stabilizer [12-14]. In patients with a concomitant elbow dislocation, radial head excision should be avoided due to associated disruption of the medial and lateral collateral ligaments of the elbow [15]. In the absence of an elbow or distal radioulnar joint dislocation these associated ligament injuries are often difficult to diagnose on clinical examination in patients with pain from a radial head fracture. However, these soft tissue injuries are present in the vast majority of patients with a comminuted radial head fracture, suggesting that radial head replacement should be considered in most patients with an acute unreconstructable fracture [16].

Radial head arthroplasty may also be useful for post-traumatic reconstruction such as radial head malunions, nonunions, and rheumatoid arthritis. They may also be considered for the management of late axial forearm instability from Essex-Lopresti injuries, valgus instability from medial collateral ligament insufficiency, and varus or posterolateral rotatory instability from lateral collateral ligament insufficiency. The success of radial head implantation for these chronic conditions has received little attention to date, with most studies focussing on the acute treatment of radial head fractures.

Silicone radial head implants offer little in the way of axial or valgus stability to the elbow relative to less-compliant metallic implants [17-19]. Silicone implants have been complicated by a high incidence of wear and fragmentation and, in some incidences, led to silicone synovitis and generalized joint damage [20-24]. Clinical experience with an uncemented monoblock metallic radial head implant has been favourable in the setting of complex instability of the elbow, in our experience and that of others [25-32]. Until recently, commercially available metallic implants have not been properly sized and have only been available as a monoblock design [33]. These have made implantation difficult and implant fit often suboptimal.

A modular metallic radial head implant (Evolve™, Wright Medical Technology, Arlington TN) has been developed based on a series of anthropometric measurements in cadaveric proximal radii and from contralateral radiographs of patients who had undergone radial head replacement arthroplasty [34]. Early clinical experience with this implant has been favourable.

Rationale for Metallic Radial Head Replacements

In a study comparing the valgus stability afforded by four different radial head implants, King et al. [19] reported that silicone radial head implants did not significantly increase the stability of the medial collateral ligament-deficient elbow. All three metallic radial head implants studied afforded improved stability, similar to the native radial head. Similarly in a study by Sellman et al. [17], the Authors demonstrated that silicone radial head implants did not improve the axial stability of the interosseous ligament-deficient forearm. Metallic radial head implants restored stability similar to the native radial head. Reconstruction of the interosseous ligament further increased stability. These in vitro biomechanical studies provide a rationale for metallic radial head replacement of an unreconstructable comminuted radial head fracture in the setting of a concomitant interosseous or medial collateral ligament injury.

Beingessner et al. [35] reported a subtle but significant alteration in elbow kinematics and stability following radial head excision in cadaveric elbows with intact ligaments. In addition to increasing the varus-valgus laxity of the elbows, the articulation was noted to track slightly more valgus when subjected to simulated active flexion. These subtle but significant alterations in kinematics and stability following radial head excision were corrected by a modular metallic radial head arthroplasty. These biomechanical data suggest that metallic radial head arthroplasty should be considered in all patients following radial head excision in patients with unreconstructable fractures regardless of the status of the collateral ligaments [1, 36]. Randomised trials are needed to determine whether the clinical outcome of metallic radial head arthroplasty is superior to radial head excision in the setting of intact collateral ligaments.

The availability of silicone implants in the 1970's resulted in the widespread use of silicone radial head arthroplasty [37]. A number of authors have reported the results of silicone radial head replacements. While the early clinical reports were favourable, implant fracture and persistent joint instability have been commonly described in more recent studies [20-23, 38]. Silicone synovitis has also been reported due to particulate debris [24]. As a consequence of problems with silicone devices, metallic implants have become more popular. Although the clinical reports of experience with metallic radial head arthroplasty are limited, they are generally encouraging. Harrington and Tountas [27] reported their preliminary experience with a monoblock titanium radial head implant. A subsequent medium-term follow-up study from this centre demonstrated the durability of this metallic implant at an average of 12 years [26]. Our experience with this uncemented spacer concept has also been encouraging and prompted the development of the current implant [30].

Design Rationale of the Evolve™ Modular Radial Head Arthroplasty

The optimal design features of a radial head implant system are unknown. Our clinical experience with early generations of metallic radial head replacements parallels that of Beredjiklian et al. [39], who studied the anatomic dimensions of the proximal radius and compared them to those of a commercially available titanium implant system. The available implants overestimated the medullary diameter of the radial neck and underestimated the thickness of the radial head, making it difficult to restore normal anatomy. We studied the anthropometric features of the proximal radius using a highly accurate measurement system, a coordinate measurement machine [34]. The native radial head was found to have a somewhat elliptical shape, and the articular dish of the radial head was variably offset from the radial neck. The medullary diameters of the radial neck and the diameter of the radial head were also measured from the radiographs of patients who had had a radial head arthroplasty. There was no correlation of the dimensions of the radial head and neck, suggesting that a modular implant design is needed to optimally size a radial head arthroplasty.

The surgical implantation of a monoblock radial head implant, where the head is fixed to the stem, may be difficult if the elbow is not unstable such as following an elbow dislocation or lateral ligament disruption. Placement of such implants requires subluxation of the proximal radius either laterally or posterolaterally. In the setting of acute fractures it is usually possible to deliver the proximal radius laterally by division of the radial collateral and annular ligaments while preserving the more important lateral ulnar collateral ligament. A homan retractor is carefully placed around the posterior aspect of the radial neck and gently levered against the ulna to facilitate lateral translation of the proximal radius. This allows the insertion of a monoblock or a pre-assembled modular implant in patients with an intact lateral collateral ligament, yet avoids iatrogenic varus or posterolateral rotatory instability of the elbow by maintaining the integrity of the lateral ulnar collateral ligament. In patients with delayed management of acute fractures or for late reconstruction there is often insufficient lateral mobility of the proximal radius to permit a monoblock or an assembled modular metallic implant to clear the capitellum. This necessitates division of the lateral ulnar collateral ligament, resulting in varus and posterolateral rotatory instability of the elbow requiring meticulous ligamentous repair and careful rehabilitation. In this setting a modular implant that allows implantation of the stem first, then the placement of the head over the stem with coupling in situ is advantageous. In situ implant assembly significantly reduces the surgical exposure needed, allowing preservation of the lateral ulnar collateral ligament, thereby simplifying the surgical procedure.

The Evolve™ prosthesis is designed to function as a spacer, hence it does not aim to achieve rigid fixation in the proximal radius. This avoids the use of cement or the need for porous surface treatments on the implant stem. The smooth round stems are highly polished, allowing for some motion of the implant within the radial neck, which allows the contact of the implant articulation with the capitellum and proximal radioulnar joint to be optimised. As previously discussed, the native radial head is not circular, rather it is variably elliptical, making an "off-the-shelf" implant difficult to precisely fit all patients. In addition, the native radial head is variably offset from the medullary canal of the radial neck, suggesting that a rigidly fixed axisymmetric implant may result in abnormal kinematics and contact pressures whilst articulating with the capitellum and proximal ulna [41]. This may lead to premature cartilage wear and secondary pain due arthrosis. A non-rigidly fixed implant such as the Evolve™ allows the articular surface to align with the capitellum and the lesser sigmoid notch as it is guided by the articular shape and the annular ligament rather than the precise motion pathway of the proximal radius. Improved articular alignment should decrease cartilage contact pressures and improve implant survival. An alternative approach to optimize radiocapitellar contact would be to obtain rigid stem fixation and then use a bipolar articulation. While a bipolar device has some

theoretical advantages over a spacer implant, it introduces the potential for polyethylene wear, which may result in implant loosening and the need for revision arthroplasty. Bipolar implants do not provide as much resistance to posterolateral subluxation of the elbow in the setting of incompetent lateral ligaments, which are commonly injured in patients with comminuted radial head fractures [42]. An implant with a rigid head/stem resists posterolateral subluxation because the articulating concave dish captures the capitellum. In contrast, a bipolar implant simply angles through the articulation if exposed to a posterolateral rotatory moment, allowing the radial head to slide off the capitellum if there is residual insufficiency of the lateral collateral ligament.

Design Features of the Evolve™ Modular Radial Head Arthroplasty

The implant is currently available in five different head diameters (20, 22, 24, 26, 28 mm) and three different thicknesses (standard, +2, +4 mm). The stems are available in five diameters (5.5, 6.5, 7.5, 8.5, 9.5 mm) and two thicknesses (standard or +4 mm). Each head can be mated to any stem using a standard morse taper, resulting in 150 potential size combinations (Fig. 1). Implant sizing is based on the extensive anatomical studies outlined above. The three head thicknesses accommodate for the variable articular height of the native head and extension of the

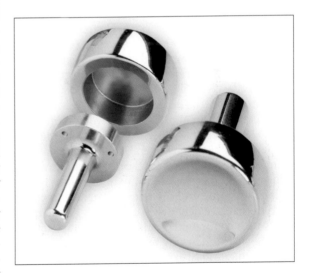

Fig. 1. Evolve™ modular radial head implant. The implant has a separate head and stem that are coupled using a morse taper. Holes in the stem base allow for fluid egress during in situ assembly (Figure reproduced with permission, Wright Medical Technology)

fractures into the proximal neck. The +4 mm stem accounts for further neck loss in acute fractures and is particularly useful in patients undergoing late reconstruction following radial head excision. The stems have drainage holes to allow proper locking of the morse taper in the presence of body fluids. The implant is manufactured in cobalt-chrome to ensure maximal biocompatibility with the articulation against the cartilage of the capitellum.

Surgical Implantation of the Evolve™ Modular Radial Head Arthroplasty

Templates are available to facilitate pre-operative implant selection based on radiographs of the injured and contralateral elbow. Pre-operative intravenous prophylactic antibiotics are administered as for any joint replacement. The patient is placed in the supine position under general or regional anaesthesia. A tourniquet is placed on the upper arm and inflated. A lateral skin incision centred over the lateral epicondyle can be used; however, the author prefers to employ a midline posterior elbow incision to avoid injury to cutaneous nerves and to provide better cosmesis than a lateral incision [43]. A full thickness lateral flap is elevated on the deep fascia. This provides access to the lateral collateral ligament, radial head, capitellum, and coronoid. A medial flap can be elevated to expose the medial collateral ligament and coronoid if needed for the management of more complex injuries. The fascial interval between the anconeus and extensor carpi ulnaris is identified and developed. The extensor carpi ulnaris is elevated slightly anteriorly off the lateral collateral ligament complex such that the radial collateral ligament and annular ligament are incised at the mid-axis of the radial head, staying anterior to lateral ulnar collateral ligament (Fig. 2). The radial collateral ligament and overlying extensor muscles are elevated anteriorly off the lateral epicondyle to expose the anterior half of the radial head. The lateral ulnar collateral ligament is preserved to prevent the development of posterolateral rotatory instability. Avulsion of the lateral collateral ligament and common extensor muscles from the lateral epicondyle is commonly noted in patients with comminuted radial head fractures and is routinely seen following an elbow dislocation, simplifying the surgical exposure of the radial head.

Excision of the fragments of the radial head can be facilitated with the use of an image intensifier and a pituitary ronguer. Copious joint irrigation should be performed to remove all loose intra-articular debris. The capitellum is evaluated for chondral injuries or

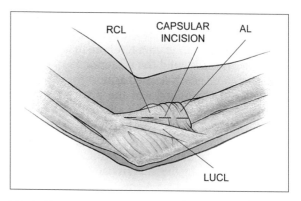

Fig. 2. Ligament incision. The incision in the lateral collateral ligament is performed just anterior to the mid-axis of the radial head staying anterior to the lateral ulnar collateral ligament (*LUCL*). Division of the radial collateral ligament (*RCL*) and annular ligament (*AL*) are usually needed for adequate exposure (Figure reproduced with permission, Wright Medical Technology)

osteochondral fractures. Associated fractures of the coronoid, olecranon, and proximal ulna are managed as indicated. Access to the coronoid is facilitated by radial head excision, such that coronoid fixation should be performed prior to radial head replacement. Valgus and axial stress tests are performed using an image intensifier to evaluate the competency of the medial collateral and interosseous ligaments. At the level of the head-neck junction, or at the level of the neck fracture, a minimal amount of radial neck is resected at a right angle to the medullary canal to make a smooth surface for load transfer to the implant. The excised radial head is reassembled in the provided sizing template to assist in the accurate sizing of the prosthesis and to ensure that all of the fragments have been removed from the elbow. The appropriate diameter and thickness of radial head implant are selected for trial implantation. Overstuffing of the radiocapitellar joint can occur if the implant is too thick, resulting in erosions of the capitellar cartilage with associated stiffness and pain [44, 45]. An implant whose diameter is too large may result in limitation of elbow motion due to impingement in flexion and may also cause abnormal capitellar contact and pain. If the native radial head is in between implant sizes, the implant diameter or thickness should, in general, be downsized, not upsized. The thickness of the selected implant should be verified by comparing it to the distance between the neck cut and the proximal aspect of the lesser sigmoid notch.

The medullary canal of the radial neck is gently rasped using hand reamers until cortical contact is achieved. A trial stem one size smaller than the rasp is inserted for a non-tight press fit. The trial head is inserted onto the trial stem using the insertion tools. The diameter, thickness, and articular tracking of the trial prosthesis are assessed visually and with the aid of an image intensifier. Ulnar variance at the wrist is checked to ensure correct prosthesis thickness. If the tracking of the implant on the capitellum is not optimal, then the stem is downsized to ensure that the congruency of the radial head on the capitellum is maintained throughout elbow flexion and forearm rotation. The need to downsize the stem is most likely when the native radial head has a large offset from the radial neck, making a loose stem necessary for an axisymmetric design.

The trial components are removed and the definitive modular Evolve™ implant is inserted either preassembled or using the in situ assembly tool. In patients with most acute fractures with an intact lateral collateral ligament and in those with a torn lateral collateral ligament (such as with an associated elbow dislocation), insertion is easily achieved after pre-assembly of the head and stem on a back table.

The key to achieving an atraumatic insertion of an assembled implant in the setting of an intact lateral collateral ligament is to divide the radial collateral and annular ligament at the mid-portion of the radial head, and using a homan retractor placed around the posterior radial neck, lever the radius laterally by gently prying against the ulna. Anterior retractors should not be used due to the proximity of the radial nerve. The lateral ulnar collateral ligament, a key stabiliser against varus and posterolateral rotatory stability, is preserved by avoiding dissection posterior to the mid-portion of the radial head [40]. If the mobility of the proximal radius is insufficient to allow insertion of an assembled implant, the stem can be inserted into the proximal radius, followed by placement of the head component into the joint space. The morse taper which connects the head to the stem is firmly compressed in situ using an assembly tool.

Following radial head replacement, the annular ligament is repaired and the radial collateral ligament is sutured to the lateral ulnar collateral ligament, which is still attached to the lateral epicondyle. If the lateral collateral ligament has been detached as a consequence of the original injury, it is carefully repaired to the lateral epicondyle using heavy nonabsorbable sutures through drill holes. The fascial interval between the anconeus and extensor carpi ulnaris should also be repaired to augment lateral stability of the elbow.

Post-operative Management

Following radial head replacement and lateral soft tissue closure, the elbow should be placed through an arc of flexion-extension while carefully evaluating el-

bow stability in pronation, neutral, and supination using an image intensifier. Pronation is generally beneficial if the lateral ligament repair is tenuous, supination if the medial ligaments are deficient, and neutral position if both sides have been damaged, either by the injury or the surgical approach [46, 47]. In patients who have an associated elbow dislocation, repair of the lateral collateral ligament is routinely performed during radial head arthroplasty. Repair of the medial collateral ligament is generally not required to restore sufficient stability to allow early active motion, and healing of the medial collateral ligament can be expected [48, 49]. However, if the elbow subluxes at greater than 40° of extension, both the medial collateral ligament and flexor pronator origin should be repaired to restore stability to allow early active motion [50]. In patients with collateral ligament injuries, the elbow should be initially splinted at 90° of flexion in the optimal position of forearm rotation. If the collateral ligaments are intact, or have been stably repaired, the elbow is splinted in near full extension prior to initiating early active motion.

Patients should commence active flexion and extension exercises within a safe arc of motion one day post-operatively. Depending on the associated injuries and patient compliance, a resting splint with the elbow maintained at 90° or a hinged brace is employed for 3-6 weeks. Active forearm rotation is performed with the elbow at 90° flexion to avoid stressing the medial and/or lateral ligamentous injuries or repairs. A static progressive extension splint is employed at night as ligamentous healing progresses and elbow stability improves, usually by 6 weeks post-operatively. No passive stretching is permitted for 6 weeks post-operatively due to the risk of heterotopic ossification. Progressive strengthening exercises are initiated once any associated fracture or ligament injuries have adequately healed, usually about 8 weeks post-operatively.

Indomethacin (25 mg, three times daily) for 3 weeks should be considered in patients undergoing radial head replacement to decrease post-operative pain and swelling, and potentially the incidence of heterotopic ossification. This medication should be avoided in the elderly and in patients with a history of peptic ulcer disease, known allergy, or other contraindications to anti-inflammatory medications.

Clinical Results of the Evolve™ Modular Radial Head Arthroplasty

Our early clinical experience with the Evolve™ modular radial head system has been favourable; however, long-term results are not yet available (Fig. 3).

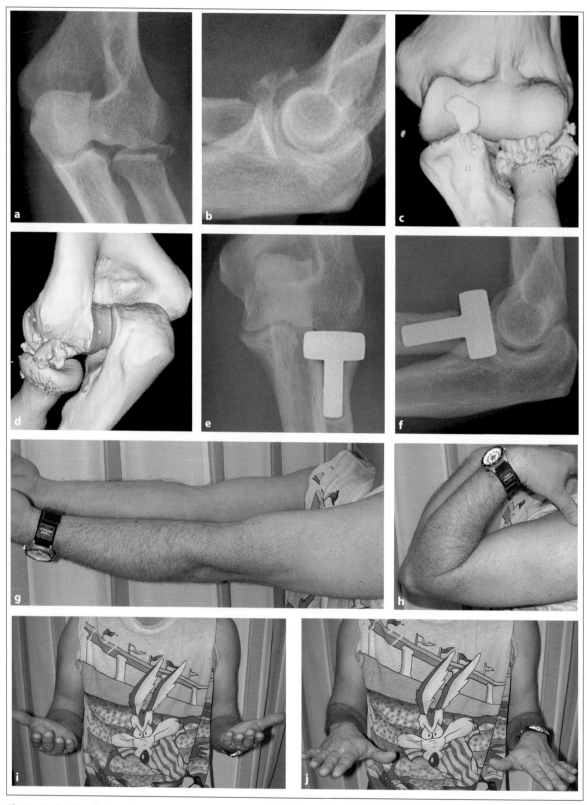

Fig. 3. Evolve™ radial head replacement. (**a, b**) Anteroposterior and lateral radiographs of a 40-year-old male painter who fell 10 feet off a scaffold. (**c, d**) The comminuted radial head fracture, small coronoid fracture, and elbow subluxation are well seen on the CT scan. (**e, f**) Radiographs one year following radial head replacement with a modular radial head implant and a lateral ligament repair. (**g- j**) The patient achieved a painless, stable elbow with an arc of flexion from 10° to 140° and full prosupination

We have recently reported on the outcome of 28 patients with comminuted radial head fractures who were treated with the Evolve™ radial head arthroplasty at our centre [51]. The patients were prospectively followed and independently evaluated postoperatively. Associated injuries included: fractures of the coronoid, olecranon, ulna, or capitellum; soft tissue injuries included elbow dislocations and isolated injuries to the medial collateral or interosseous ligaments. Patient satisfaction with their surgery was 9.7 out of 10. The Mayo Elbow Performance Score was an average of 82. Stability was restored to the elbow and forearm of all patients. There were no implant failures and no mechanical symptoms. Asymptomatic nonprogressive stem lucencies were commonly observed. No implants have been removed to date.

Ring et al. [52] reported their preliminary experience with the Evolve™ radial head arthroplasty in patients with complex elbow instability and associated comminuted radial head fractures. Thirty-two patients were followed an average of 18 months post-operatively. They reported restoration of elbow stability in all but one patient. Two patients had the prosthesis removed, one due to infection and another at the time of an elbow contracture release due to possible overstuffing. They reported no apparent problems with the prosthesis and no pain referable to the implant.

The outcome from these early clinical series has encouraged the continued utilization of the Evolve™ metallic radial head arthroplasty for unreconstructable radial head fractures at our centre. It is relatively simple to use and has proven to be successful in clinical practice.

References

1. King GJ (2005) Fractures of the head of the radius. In: Green DP, Hotchkiss RN, Pederson WC, Wolfe SW (eds), Green's Operative Hand Surgery. Elsevier Churchill Livingstone, Philadelphia, pp 845-887
2. Holdsworth BJ, Clement DA, Rothwell PN (1987) Fractures of the radial head. The benefit of aspiration: a prospective controlled trial. Injury 18:44-47
3. Mason ML (1954) Some observations on fracture of the head of the radius with a review of one hundred cases. Br J Surg 42:123-132
4. Wexner SD, Goodwin C, Parkes JC et al (1985) Treatment of fractures of the radial head by partial excision. Orthop Rev 14:83-86
5. Murray RC (1940) Fractures of the head and neck of the radius. Br J Surg 27:106-118
6. Castberg T, Thing E (1953) Treatment of fractures of the upper end of the radius. Acta Chir Scand 1051:62-69
7. Esser RD, Davis S, Taavao T (1995) Fractures of the radial head treated by internal fixation: Late results in 26 cases. J Orthop Trauma 9:318-323
8. Geel CW, Palmer AK, Ruedi T, Leutenegger AF (1990) Internal fixation of proximal radial head fractures. J Orthop Trauma 4:270-274
9. King GJ, Evans DC, Kellam JF (1991) Open reduction and internal fixation of radial head fractures. J Orthop Trauma 5:21-28
10. Ring D, Quintero J, Jupiter JB (2002) Open reduction and internal fixation of fractures of the radial head. J Bone Joint Surg Am 84:1811-1815
11. Shmueli G, Herold HZ (1981) Compression screwing of displaced fractures of the head of the radius. J Bone Joint Surg Br 63:535-538
12. Roberts PH (1969) Dislocation of the elbow. Br J Surg 56:806-815
13. Adler JB, Shaftan GW (1962) Radial head fractures, is excision necessary? J Trauma 4:115-136
14. Johnston GW (1962) A follow-up of one hundred cases of fracture of the head of the radius with a review of the literature. Ulster Med J 31:51-56
15. Josefsson PO, Johnell O, Wendeberg B (1987) Ligamentous injuries in dislocations of the elbow joint. Clin Orthop Relat Res 221:221-225
16. Davidson PA, Moseley Jr JB, Tullos HS (1993) Radial head fracture. A potentially complex injury. Clin Orthop Relat Res 297:224-230
17. Sellman DC, Seitz Jr WH, Postak PD, Greenwald AS (1995) Reconstructive strategies for radioulnar dissociation: A biomechanical study. J Orthop Trauma 9:516-522
18. Pribyl CR, Kester MA, Cook SD et al (1986) The effect of the radial head excision and prosthetic radial head replacement on resisting valgus stress at the elbow. Orthopedics 9:723-726
19. King GJ, Zarzour ZD, Rath DA et al (1999) Metallic radial head arthroplasty improves valgus stability of the elbow. Clin Orthop Relat Res 368:114-125
20. Gordon M, Bullough PG (1982) Synovial and osseous inflammation in failed silicone-rubber prostheses: a report of six cases. J Bone Joint Surg Am 64:574-580
21. Martinelli B (1985) Silicone-implant replacement arthroplasty in fractures of the radial head. A follow-up report. Bull Hosp Jt Dis Orthop Inst 45:158-161
22. Mayhall WS, Tiley FT, Paluska DJ (1981) Fracture of silastic radial-head prosthesis. Case report. J Bone Joint Surg Am 63:459-460
23. Trepman E, Ewald FC (1991) Early failure of silicone radial head implants in the rheumatoid elbow. A complication of silicone radial head implant arthroplasty. J Arthroplasty 6:59-65
24. Vanderwilde RS, Morrey BF, Melberg MW, Vinh TN (1994) Inflammatory arthritis after failure of silicone rubber replacement of the radial head. J Bone Joint Surg Br 76:78-81
25. Edwards GE, Rostrup O (1960) Radial head prosthesis in the management of radial head fractures. Can J Surg 3:153-155
26. Harrington IJ, Sekyi-Otu A, Barrington TW et al (2001) The functional outcome with metallic radial head implants in the treatment of unstable elbow fractures: A long-term review. J Trauma 50:46-52

27. Harrington IJ, Tountas AA (1981) Replacement of the radial head in the treatment of unstable elbow fractures. Injury 12:405-412

28. Judet T, Garreau DL, Piriou P, Charnley G (1996) A floating prosthesis for radial-head fractures. J Bone Joint Surg Br 78:244-249

29. Knight DJ, Rymaszewski LA, Amis AA, Miller JH (1993) Primary replacement of the fractured radial head with a metal prosthesis. J Bone Joint Surg Br 75:572-576

30. Moro JK, Werier J, MacDermid JC et al (2001) Arthroplasty with a metal radial head for unreconstructible fractures of the radial head. J Bone Joint Surg Am 83:1201-1211

31. Popovic N, Gillet P, Rodriguez A, Lemaire R (2000) Fracture of the radial head with associated elbow dislocation: Results of treatment using a floating radial head prosthesis. J Orthop Trauma 14:171-177

32. Smets S, Govaers K, Jansen N et al (2000) The floating radial head prosthesis for comminuted radial head fractures: a multicentric study. Acta Orthop Belg 66:353-358

33. Gupta GG, Lucas G, Hahn DL (1997) Biomechanical and computer analysis of radial head prostheses. J Shoulder Elbow Surg 6:37-48

34. King GJ, Zarzour ZD, Patterson SD, Johnson JA (2001) An anthropometric study of the radial head: implications in the design of a prosthesis. J Arthroplasty 16:112-116

35. Beingessner DM, Dunning CE, Gordon KD et al (2004) The effect of radial head excision and arthroplasty on elbow kinematics and stability. J Bone Joint Surg Am 86:1730-1739

36. Johnson JA, Beingessner DM, Gordon KD et al (2005) Kinematics and stability of the fractured and implant reconstructed radial head. J Shoulder Elbow Surg 14:S195-S201

37. Swanson AB, Jaeger SH, La Rochelle D (1981) Comminuted fractures of the radial head The role of silicone-implant replacement arthroplasty. J Bone Joint Surg Am 63:1039-1049

38. Carn RM, Medige J, Curtain D, Koenig A (1986) Silicone rubber replacement of the severely fractured radial head. Clin Orthop Relat Res 209:259-269

39. Beredjiklian PK, Nalbantoglu U, Potter HG, Hotchkiss RN (1999) Prosthetic radial head components and proximal radial morphology: a mismatch. J Shoulder Elbow Surg 8:471-475

40. O'Driscoll SW, Morrey BF, Korinek S, An KN (1992) Elbow subluxation and dislocation. A spectrum of instability. Clin Orthop Relat Res 280:186-197

41. Liew VS, Cooper IC, Ferreira LM et al (2003) The effect of metallic radial head arthroplasty on radiocapitellar joint contact area. Clin Biomech 18:115-118

42. Schneeberger A, Sadowski MM, Jacob HAC (2004) Coronoid process and radial head as posterolateral rotatory stabilizers of the elbow. J Bone Joint Surg Am 86:975-982

43. Dowdy PA, Bain GI, King GJ, Patterson SD (1995) The midline posterior elbow incision. An anatomical appraisal. J Bone Joint Surg Br 77:696-699

44. Van Glabbeek F, Van Rift R, Baumfeld J et al (2005) Detrimental effects of overstuffing or understuffing with a radial head replacement in the medial collateral ligament deficient elbow. J Bone Joint Surg Am 86:2629-2635

45. Birkedal JP, Deal DN, Ruch DS (2004) Loss of flexion after radial head replacement. J Shoulder and Elbow Surg 13:208-213

46. Armstrong AD, Dunning CE, Faber KJ et al (2000) Rehabilitation of the medial collateral ligament-deficient elbow: an in vitro biomechanical study. J Hand Surg Am 25:1051-1057

47. Dunning CE, Zarzour ZD, Patterson SD et al (2001) Muscle forces and pronation stabilize the lateral ligament deficient elbow. Clin Orthop Relat Res 388:118-124

48. Pugh DM, Wild LM, Schemitsch EH et al (2004) Standard surgical protocol to treat elbow dislocation with radial head and coronoid fractures. J Bone Joint Surg Am 86:1122-1130

49. McKee MD, Pugh DM, Wild LM et al (2005) Standard surgical protocol to treat elbow dislocations with radial head and coronoid fractures. Surgical technique. J Bone Joint Surg Am 87:22-32

50. Hildebrand KA, Patterson SD, King GJ (1999) Acute elbow dislocations: simple and complex. Orthop Clin North Am 30:63-79

51. Faber KJ, MacDermid JC, King GJW (2004) Modular metal radial head arthroplasty is an effective treatment for comminuted radial head fractures. Ninth Conference of the International Societies for Surgery of the Hand, Budapest Hungary (*unpublished*)

52. Parisien R, Doornberg J, Ring D (2005) Fracture-dislocations of the elbow: Replacement of the fractured radial head with a modular prosthesis. American Shoulder and Elbow Surgeons Annual Meeting, Washington DC (*unpublished*)

CHAPTER 17

Radial Head Prosthetic Replacement with the Avanta Implant

B.F. MORREY

Introduction

The first English reference we can find to prosthetic replacement of the radial head is that of Speed in 1941 [1] describing a Vitallium implant employed in three patients. Cherry [2] discussed limited experience with an acrylic implant a decade later and the use of a silicone radial head implant was popularized by Swanson [3]. The logical reason to use a radial head implant is to restore function. Success may be measured by the effectiveness to restore axial or angular (valgus) stability; by enhanced strength, or ultimately by relief of pain. Morrey et al. [4] have shown the radial head is an important stabilizer of the elbow if the medial collateral ligament is deficient or in the presence of deficient distal radio-ulnar stability. King et al. [5] subsequently demonstrated that such instability can be effectively addressed by a metallic, but not by a Silastic, radial head implant.

Indications

A "complicated" radial head fracture is considered the indication for the use of the prosthesis. This circumstance is present in a number of clinical settings [6, 7]:

1. dislocation of the elbow with radial head fracture (Type IV fracture);
2. concurrent medial collateral ligament disruption;
3. concurrent or residual lateral ulnar collateral ligament dysfunction;
4. Monteggia variant with olecranon and radial head fracture;
5. fracture of the coronoid;
6. with axial radial instability (Essex Lopresti);
7. as a reconstruction option.

Hence, if the elbow dislocates the collateral ligaments are torn, and if the radial head is excised the elbow is grossly unstable. In this setting replacement with a radial head prosthesis will enhance stability and allow early motion (Fig. 1). Increased valgus angulation, probably due to concurrent medial ligament injury [4, 7-9], may also be addressed with use of a prosthetic radial head [3, 10]. Instability of the proximal radius associated with severe fractures or excessive excision [1, 10, 11] may be lessened with use of an implant. With large Type II coronoid fractures considerably enhanced stability is offered by the radial head, hence the prosthesis may provide some element of stability in this clinical setting (Fig. 2). Finally, the implant stabilizes the radius if the head is removed in the presence of interosseous membrane and DRUJ disruption.

Prosthetic Design

The early prostheses were made of Vitallium [1, 11] and acrylic [2], but the Silastic device described by Swanson was certainly the most commonly used in this country [12-14] and abroad [10, 15]. However, the host of complications coupled with the poor mechanical properties of Silastic to withstand axial load has dramatically lessened the use of this

Fig. 1. The radial head adds little stability if the MCL is intact. If the medial collateral ligament is torn, the radial head assumes an important secondary stabilizing role

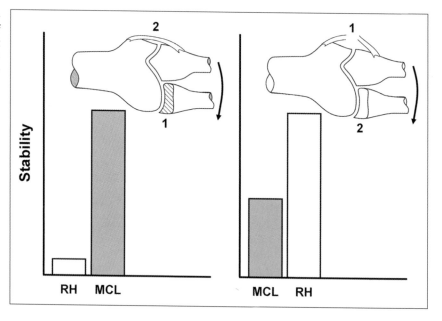

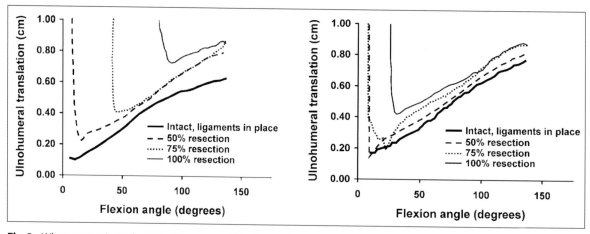

Fig. 2. When approximately 50% of the coronoid is absent, the radial head assumes an important role in elbow stability

material as a prosthetic radial head replacement. Gupta et al. [16] recently assessed the mechanical properties of cobalt-chrome, titanium alloy, alumina ceramic, and ultra-high – molecular-weight polyethylene (UHMPE). Any of the rigid implants were shown to be theoretically superior to the Silastic device, and several are now commercially available (Fig. 3). The effectiveness of metallic implants has been confirmed in our laboratory [17] and by several clinical experiences [18-20].

The articulated bipolar design of Judet et al. [21] is a real advance in design concept (Fig. 4). Yet, concern does exist regarding the extent of the exposure necessary to implant the device due to the length of the stem and the dimension of the radial

head implant sometimes requires excision of normal proximal radius. Because of the increasing recognition of "complex instability" or fracture dislocation and because of the theoretical advantages of radial head replacement in this setting, renewed interest has been generated in prosthetic replacement and hence in improved implant designs. These newer designs feature several size options, flexibility at the articulation, and enhanced instrumentation to allow accurate and reproducible implantation. At the Mayo Clinic, we have developed a replacement that is designed to be inserted with less soft tissue release and provide the flexibility of surgery options necessary to treat the pathology that occurs at this joint (see Fig. 3c).

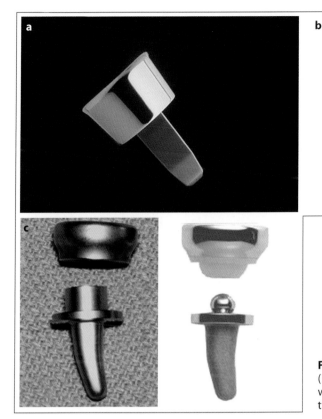

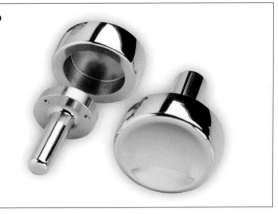

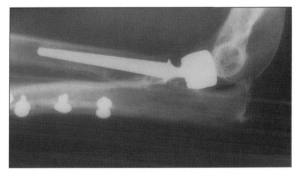

Fig. 3. Metallic implants are now available as monoblock (Wright) (**a**), modular Evolve™ (Wright) (**b**), and modular with rHead Recon™ or without rHead™, a bipolar articulation, (Avanta) (**c**)

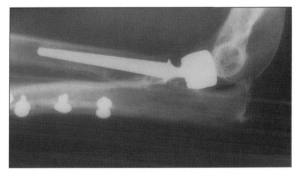

Fig. 4. The articulated "bipolar" device designed by Judet represents a real advance in the concept of radial head replacement (Tornier SA, Saint-Ismier, France)

Technique (rHead™, Avanta)

The procedure to insert the rHead™ is described below. Similar features are applicable to other designs as well.

Exposure

A supine position and capsular exposure through Kocher's interval is employed (Fig. 5). The lateral capsule is entered slightly anteriorly to the collateral ligament and the annular ligament and capsule are reflected anteriorly and posteriorly to expose the radial head. A portion of the lateral collateral ligament and anterior capsule can be reflected from the lateral epicondyle and anterior humerus to facilitate exposure if necessary. Efforts are made not to detach the lateral ulnohumeral ligament but if greater exposure is required, the ligament is reflected from its humeral origin and securely reattached at the completion of the procedure. If the ligament has been disrupted, then the exposure progresses through the site of disruption to expose the radiohumeral joint. The common extensor tendon and anterior capsule are retracted as needed for adequate exposure.

Resection Guide

Congruous prosthetic articulation requires an accurate resection that provides precise implant placement. A resection guide has thus been developed to replicate the anatomic axis of forearm rotation using the capitellum and ulnar styloid as landmarks. Since accurate restoration of length is of critical importance, the cutting guide is adjustable proximally or distally for the desired amount of radial head resec-

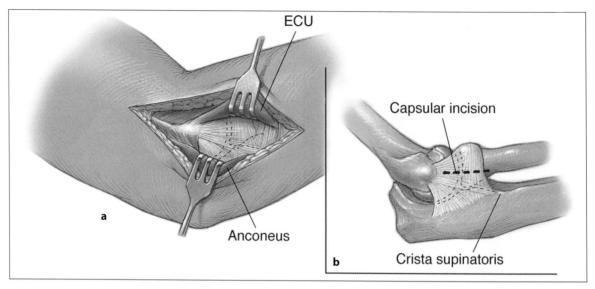

Fig. 5. The patient is placed in a supine position with the arm brought across the chest. (**a**) A Kocher incision is made and the interval between the anconeus and extensor carpi ulnaris is developed. (**b**) If the collateral ligament is intact, reflection from the humeral attachment to a variable extent may be necessary for adequate exposure and implant insertion

tion. This is a very sensitive variable as variation of as little as 2 mm can alter elbow kinematics [22, 23].

still compatible with implant insertion and length restoration options for the design being used.

Resecting the Radial Head

During resection forearm rotation should be assessed to insure that the cut is perpendicular to the axis of rotation (Fig. 6). The distal extent of resection is the minimal amount that is consistent with the restoration of function as dictated by the fracture line or previous radial head resection but

Intramedullary Preparation

Varus stress and rotation of the forearm allow exposure of the medullary canal especially if the elbow is unstable. If this does not allow adequate exposure of the proximal radius, careful reflection of the origin of the collateral ligament from the lateral epicondyle may be necessary to permit adequate

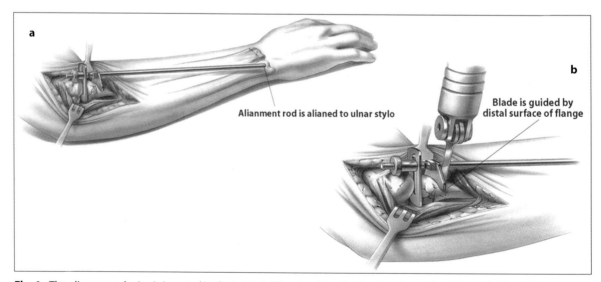

Fig. 6. The alignment device is inserted in the joint. (**a**) The distal portion is placed over the ulnar styloid, and the proximal portion rests against the capitellum. (**b**) An oscillating saw is used to resect the neck perpendicular to the axis of rotation

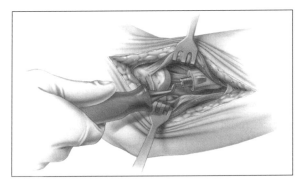

Fig. 7. Insertion of the broach down the canal is facilitated by the curvature, which matches the stem of the implant

access to the medullary canal. The canal is entered with a starter awl using a twisting motion, followed by the curved broach (Fig. 7) until the largest sized stem is accommodated.

Trial Reduction

The appropriate sized trial stem is inserted with a rotating motion to direct the stem down the canal (Fig. 8). The trial head is then applied. Tracking, both in flexion and extension and forearm rotation, should be carefully assessed. If the collateral ligament has been released its function is simulated during the trial reduction. Malalignment of the radial osteotomy cut will cause improper seating of the implant and hence abnormal tracking during flexion-extension and/or forearm pronation and supination.

Implanting the Final Components

Once proper size, alignment, and positioning of the implant have been determined, the prosthetic stem is inserted with a rotational motion down the

medullary canal of the radius and tapped in place with the impactor. Bone cement (PMMA) may occasionally be used if secure press-fit fixation is not attainable but I try to avoid the use of PMMA in virtually all settings. The modular head is next placed over the taper using longitudinal distraction and/or varus stress to separate the radiocapitellar interface sufficiently to permit the radial head to be inserted. The radial head implant is secured using the impactor. Alignment is again assessed. Alternatively the head may be coupled with the stem prior to insertion if the trial insertion suggests that this is the best strategy for this particular patient. Since we use the bipolar articulation for all acute and reconstructive indications, this is assembled prior to insertion.

Closure

Reconstitution of the LUCL is essential at closure. If the ligamentous tissue appears inadequate, it should be reinforced with a No. 5 nonabsorbable Bunnell or Krakow stitch (Fig. 9). For reconstruc-

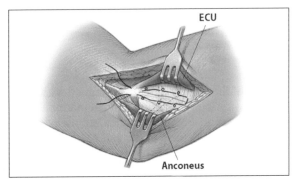

Fig. 9. Formal repair/reconstruction of the LUCL is necessary to assure proper stability in those clinical instances in which the radial head implant is inserted

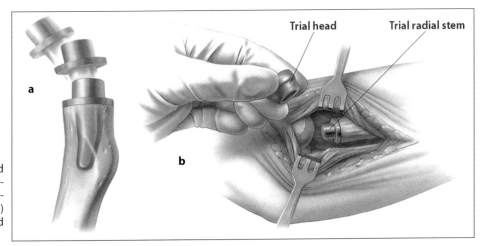

Fig. 8. (a) The curved trial stem of the implant is readily inserted down the canal. (b) The appropriate sized head is applied

tion applications, a formal LUCL substitute with tendon allograft (palmaris longus) or autograft (plantaris) may be necessary.

Aftercare

The goal of radial head replacement and soft tissue repair/reconstruction is to achieve elbow stability. Passive flexion and extension with the forearm in pronation to protect the lateral ligament is allowed on the second day assuming the elbow is stable. The Mayo Elbow Brace™ (AirCast, New Jersey) is applied to facilitate motion and protect the ligament repair (Fig. 10). Flexion/extension is allowed without restriction by day five, but we position the forearm in pronation for three weeks.

Long term aftercare requires surveillance as with any prosthetic replacement. If the implant is asymptomatic and tracks well, routine implant removal is not necessary.

Results

Early Experience

The use of the Silastic implant is plagued with complications ranging from mechanical inadequacy to adverse response from particulate debris and hence is no longer used to any extent [11, 24].

The Vitallium metallic replacement has provided satisfactory results in a limited number of uncomplicated radial head fractures [25]. An early detailed description by Harrington et al. [6] of the use of 15 Vitallium and two Silastic replacements for unstable elbow joints documented eight excellent, six good,

two fair, and one poor result. These investigators wisely recommend use of the implant specifically in radial head fractures complicated by instability.

Edwards and Rostrup [26] compared 14 patients with simple radial head fractures treated by excision to 11 metallic prosthetic replacements. He also showed satisfactory results in 76% of those with the device. Judet et al. [21] report on 12 patients followed at least 2 years with all five inserted for acute fractures and all had a satisfactory outcome.

Recent Experience

Favorable outcomes are being reported with recent current designs (Fig. 11) particularly for the Judet (Tournier, France) bipolar implant. With a mean 25 month assessment, a Belgium group reported that 10 of 13 (77%) patients treated for the acute fracture with the Judet device experienced satisfactory outcomes after Mason III fractures [27]. A subsequent study reported eight of 11 satisfactory outcomes at a mean of 32 months [28]. Most recently 13 of 15 (87%) patients with fracture dislocations were deemed satisfactory at a mean of 18 months [29].

Less is known regarding the modular non-articulated designs. Management of 15 fracture dislocations and 10 Mason III fractures revealed satisfactory results at a mean of 39 months in 17 (71%) patients.

In summary, the available data suggest that a radial head prosthesis is useful in fractures associated with elbow or wrist instability. Current data suggest the radial head implant is successful in 70% to 85% of patients managed acutely with Mason III fractures and when the fracture occurs with an associated injury. Yet, concern persists regarding the effectiveness when addressing problems of extensive resection, of implant malalignment and instability which occur when used for reconstructive procedures.

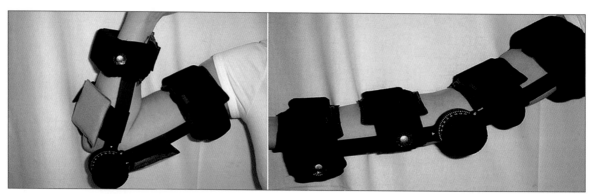

Fig. 10. The Mayo Elbow Brace™ (AirCast, New Jersey) is routinely used after surgery to protect the collateral ligament repair and to allow stretching of the soft tissues if this becomes necessary

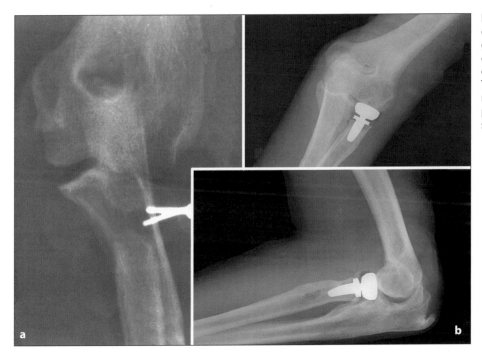

Fig. 11. (**a**) A fracture/dislocation has progressed to nonunion of the radial head and elbow subluxation. (**b**) Treatment with the rHead Recon™ implant and MCL reconstruction

Complications

Numerous adverse effects have been associated with radial head implants. Fatigue failure has occurred with both the acrylic [26] and the Silastic [12, 30] prostheses. Fatigue failure of implants made of Silastic appears to account for most of the poor results. The inadequate material properties of the Silastic device for use at the radial head are generally accepted and have been confirmed by recent studies [24, 31]. Furthermore, synovitis reported with Silastic finger implants also occurs at the elbow [32, 33]. Worsing and et al. [33] observed clinical and experimental evidence of foreign-body giant cell reaction elicited by particulate Silastic debris. We have observed an articular reaction from silastic identical to that seen in rheumatoid arthritis [34]. Thus, because of their inadequate material properties and demonstrable adverse biologic characteristics, Silastic replacements should not be used at the elbow.

Metallic implants have gained considerable popularity in recent years. Malalignment, dislocation, and loosening are possible with all radial head devices [6]. Malalignment causes deterioration and arthritis at the metallic/capitellar articulation. Instability is usually due to malalignment or inadequate repair of the lateral ulnar collateral ligament. As we await the long-term outcome data of the current generation of modular/metallic radial head implants, incongruity, articular compatibility, loosening, and instability are of greatest concern.

References

1. Speed K (1941) Ferrule caps for the head of the radius. Surg Gynecol Obstet 73:845
2. Cherry JC (1953) Use of acrylic prosthesis in the treatment of fracture of the head of the radius. J Bone Joint Surg Br 35:70
3. Swanson AB (1973) Flexible implant resection arthroplasty in the hand and extremities. CV Mosby Co, St. Louis
4. Morrey BF, Tanaka S, An KN (1991) Valgus stability of the elbow: a definition of primary and secondary constraints. Clin Orthop 265:187-195
5. King GJ, Zarzour ZDS, Rath DA et al (1999) Metallic radial head arthroplasty improves valgus stability of the elbow. Clin Orthop Relat Res 368:114-125
6. Harrington IJ, Sekyi-Otu A, Barrington TW et al (2001) The functional outcome with metallic radial head implants in the treatment of unstable elbow fractures: a long-term review. J Trauma 50:46-52
7. Hotchkiss RN (1997) Displaced fractures of the radial head: internal fixation or excision? J Am Acad Orthop Surg 5:1-10
8. Johansson O (1962) Capsular and ligament injuries of the elbow joint. Acta Chir Scand Suppl 287:1-159
9. Schwab GH, Bennett JB, Woods GW, Tulloos HS (1980) The biomechanics of elbow instability: the role of the medial collateral ligament. Clin Orthop 146:42
10. Mackay I, Fitzgerald B, Miller JH (1979) Silastic replacement of the head of of the radius in trauma. J Bone Joint Surg Br 61:494
11. Taylor TKF, O'Connor BT (1964) The effect of the radius in adults. J Bone Joint Surg Br 46:83
12. Mayhall WST, Tiley FT, Paluska DJ (1981) Fractures of the Silastic radial head prosthesis. J Bone Joint Surg Am 53:459

13. Morrey BF, Askew L, Chao EY (1981) Silastic prosthetic replacement for the radial head. J Bone Joint Surg Am 53:454

14. Swanson AB, Jaeger SH, LaRochelle D (1981) Comminuted fractures of the radial head: the role of silicone-implant replacement arthroplasty. J Bone Joint Surg Am 63:1039

15. Martinelli B (1975) Fractures of the radial head treated by substitution with the Silastic prosthesis. Bull Hosp Joint Dis 36:61

16. Gupta GG, Lucas G, Hahn DL (1997) Biomechanical and computer analysis of radial head prostheses. J Shoulder Elbow Surg 6:37-48

17. Pomianowski S, Morrey BF, Neale PG et al (2001) Contribution of monoblock and bipolar radial head prostheses to valgus stability of the elbow. J Bone Joint Surg Am 83:1829-1834

18. Knight DJ, Rymaszewski LA, Amis AA, Miller JH (1993) Primary replacement of the fractured radial head with a metal prosthesis. J Bone Joint Surg Br 75:572-576

19. Moro JK, Werier J, MacDermid JC et al (2001) Arthroplasty with a metal radial head for unreconstructible fractures of the radial head. J Bone Joint Surg Am 83:1201-1211

20. Wick M, Lies A, Muller EJ et al (1998) Prostheses of the head of the radius. What outcome can be expected? Unfallchirurg 101:817-821

21. Judet T, de Loubresse CG, Piriou P, Charnley G (1996) A floating prosthesis for radial-head fractures. J Bone Joint Surg Br 78:244-249

22. van Glabbeek F, van Riet R, Verstreken J (2001) Current concepts in the treatment of radial head fractures in the adult. A clinical and biomechanical approach. Acta Orthop Belg 67:430-441

23. van Riet RP, Morrey BF, O'Driscoll SW, van Glabeek F (2005) Associated injuries complicating radial head fractures: a demographic study. Clin Orthop Relat Res 441:351-355

24. Carn RM, Medige J, Curtain D, Koenig A (1986) Silicone rubber replacement of the severely fractured radial head. Clin Orthop 209:259

25. Carr CR, Howard JW (1951) Metallic cap replacement of radial head following fracture. West J Surg 59:539

26. Edwards GE, Rostrup O (1960) Radial head prosthesis in the management of radial head fractures. Can J Surg 3:163

27. Smets S, Govaers K, Jansen N et al (2000) The floating radial head prosthesis for comminuted radial head fractures: a multicentric study. Acta Orthop Belgica 66:353-358

28. Popovic N, Gillet P, Rodriguez A, Lemaire R (2000) Fracture of the radial head with associated elbow dislocation: Results of treatment using a floating radial head prosthesis. J Orthop Trauma 14:171-177

29. Holmenschlager F, Halm JP, Piatek S et al (2002) Comminuted radial head fractures. Initial experiences with a Judet radial head prosthesis. Unfallchirurg 105:344-352

30. Morrey BF, Chao EY, Hui FC (1979) Biomechanical study of the elbow following excision of the radial head. J Bone Joint Surg Am 61:63

31. Trepman E, Ewald FC (1991) Early failure of silicone radial head implants in the rheumatoid elbow. J Arthroplasty 6:59

32. Gordon M, Bullough PG (1982) Synovial and osseous inflammation in failed silicone-rubber prostheses. J Bone Joint Surg Am 64:574

33. Worsing RA, Engber WD, Lange TA (1982) Reactive synovitis from particulate Silastic. J Bone Joint Surg Am 64:581

34. VanderWilde RS, Morrey BF, Melberg MW, Vinh TN (1994) Inflammatory arthrosis of the ulno-humeral joint after failed Silicone radial head implant. J Bone Joint Surg Br 76:78-81

CHAPTER 18

Radial Head Replacement with a Pyrocarbon Head Prosthesis: Preliminary Results of a Multicentric Prospective Study

Y. ALLIEU, M. WINTER, J.P. PEQUIGNOT, P. DE MOURGUES

Introduction

The treatment options for radial head fractures are conservative treatment, open reduction and internal fixation, radial head excision, and radial head prosthesis. The importance of the radial head in elbow biomechanics is now well known. The radial head is of prime importance for the elbow stability, especially when radial head fractures are associated with elbow dislocation. Consequently according to all of the extent reports, the radial head must be conserved and its excision is contraindicated when there is elbow instability.

All of the reporting authors stress the importance of early elbow mobilization in order to avoid stiffness, and as a result conservative treatment is only indicated if this mobilization is possible. Rigid internal fixation must be carried out in all possible cases. In comminutive fractures when this synthesis is impossible, radial head excision must be completed by radial head arthroplasty in all cases with medial ligament injury and elbow instability. Radial head prosthesis is also indicated for pain and mobility reduction in selective cases of degenerative radio-ulnar proximal arthritis, rheumatoid arthritis, radial head fracture sequel-

lae, and radial head resection with complications in the elbow and/or distal radio-ulnar joint.

The purpose of this chapter is to present a new radial head arthroplasty in pyrocarbon, and its preliminary results.

Prosthesis Design

The prosthesis MoPyc (Radial Head Prosthesis MoPyc, Laboratory Bioprofile, Grenoble) is modular and formed with three components: head, neck and stem (Fig. 1). The head, made of pyrocarbon, has a spherical shape in order to fit in the proximal radial notch. The proximal part is concave to fit into the capitellum. The neck and the stem are made of TAGV (Titanium alloy). The neck has a 15° angulation to restore the anatomical axis. The orientation of the neck is critical and facilitated by an anallary guide. The stem (titanium) is cementless, fixed due to an expansion device controlled by a dynamic screw allowing primary fixation.

There are three sizes for the head, four sizes for the neck (5-, 7-, 9-, and 11-mm lengths), and four sizes for the stem. This extensive modularity (48 possibilities of stem/neck/head combinations) allows anatomic adaptability and minimal bone resection.

Pyrolitic Carbon

As mentioned above, the prosthesis head is made of pyrolitic carbon, which is formed by the pyrolysis of a hydrocarbon gas. It is deposited as a coating onto high-strength graphite substrates.

Pyrolytic carbon was first used for artificial heart valves in 1969. Since then, several millions of heart

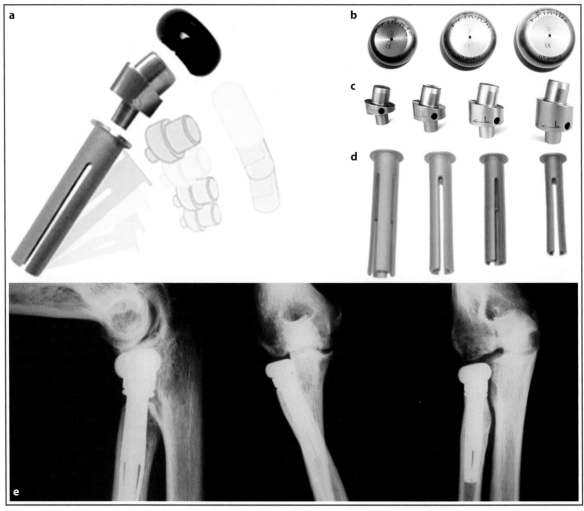

Fig. 1. The MoPyc prosthesis. (**a**) The modular prosthesis with an angulated neck and pyrocarbon head. (**b**) Pyrocarbon head in three sizes. (**c**) Angulated neck in four sizes. (**d**) Stem in four sizes. (**e**) X-ray control in pronation and supination

valves in the world have been made of pyrocarbon. Pyrocarbon was more recently used in the orthopedic field for MCP arthroplasties [1, 2], the PIP arthroplasties [3], and for the proximal scaphoid implant [4].

Pyrocarbon is extremely biocompatible (Table 1). Pyrocarbon biocompatibility has been proven for more than 34 years in heart valves in contact with blood and for more than 20 years in finger joint implants.

Pyrolytic carbon also has very attractive mechanical properties. It has high wear resistance, and the polishing of pyrocarbon can be superior to the other materials used in the orthopedic field (Ra = 0.03 μm) allowing perfect gliding on lateral condyle without damage or wear.

Moreover, pyrocarbon, contrary to other materials has more or less the same mechanical properties as bone. Its density and elasticity modulus are very close to that of bone and allow a good transmission of mechanical strength between bone and implant.

With an alumina implant in contact with bone, the bone sustains 100% of the constraints; with a silicone implant the silicone sustains the constraints and fails; with pyrocarbon, the elasticity modulus are matched and constraints are shared. Thanks to its mechanical properties, pyrocarbon is adapted to the contact with the cartilage. Cook et al. [1, 2] carried out prosthetic replacement of femur heads in 45 dogs with three types of prostheses: pyrocarbon, chrome-cobalt, and titanium. The dogs were implanted for a period ranging from 2 weeks to 18 months. The acetublar joint cartilage was analyzed. The results showed the superiority of pyrocarbon compared to the metallic implants. In terms of survival of joint cartilage at 18 months, pyrocarbon showed 92% of survival against 20% for metallic implants with important lesions.

Materials and Methods

The multicentric prospective study was based on 30 implantations of the prosthesis from November 2002 to September 2004. The mean age of the patients was 50 years (range 17-82 years). There were 19 men and 11 women. The dominant arm was injured in 43.3% of the cases. The mean follow-up was 18 months (range 6-29 months). The surgeons were all seniors.

Etiology

In 25 cases, the etiology was a fracture of the radial head; 18 were recent fractures (Group A), with seven Mason III and 11 Mason-Johnston IV fractures. Two ulnar fractures and two coronoid fractures were associated. An elbow dislocation or subluxation was associated in 11 cases (Mason-Johnston IV). No distal radio ulnar joint instability was noted among the patients. The mean time to surgery in Group A was 2.4 days (range 0-7 days). Seven cases were fracture sequellae (Group B), with three initial radial head resections, one initial radial head replacement with a floating prosthesis (CRF), and three malunions after orthopaedic treatment for displaced radial head fractures. Five cases were nontraumatic (Group C); three of them were isolated humero-radial degenerative arthritis, with no obvious traumatic cause, but the three patients were heavy-load workers, presenting a risk of microtraumatic lesions. Two of them had rheumatoid arthritis, with major lesions on the lateral aspect of the elbow joint.

Surgical procedure

Approach

The forearm was operated in a pronated position in order to avoid neurological damage to the posterior interosseous nerve, as described by Diliberti et al. [5]. A straight lateral approach was done to gain access to the radial head, through the extensor radialis longus and extensor digiti communis or directly through the epicondylar muscle to the protrusion of the radial head in acute injury. Indeed, compared to the classical Kocher's approach (between aconeus and extensor carpi ulnaris muscle), this approach is respectful to the humero ulnar part of the collateral lateral ligament, whose importance was highlighted by Seki et al. [6]. We favor this approach because there are no risks of vasculo-nervous lesions of the anconé, and risks of devascularization of the radial head are more limited compared to the posterolateral approach. Moreover, access to the coronoid process is easier through this approach [7]. Once the access to the joint was done, the annular ligament was opened in an oblique way in order to be able to lengthen it during closure.

Radial Head Resection

A cutting guide was used in order to achieve a good resection, which must be perpendicular to the axis of the radius (Figs. 2, 3).

The parts of the broken head were reassembled on a table in order to ensure that the whole head had been resected and to choose the size of the prosthetic head. If a coronoid fracture or an anterior capsule tear was present, the surgeon repaired it at this time. The level of resection was not imposed, knowing that the prosthesis neck is available in three different sizes.

Introduction of the Stem

After resection of the radial head, the radial shaft was prepared. Each broach is color-coded, corresponding to the same trial stem size. The broach sizes go from 5 to 10 millimeters. Then the trial stem was introduced and left temporarily in place.

Choice of the Neck and Positioning of its Angulation

The positioning and the height of the prosthesis are essential for the success of the implantation.

Table 1. Properties of pyrocarbon

	Silicon	PE	Bone	Pyrocarbon	TA6G Metal	CoCr Metal	Alumine
Elasticity (GPa)	0.004	1	15-20	20-25	110	200-340	407
Density (g.cm-3)	1.1	0.9-1.1	2.0	1.7-2.0	4.5	8.3-9.2	3.5

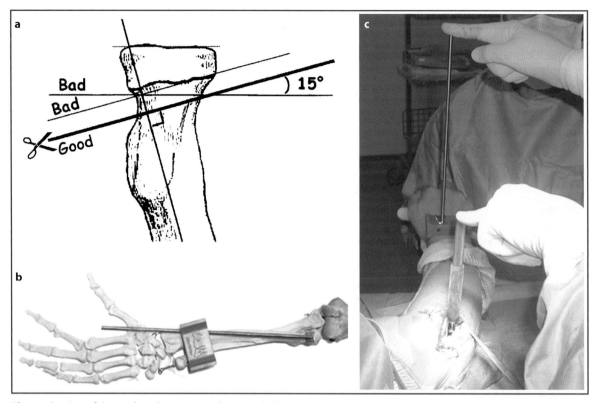

Fig. 2. Cutting of the neck and cutting guide. (**a**) Radial head resection after cutting of the neck perpendicular to the axis of the radius. (**b**) The cutting guide. (**c**) Intra-operative use of the cutting guide

Four sizes of neck are available. The head had to reach the limit between the trochlear notch and the radial notch of the ulna. Regarding the position of the angulation, in a pronated position, the angulation had to be in the same plane as the first metacarpal bone, enabling the radius to cross over the ulna while pronating. In a supinated position, the radial head had to "watch" in the direction of the capitellum.

X-rays were performed to check the proper choice of the elements sizes, the positioning of the neck, and the height of the prosthesis. According to Van Glabbeek et al. [8, 9], the height of the prosthesis must not exceed 2.5 mm of over or understuffing. Anteroposterior X-rays were done in pronated and supinated position.

Implantation of the Prosthesis

After removal of the trial elements, the stem was inserted. The expansion screw was then applied with the expansion screw driver. After stem locking, the head and the neck were assembled together with a special device on the table, and inserted together on the stem. At this stage, another X-ray

control was done in order to check the good positioning of the prosthesis.

Associated Procedures

For recent fractures (Group A), associated procedures included ulnar osteosynthesis in cases of Monteggia fractures (cases 5 and 6), coronoid reconstruction (case 2, Table 3), or lateral ligament reparation (cases 4, 5, 10, 12, 14, 15, 18, 20, 28) (Table 2).

For fracture sequellae (Group B), arthrolysis was performed at the same time before prosthesis implantation if necessary (case 8). In case 17 of revisional procedure after anterior RHP (CRF), an ulnar shortening was done after the arthroplasty. In cases of rheumatoid arthritis (Group C), a synovectomy was performed in the same stage (cases 13 and 16).

Post-operative Care

When elbow stability was achieved by the prosthesis, a removable extension wrist splint was worn for 1-2 weeks in order to rest the lateral epi-

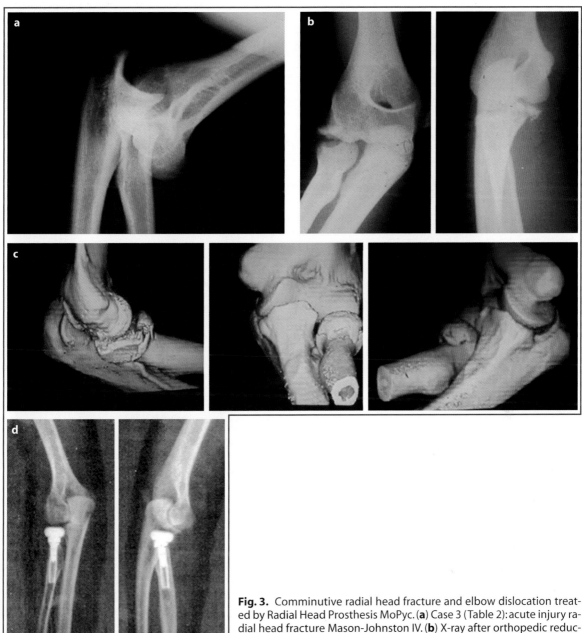

Fig. 3. Comminutive radial head fracture and elbow dislocation treated by Radial Head Prosthesis MoPyc. (**a**) Case 3 (Table 2): acute injury radial head fracture Mason-Johnston IV. (**b**) X-ray after orthopedic reduction. (**c**) Scan after orthopedic reduction. (**d**) Post-operative control after MoPyc radial head prosthesis

condylian muscles. In cases of instability, a removable brachio-antibrachial 90° resting splint was worn for a maximum of 3 weeks (8 weeks in Group A, 6 in Group B, 3 in Group C). The average duration of immobilization was 10 days. Early mobilization began with a hand therapist, even in cases of residual instability. Forearm rotation was not allowed in extension for the first 3 weeks. Active motion began after 3 weeks. Patients were supervised by the therapist for 2 months.

Clinical Patient Review

The evaluation of the patients included a personal interview, a physical examination, and the assessment of current X-rays. Each surgeon had to send the results of the evaluation at each review. The ranges of motion were measured on both sides with a goniometer. The grip strength was measured with a Jamar-type dynamometer on both sides.

Table 2. Data of the 30 cases

Case	Age	Sex	Profession	Dominant side	Etiology	Associated fractures
1	49	M	Office worker	No	Sequellae RHF malunion 60 mos after	
2	39	M	Manual worker	No	Acute injury RHF Mason-Johnston 4	Coronoid fracture Regan-Morrey 1
3	39	M	Office worker	No	Acute injury RHF Mason-Johnston 4	
4	38	M	Manual worker	No	Acute injury RHF Mason 3	
5	82	F	Retired	No	Acute injury RHF Mason-Johnston 4	Ulnar fracture
6	47	M	Office worker	No	Acute injury RHF Mason-Johnston 4	Ulnar fracture
7	73	M	Retired	No	Humero-condylar degenerative arthrosis	
8	53	F	Manual worker	Yes	Sequellae RHF malunion 12 mos after	
9	48	F	Office worker	No	Sequellae RHF malunion 2.5 mos after	
10	80	F	Retired	Yes	Acute injury RHF Mason-Johnston 4	
11	57	M	Office worker	No	Sequellae RHF malunion 6 mos after	
12	59	M	Retired	No	Acute injury RHF Mason 3	
13	60	F	-	Yes	Rheumatoid arthritis	
14	55	F	-	Yes	Acute injury RHF Mason-Johnston 4	Coronoid fracture Regan-Morrey 1
15	32	M	Manual worker	No	Acute injury RHF Mason-Johnston 4	
16	68	F	Retired	Yes	Rheumatoid arthritis	
17	33	M	Office worker	No	Revisional procedure of another RHP C.R.F.)	
18	45	M	Office worker	Yes	Acute injury RHF Mason 3	
19	59	M	Retired	Yes	Humero-condylar degenerative arthrosis	
20	42	M	Office worker	No	Acute injury RHF Mason 3	
21	40	M	Manual worker	Yes	Sequellae RH Resection	
22	42	M	Heavy manual worker	Yes	Acute injury RHF Mason 3	
23	61	F	Retired	Yes	Sequellae anterior RHR	
24	23	F	Office worker	Yes	Acute injury RHF Mason-Johnston 4	
25	52	F	Office worker	No	Acute injury RHF Mason-Johnston 4	
26	17	F	Student	No	Acute injury RHF Mason-Johnston 4	
27	53	M	Manual worker	Yes	Humero-condylar arthrosis	
28	41	M	Manual worker	No	Acute injury RHF Mason 3	
29	72	M	Retired	No	Acute injury RHF Mason 3	
30	50	M	Office worker	Yes	Acute injury RHF Mason-Johnston 4	

RHF, Radial head fracture; *RH*, Resection: Radial Head Resection Density (g. cm-3)

The Broberg and Morrey score [10] and the Mayo Elbow Performance Score [11] were used to evaluate the disability of the elbow. Anteroposterior and lateral X-rays of the elbow were done at each review, in pronation and supination to evaluate the integration of the prosthesis and the status of the elbow joint. Anteroposterior and lateral X-rays of the wrists were also done to evaluate the radio ulnar index.

Results

The details of each patient are presented in Tables 2 and 3.

Mobility. The average flexion was 122° (loss of 11.5% compared to the noninjured side). The average extension was -15°. The average pronation was 74° (90% of the noninjured side). The average

Table 3. Operative treatment and results of the 30 cases

Case	Operative treatment RHP Associated procedures	Follow-up (years)	Post-operative Flex-Ext ROM	Post-operative Prono-Supination	Post-operative mobility in Broberg-Morrey Score
1	-	1.19	123	75/60	37
2	Coronoid O.R.I.F.	1.73	90	60/90	31
3	Ligament repair	1.15	140	85/85	40
4	Ligament repair	1.12	60	80/80	25
5	Ulnar ORIF Ligament repair	2.30	100	70/70	33
6	Ulnar ORIF	1.67	95	0/0	19
7	Epicondylar muscle lengthening	1.05	100	70/60	32
8	Arthrolysis	1.11	100	80/50	31
9	-	0.49	110	70/80	35
10	Ligament repair	1.21	105	80/70	34
11	Humero-condylar synovectomy and ligamentous plasty	1.51	95	85/70	32
12	Ligament repair	2.06	120	80/70	37
13	Synovectomy Ligament repair	1.79	130	80/70	39
14	Ligament repair	1.74	130	70/80	39
15	Ligament repair	1.68	90	70/80	31
16	Synovectomy	1.57	130	80/70	39
17	Ulnar shortening	1.34	110	80/70	35
18	Ligament repair	1.19	135	80/80	40
19	Ligamentous plasty	1.17	90	80/80	31
20	Ligament repair	0.75	135	80/80	40
21	-	2.37	115	90/90	36
22	-	2.35	120	90/90	37
23	Radial nerve neurolysis	2.12	100	80/80	33
24	-	0.89	110	90/90	35
25	-	2.27	95	70/80	32
26	-	0.65	95	80/80	32
27	-	1.35	90	80/80	31
28	Ligament repair	1.37	125	90/90	38
29	-	1.58	68	0/0	14
30	-	1.21	110	80/90	35

supination was 72° (86% of the noninjured side). You can see the point value of motion according to the Broberg and Morrey score [10] on Table 4.

Average strength. The average grip strength was 90% of the noninjured side.

Pain. Pain was classified as slight, moderate, or important. At the latest follow-up, six patients presented with slight pain at rest, eight presented with slight pain during daily activities. During heavy work, 10 patients presented with slight pain, and 13 presented with moderate pain.

The average Broberg and Morrey score (Table 4, Fig. 4) was 88/100 (77% of the patients had excellent or good results). The average Mayo Elbow Performance Score (MEPS) was 95/100 (97% of the patients had excellent or good results) (Fig. 5).

Twenty-three patients returned to their previous work; one patient had not returned to work yet. Six patients were retired or without professional activity. No clinical instability was found at the latest review.

Complications: Case 1 (Group B) presented post-operative ossifications without any consequence on mobility. Case 4 (Group A) sustained an arthrolysis 6 months after the implantation, with fair results in circumstances of worker compensation. Cases 6 and 29 (Group A) presented heterotopic ossifications leading to a radio-ulnar synostosis. At the latest review, an arthrolysis was planned in each case. Case 24 (Group A) had an understuffed implant with unstable elbow which was changed a few weeks after the first operation, with a good final result. Case 26 (Group A)

Table 4. Broberg and Morrey's Score: functional rating index

Variable	Point Value
Motion	
Degree of flexion (0.2 x arc)	27
Degree of pronation (0.1 x arc)	6
Degree of supination (0.1 x arc)	7
Strength	
Normal	20
Mild loss (appreciated but not limiting, 80% of opposite side)	13
Moderate loss (limits some activity, 50% of opposite side)	5
Severe loss (limits everyday tasks, disabling)	0
Stability	
Normal	5
Mild loss (perceived by patient, no limitation)	4
Moderate loss (limits some activity)	2
Severe loss (limits everyday tasks)	0
Pain	
None	35
Mild (with activity, no medication)	28
Moderate (with or after activity)	15
Severe (at rest, constant medication, disabling)	0

Total score to qualitative groups was as follows: 95 to 100 points, excellent; 80 to 94 points, good; 60 to 79 points, fair; 0 to 59 points, poor

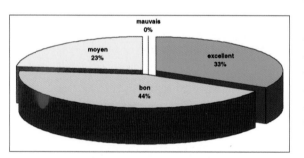

Fig. 4. Results of the 30 cases according to Broberg-Morrey score

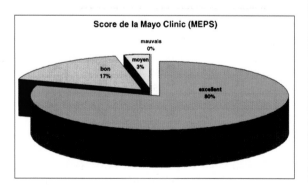

Fig. 5. Results of the 30 cases according to the Mayo Elbow Performance Score (MEPS)

demonstrated a tendency to posterior subluxation during heavy work, but this phenomenon decreased with time.

Radiological Assessment

In three cases we noted a 2 to 3-mm osteolysis under the neck (stress shieldings) without clinical symptoms (Fig. 6).

In two cases we note a peri-prosthesis stem lucency without clinical signs either. Five patients presented a pre-operative capitellar erosion (case 20, Group A and case 21, Group B). The two patients with rheumatoid arthritis (Group C) also presented elbow degenerative arthritis (cases 13 and 16). In case 17 we noted capitello-humeral erosion after Judet-CRF radial head prosthesis placed too high. No progression of the radiological sign was noted at the last follow-up. We noted no radiological instability of the elbow in any of the cases. When evaluated (in 15 cases) the ulnar variance on wrist X-ray was normal.

Discussion and Conclusions

The objective of this prospective study was to evaluate the preliminary results of this new implant in terms of reliability of implantation, clinical and radiological results. The multicentric aspect of this study can give rise to criticism, but all of the surgical procedures were performed by senior surgeons

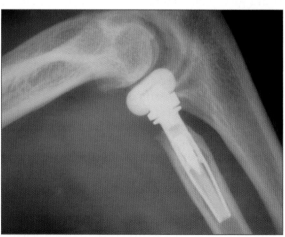

Fig. 6. Light osteolysis under the neck one year after (stress shieldings)

and the criteria of results evaluation was the same for all the cases.

Regarding the indication in all of the cases, the implantation of the prosthesis was decided if a stable reconstruction of the radial head by rigid osteosynthesis allowing an early elbow mobilization was not possible. In cases of combined coronoid or anterior capsular lesions as described recently by Pugh et al. [7], the reparation of these lesions is done by the lateral approach, taking benefit of the radial head resection to gain access to the anterior aspect of the joint.

We do not report treatment of persistent instability by repairing the medial collateral ligament using a medial approach or by using external elbow fixator [12].

In case of sequellae of radial head resection the restitution of the initial radial head when there is radial ascension might lead to a painful overstuffing of the prosthesis. Consequently the implantation must be carried out in place. If necessary an ulnar procedure must be associated to avoid ulno-carpal conflict (case 17). In one case of rheumatoid arthritis (case 13) elbow synovectomy was performed in the same stage before prosthesis implantation. The pyrocarbon head prosthesis was a new material which presents several advantages.

The literature has shown that silicone rubber implants presented no benefit compared to simple radial head resection [13]. Moreover, these implants have shown many complications due to silicone rubber. Monoblock metallic implants are nowadays commonly used to replace the radial head [14-26]. Judet et al. [19] described a floating prosthesis which presents a mobile head and an angulated neck with good results. Moreover, Pomianowski et al. [27] have shown that monoblock implants give better stability of the elbow. In cases of wide resection of the radial head, the restitution of proximal radius shape is mandatory, so the prosthesis should be angulated at 15° (average neck-shaft angle) [28]. Furthermore, the head of the implant must match with the concave radial notch of the ulna, presenting a convex peripheral shape in addition to a concave proximal surface to articulate with the capitellum.

The prosthesis used in this study answers those conditions: monoblock, angulated neck, convex shape of the peripheral aspect of the head, and concavity of its proximal aspect. Stem, neck, and head are available in different sizes, allowing 48 combinations for perfect adaptation in each individual case.

Radial head replacement is a unilateral arthroplasty. Consequently, the contact between native cartilage and the prosthesis might lead to lesions of the capitellum and the radial notch [29-31]. Pyrolytic carbon has shown excellent abilities in articulating with bone and cartilage [1, 2].

Radial head prosthesis has three goals. First, it must restitute the height of the radius, in order to obtain stability of the elbow [8, 9]. Second, it must permit good rotation of the forearm. Third, it must prevent proximal migration of the radius. Various reports have shown that a silastic implant does not ensure these goals, contrary to metallic implants [11, 17-19, 21, 22]. But metallic implants might alter the capitellum, according to a recent report [31]. This report shows that pyrocarbon is an elegant solution to preserve the capitellum and the radial notch. Moreover, we believe that monoblock implants are preferable to floating implants, and that the convex shape of the peripheral aspect of the prosthetic head ensures a better forearm rotation.

Radial head replacement is not free from complications. Indeed, the surgeon must avoid over or understuffing, and malrotation of the implant.

Our results are similar to those of the other series in the literature: Mackay [32], Harrington and Tountas [16], Knight [21], Judet [19], Popovic [24], Smets [26], Harrington [17], Moro [22], Holmenschlager |18], Alnot [33], and Skalski [25]. A long-term study based on the same patients and with additional cases will perhaps confirm our preliminary good results with this new pyrocarbon head prosthesis.

References

1. Cook SD, Thomas KA, Kester MA (1989) Wear characteristics of the canine acetabulum against different femoral prostheses. J Bone Joint Surg Br 71:189-197
2. Cook SD, Beckenbaugh RD, Redondo J et al (1999) Long term follow-up of pyrolytic carbon metacarpophalangeal implants. J Bone Joint Surg Am 81, 5:635-648
3. Moutet F, Guinard D, Gerard P et al (1994) Un nouvel implant articulaire digital titane-carbone. A propos des 15 premiers cas. Ann Chir Main Menb Super 13:345-353
4. Pequignot JP, Lussiez B, Allieu Y (2000) Implant adaptatif du scaphoïde proximal. Chir Main 2:276-285
5. Diliberti T, Botte M, Abrams R (2000) Anatomical considerations regarding the posterior interosseous nerve during posterolateral approaches to the proximal part of the radius. J Bone Joint Surg Am 82:809-813
6. Seki A, Olsen B, Jensen S et al (2002) Functional anatomy of the lateral collateral ligament complex of the elbow: configuration of Y and its role. J Shoulder Elbow Surg 11:53-59
7. Pugh D, Wild LM, Schemitsch E et al (2004) Standard surgical protocol to treat elbow dislocations with radial head and coronoid fractures. J Bone Joint Surg Am 86:1122-1130

8. Van Glabbeek F, Van Riet R, Baumfeld JA et al (2004) The kinematic importance of radial neck length in radial head replacement. Medical Engineerings 16:114-121

9. Van Glabbeek F, Van Riet R, Baumfeld JA et al (2004) Detrimental effects of overstuffing or understuffing with radial head replacement in the medial collateral ligament deficient elbow. J Bone Joint Surg Am 12:2629-2635

10. Broberg MA, Morrey BF (1986) Results of delayed excision of the radial head after the radial head fracture. J Bone Joint Surg Am 68:669-674

11. Morrey BF (1993) Radial head fracture. The elbow and its disorders. WB Saunders Co, Philadelphia, pp 383-404

12. Pennig D, Gausepohl T, Mader K (2000) Trans-articular fixation with the capacity for motion in fracture dislocations of the elbow. Injury 31: 35-44

13. King GJW, Zarzour Z, Rath D et al (1999) Metallic radial head arthroplasty improves valgus stability of the elbow. Clin Orthop 368:114-125

14. Carr CR (1971) Metallic cap replacement of the radial head. J Bone Joint Surg Am 53:1661

15. Charnley G, Judet T, de Loubresse C, Piriou P (1996) Articulated radial head replacement and elbow release for post head-injury heterotopic ossification. J Orthop Trauma 10:68-71

16. Harrington IJ, Tountas AA (1981) Replacement of the radial head in the treatment of unstable elbow fractures. Injury 12:405-412

17. Harrington IJ, Sekiyi-Out A, Barrington T et al (2001) The functional outcome with metallic radial head implants in the treatment of unstable elbow fractures: a long term review. J Trauma 50:46-52

18. Holmenschlager F, Halm JP, Winckler S (2002) Les fractures fraîches de la tête radiale: résultats de la prothèse à cupule flottante de Judet. Rev Chir Orthop 88:387-397

19. Judet T, de Loubresse C, Garreau C et al (1996) A floating prosthesis for radial head fractures. J Bone Joint Surg Br 2:244-249

20. King GJ (2004) Management of radial head fracture with implant arthroplasty. J Hand Surg Am 1:11-26

21. Knight DJ, Rymaszewski LA, Amis AA, Miller JH (1993) Primary replacement of the fractured radial head with a metal prosthesis. J Bone Joint Surg Br 75:572-576

22. Moro JK, Werier J, McDermid J et al (2001) Arthroplasty with a metal radial head for unreconstructible fractures of the radial head. J Bone Joint Surg Am 83:1201-1211

23. Miller JH, Kaye JC, Amis AA (1986) Vitallium replacement of the radial head in trauma. J Bone Joint Surg Br 68:665-666

24. Popovic N, Gillet P, Rodriguez A, Lemaire R (2000) Fracture of the radial head with associated elbow dislocation: results of treatment using a floating radial head prosthesis. J Orthop Trauma 14:171-177

25. Skalski K, Swieskowski W, Pomianowski S et al (2004) Radial head prosthesis with a mobile head. J Shoulder Elbow Surg 13:78-85

26. Smets S, Govaers K, Jansen N et al (2000) The floating radial head prosthesis for comminuted radial head fractures: a multicentric study. Acta Orthop Belg 66:353-358

27. Pomianowski S, Morrey BF, Neale P et al (2001) Contribution of monoblock and bipolar radial head prostheses to valgus stability of the elbow. J Bone Joint Surg Am 12:1829-1834

28. Gupta G, Lucas G, Hahn D (1997) Biomechanical and computer analysis of radial head prostheses. J Shoulder Elbow Surg 6:37-48

29. Beredjikian P, Nalbantoglu U, Potter H, Hotchkiss R (1999) Prosthetic radial head components and proximal radial morphology: a mismatch. J Shoulder Elbow Surg 8:471-475

30. Liew V, Cooper I, Ferreira L et al (2003) The effect of metallic radial head arthroplasty on radiocapitellar joint contact area. Clinical Biomechanics 18:115-118

31. Van Riet R, Van Glabbeek F, Verbogt O, Gielen J (2004) Capitellar erosion caused by a metal radial head prosthesis. J Bone Joint Surg Am 5:1061-1064

32. Mackay I, Fitzgerald B, Miller JH (1979) Silastic replacement of the head of the radius in trauma. J Bone Joint Surg Br 61:494-497

33. Alnot JY, Katz V, Hardy P, le GUEPAR (2003) La prothèse de tête radiale GUEPAR dans les fractures récentes et anciennes. Rev Chir Orthop 89:304-309

Introduction

The elbow is affected more frequently than any other joint by post-traumatic loss of motion. It is not clear why the elbow tends to develop stiffness after trauma. Its anatomic complexity certainly plays a relevant role:

- the presence of the three most congruous joints in a single capsule and a synovial space;
- the lateral collateral ligament (LCL) and the medial collateral ligament (MCL) often taut through the whole range of motion (ROM);
- a very close relationship with tendons, muscles and skin;

Several treatment options have been proposed for stiff elbow. In case of failure of non-operative treatment, surgical attempt may be indicated. The patient selection and the best surgical technique choices depend on:

- the type of injury and tissues involved;
- the surgeon's skill in recovering joint stability and restoring anatomical articular surfaces after intra-articular fractures through rigid fixation;
- the patient's ability during the postsurgical rehabilitation program to recover early active and passive motion.

Etiology

In elbow post-traumatic stiffness, the pre-operative assessments should identify the articular and periarticular tissues involved and more specifically, it should determine how much the articular surfaces and osteoarticular congruity are preserved. We will focus on the most important conditions and the tissue reactions after trauma in order to understand the causes of joint stiffness.

A logical surgical plan is based upon a deep knowledge of the anatomical obstacles and the associated lesions that the trauma provoked with:

- the periarticular soft tissue contractures;
- heterotopic ossification (HO);
- the osteoarticular incongruity.

The Periarticular Soft Tissue Contractures

The Skin Contracture

Serious skin burns, post-traumatic contractured wounds, or hypertrophic scars often cause a skin retraction of the anterior surface of the elbow.

The excision of full thickness eschar can solve the elbow extension restraint and the large exposition areas of the deep structures (especially the tendons) can be covered by skin grafts or local and regional island flaps.

An aggressive passive motion therapy after burns was identified as a contributing factor in the development of HO and it should be avoided [1-2], particularly in patients with an altered level of consciousness. This late painful and functionally limiting sequela of burn injuries is very common for the elbow joint.

Contractures Due to Imbalanced Muscles

Spastic flexion deformity of the elbow often follows a cerebral vascular accident in adults or spastic hemiplegia in children. If the deformity becomes severe, the correction of the elbow flexion could be achieved by lengthening the biceps and brachial muscle-tendons.

Neurological lesions (such as poliomyelitis or obstetrical palsy in children and brachial plexus lesions in adults) can be associated with chronic and static paresis of the elbow. The flexor muscles' paresis is often associated with extensor muscles' contracture and the elbow flexor muscles' contracture is associated with the elbow extensor muscles' paresis.

Before the surgical active restoration of elbow flexion/extension through muscle-tendon transfer, we have to recover the passive ROM by triceps or biceps tendons lengthening. The capsular release is often necessary.

Capsular and Ligament Contractures

The most common cause of extrinsic contracture with no osteoarticular damage is the simple elbow dislocation.

Josefsson [3] established the relationship between joint stiffness and a long immobilization after reduction.

In a retrospective study Melhoff et al. [4] found the relationship between the time of immobilization and the capsular contracture with no degenerative joint disease. Authors recommend active and passive gentle motion as soon as the pain allows it.

The simple elbow dislocation is a spectrum of instability which is described by O'Driscoll in the circle concept [5]. The capsule-ligamentous disruption occurs in three stages:
- in stage 1 and stage 2 the MCL is intact;
- in stage 3 MCL is torn.

In the traumatic clinical evaluation we have to distinguish stage 1 or 2 from stage 3. Thus, we can decrease the risk of acute redislocation through a correct choice of treatment.

In a few cases of "stage 3" elbow dislocation the immediate mobilization is allowed only after an elbow reduction and surgical ligaments repair.

The brace in the post-surgical treatment is useful to protect the ligament reconstruction.

In particular cases we can use the elbow external fixator in order to retain joint stability during early motion.

The results of surgical treatment *versus* nonsurgical treatment of elbow dislocation do not support the surgical choice for simple elbow dislocation if the stability after reduction could be achieved by closed means.

The soft tissue structures surrounding the elbow joint react in a unique way after an injury, with significant capsular, ligament, and muscle disruption.

In the first hours after the trauma there is an important bleeding from the capsule and from the highly vascularized brachialis muscle (which lies directly on the capsule). In the first weeks, edema and early scar tissue formation are the main causes of stiffness.

In the absence of motion the capsular or ligament scar tissue often becomes organized and the retracted fibrosis tissue involving the muscular or tendinous tissue becomes HO. Early motion, without aggressive therapy, helps to prevent elbow stiffness.

During the development of elbow stiffness, the medial and lateral collateral ligaments, which are often injured, tend to be contracted and undergo a process of ossification.

Linscheid and Wheeler [6] reported true HO in 4.5% out of 110 elbow dislocations, whereas more than 25% had calcification in the collateral ligaments.

Injuries to the collateral ligaments are not frequently recognized until the development of posttraumatic ossification at the original ulno-humeral insertion. A secondary shortening of the MCL can provoke an important elbow stiffness: a retracted MCL posterior band can cause a flexion contracture beyond 60°, while a tauter anterior part can provoke an extension contracture beyond 80°.

In case of a scarred and retracted LCL (with or without ossification) the elbow motion is decreased in flexion and extension until ankylosis.

This can be understand if we remember that the LCL (radial and ulnar band) are taut throughout flexion and extension.

In the current literature the role of the collateral ligaments in keeping elbow stiffness is not well documented [7].

The Heterotopic Ossification

Ectopic para-articular bone formation is a sequela of a traumatic event in which highly organized bone is formed and substitutes the surrounding injured soft tissues. The etiology is still unclear and misunderstood. Probably after trauma the mesenchymal cells or fibroblasts in presence of a bone morphogenic protein differentiate and proliferate into cartilage and osteoblasts [8, 9]. Direct trauma and its magnitude is the most frequent cause of HO. In the simple dislocation Thompson and Garcia [10] reported a 3% incidence of HO. In the complex instability with radial head (RH) fracture, the incidence of HO rose from 15% to 20%.

Bromberg and Morrey [11] reported a 9% incidence of HO after delayed excision of the fractured RH. An elbow trauma combined with a central nervous system injury increases the development of HO. In the literature the incidence of HO is reported from 76% [6] to 33% [12] in a series of head-injured patients with elbow and forearm trauma.

The development of HO is typically localized where the tissue is swollen and hyperemic. The development of the HO is hastened by the progressive loss of motion after trauma associated with immobility or with muscle contraction for the neurological lesions [13]. HO usually begins approximately 2 or 3 weeks after surgery or neurological insult, when aggressive manipulation is performed in order to avoid the progressive joint loss of motion.

Hastings and Graham [14] proposed a radiographic and clinical classification distinguishing three classes of elbow HO:
- class I: HO with no functional limitation;
- class II: HO with:
  - IIA limited flexo-extension;
  - IIB limited prono-supination;
  - IIC limited flexo-extension and prono-supination;
- class III: ankylosis.

While Garland identified two separate sites of HO in the elbow [15], anterior and posterior, Hastings and Graham [14] recognized the location of HO in anterior, posterior, and lateral sites of the elbow joint. In each area any tissue can be involved and HO can arise from:

In anterior site:
- coronoid;
- humero-ulnar;
- humero-radial;
- periarticular soft tissue such as capsule or brachial muscle.

In the posterior site:
- olecranon;
- humero-ulnar;
- olecranon fossa.

In the lateral sites:
- MCL;
- LCL.

The Osteoarticular Incongruity

Complications after distal humeral fractures are frequent for inadequate reduction or unstable internal fixation.

The mechanical limitation for osteoarticular deformity is likely to be associated with loss of mobility, capsular contracture, and HO.

A proper understanding of the anatomy and biomechanics of the elbow joint helps the surgeon to avoid malunion of the extra-articular or intra-articular fractures in the operative management. The complex bone anatomy has to be restored in the coronal, sagittal, and horizontal planes. The limitation of elbow movement is the most common complication if the surgeon does not recover the shapes and sizes of the articular surfaces as well as the articular anatomical axis in the humerus and proximal ulna and radius. In the distal humerus, the medial and lateral columns form a triangular "spool-shaped" construct of the articular surface [16].

The goal of fracture treatment is to restore the normal anatomical shape with relationship between:
- the size of the trochlea and the capitellum, which should be adequate to the olecranon notch size and to the proximal concavity of the RH;
- the anatomical axis of the ulno-trochlear and radio-capitellum articulations in the sagittal, coronal, and transverse planes.

The axis of the articular condyles in relation to the long axis of the humerus presents:
- 30° of anterior rotation in the sagittal plane;
- 5°-7° of internal rotation in the transverse plane;
- 6°-8° of valgus inclination in the frontal plane;
- 4°-8° of anterior offset of flexion-extension axis (the distance between the flexion-extension axis and the long axis of the humerus).

In this way the semilunar notch of the proximal ulna with 30° posterior orientation matches the trochlea. The medial column of the distal humerus diverges about 45° from the sagittal axis and the lateral column about 20°, projecting anteriorly and becoming the capitellum articular surface. The anatomical column surgical reconstruction enables easy recovery of the correct position of the articular surfaces.

The main causes that decrease elbow movement after distal humerus fractures are:
- malunions and nonunions;
- HO;
- contracture of the periarticular soft tissues.

Supracondylar and Intercondylar Fractures

(A) Malunion
In the sagittal plane, the anterior or posterior malalignment of the lateral column and capitellum with respect to the medial column and the trochlea changes the bone articular geometry. The

anatomical axis of the elbow rotation changes in two axes: the first one of the ulno-trochlear joint and the second one for the malaligned radio-capitellum joint.

In the supracondylar fractures' malunion, the elbow stiffness is often due to the loss of the anterior rotation of the articular condyles.

The loss of the condyles' antiversion, about 10°-20°, is well tolerated and the patient preserves a full elbow motion; when the loss of the antiversion is more than 30° the elbow loses its flexion for about 30°-40° ("The gun stock deformity") (Fig. 1).

In the frontal plane, the loss of the elbow valgus tilt can often provoke a cubitus varus in children with limitation of the elbow movement, and in

particular, the full elbow extension is due to the olecranon impingement in the olecranon fossa. In these cases a possible secondary posterolateral rotatory instability can occur later [5]. Elbow stiffness can occur when the displaced condylar fractures are not reduced. The common radiological aspect of the unreduced condylar fractures is an inverted V-shaped angular deformity. The anatomical deformity of the trochlea implies a secondary loss of the flexo-extension motion. In children, this condition is compatible with an elbow full motion in the adult age.

The exuberant callus with HO can occlude the coronoid or olecranon fossa with limitation of elbow ROM.

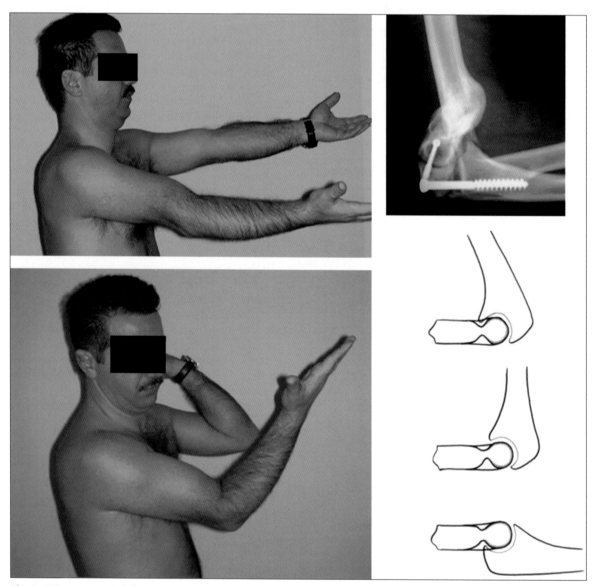

Fig. 1. "The gun stock deformity". The lost of the condyles antiversion, more than 30° is not tolerated and the elbow loses its flexion for coronoid impingement preserving a full extension

(B) Nonunion

The supracondylar nonunion is a rare complication, but this level represents a typical localization in distal humerus fractures. Nonunion is due to the inability to achieve a stable rigid fixation combined with early mobilization. Pain is often presented.

Intra-Articular Comminuted Fractures

(A) Malunion

A failed reposition of the articular fragments gives a distorted anatomy of the trochlea and capitellum. The humeral joint loses the congruent bone interfaces of the ulno-trochlea and radius-capitellum joints. If the surgeon is not able to restore the anatomy of the trochlea and its relationship to the olecranon and coronoid surfaces, the loss of function becomes very disabling.

Care must be taken not to narrow the dimension of the trochlea and the anatomical position of the capitellum because this may prevent the proper seating of the articular surfaces of the olecranon and the RH (Fig. 2).

In comminuted fractures the bone is often missing or it is not possible to use a bone articular fragment to recover the correct size and shape of the trochlea: a cortico-cancellous bone graft or an interposition bicortical graft from iliac crest can be used to re-establish the intercondylar anatomic proportion.

The malunion of the distal articular surfaces produces a mechanical obstacle of ulna-trochlear motion with a secondary limitation of both flexion and extension: osteoarthritis is prone to develop and increase the elbow stiffness and pain. In the

post-operative assessment, the surgeon has to evaluate the anatomic state of the articular surfaces, after this injury, because forced motion and manipulation under anesthesia can increase joint damage and soft tissue fibrosis or HO. In this way the motion decreases rather than increases.

(B) Nonunion

Nonunion is rare after the operative treatment of intra-articular fractures of the distal humerus. The fracture comminution or inappropriate initial treatment are involved in the nonunion development. In addition, the surgical trauma and the presence of intra-articular synovial fluid can compromise the fragments' blood supply [17].

In the Mayo experience, most nonunions are extra-articular, and only 7% developed a pseudarthrosis [18]. The patients often complain of pain and instability, and a high percentage present with motion loss [19].

Condyle Fractures

The malunion or nonunion of a single column can lead to an elbow deformation. Displaced lateral condyle fractures may cause a cubitus valgus deformity and ulnar nerve entrapment, while the displaced medial condyle fractures produce cubitus varus with a loss of ROM.

When the malunion or nonunion condylar fractures occur in children, the deformed elbow is often associated with an excellent function when they become adults. These patients usually develop arthritis with pain and loss of motion in the sixth or seventh decade of their life [20].

Capitellum Fractures

The capitellum malunion often results from a misdiagnosis of the fracture after a trauma.

Anteroposterior or lateral view low-quality radiographs often do not facilitate detection of a fracture when the small fragments are located in the superior part of the joint. The capitellum fractures in this nonanatomical position can lead to elbow stiffness at 90° flexion for impingement of the RH with capitellum malunion (Fig. 3).

Olecranon Fractures

Elbow stiffness after surgical reduction and internal fixation is often caused by an inadequate understanding of the anatomy of the articular olecra-

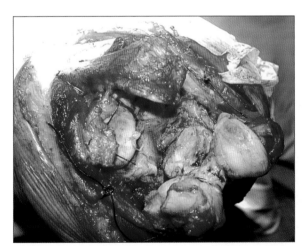

Fig. 2. The anatomical position of the capitellum and the correct size and shape of the trochlea must be recovered in the fracture of the distal humerus to prevent the proper seating of the articular surface of the olecranon and radial head

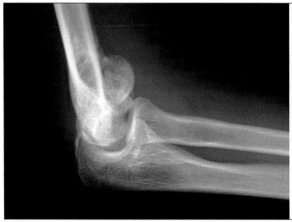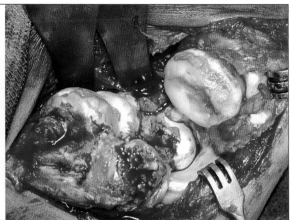

Fig. 3. The capitellum fracture can lead to elbow stiffness for impingement of the radial head with the capitellum malunion

non surface. After the fracture reduction, the surgeon should evaluate the alterations of the shape and size of the articular anatomy and the presence of bone impingement between olecranon and trochlea during the flexion-extension movement.

In a different way, in comminuted fractures it is useful to set in line the posterior cortex of the ulna (length, size, and shape) whereas the articular cartilage often presents fragments which are difficult to set in a correct anatomical position, especially in the midportion of the sigmoid notch.

The reduction and the internal fixation with K wires and use of the tension-band technique will narrow the olecranon-coronoid distance, thus reducing the olecranon-trochlea movement. The loss of elbow extension is often about 30°, while the flexion is rarely reduced. This occurs in from 50% to 75% of patients [21]. An inadequate fracture reduction is the main factor for post-traumatic degenerative arthritis: an incidence from 2% [22] to 20% [23] is reported in long-term follow-ups.

The main predisposing factor for an olecranon nonunion is an inadequate fixation with early motion; the patient preserves a false motion between the bone ends with less pain. After the surgical treatment of the olecranon nonunion, with bone grafting and the osteosynthesis of the avulsion fragment, the surgeon has to limit the postoperative active motion if the fragment is osteoporotic. When the rigid internal fixation is achieved with a plate, the main complication is necrosis of the injured olecranon skin.

Radial Head Fractures

The most common complications of the RH fractures are:

- Malunion or nonunion of the displaced or comminuted fractures:
  - the distorted anatomy of the RH can lead to incongruity with the lesser sigmoid notch of the ulna and with the capitellum (Fig. 4);
  - the angular deviation of the RH with subluxation of the proximal radio-ulnar joint will lead to a mechanical block.
- Heterotopic Ossification.

It often occurs in case of serious injury of the periarticular soft tissues or because of a delayed treatment.

When malunions, nonunions, and HO occur, the patients lose the forearm prono-supination and the elbow flexion-extension, and present with pain and radiographic degenerative arthritis.

Classification

A classification system is important in the diagnosis, prognosis, and treatment of elbow stiffness. Morrey [24] classified the post-traumatic stiffness into three groups: extrinsic, intrinsic, and mixed contractures.

- Extrinsic contracture:
  - it involves the contracture of the soft tissue (posterior and anterior capsule and ligaments and muscles surrounding the joint). Other extrinsic causes include a bone bridge across the joint for HO.
- Intrinsic contracture:
  - it is present after intra-articular fractures when there is intra-articular adhesion for articular cartilage damage or for distorted anatomy of the articular surface.

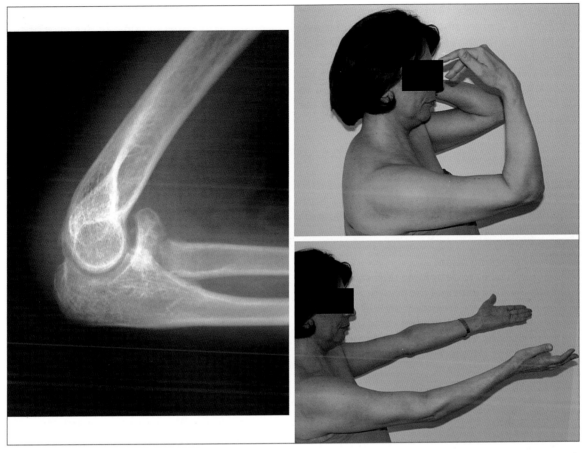

Fig. 4. The malunion or nonunion of the radial head fractures can lead to an incongruity with the lesser sigmoid notch and with the capitellum, producing a mechanical block

- Mixed contracture:
  - it is considered when intrinsic and extrinsic contractures are present.

In regard to causes of elbow stiffness, the Morrey's classification clearly identifies the etiological factors which are responsible for the joint stiffness and their precise localization in the extra-articular or intra-articular areas, but in each case the following must be taken into consideration:

- the extrinsic contracture could lead to intra-articular adhesion or to a secondary osteoarthritis;
- the intrinsic contracture is always associated with extrinsic contracture.

In our clinical experience, in the pre-operative clinical assessment we accept that in any case of stiff elbow the capsule contracture is always present and two associated lesions can modify the prognosis and the surgical management:

- the presence of HO;
- the state of the osseous articular anatomy.

In this way, after a comparison between the pre-operative clinical diagnosis and the intra-operative anatomo-pathological lesions, we propose a classification where three grades of elbow stiffness are distinguished.

We believe that the most important factors in determining outcome are the grades and extension of the tissue involved in the joint stiffness.

We can differentiate three different grades of clinical features related to the progressive injured patterns:

- Grade 1. A contracture of the capsular ligaments and periarticular muscle-tendons is present; the osteoarticular is preserved and HO is not present.
- Grade 2. A contracture of the soft tissues is associated with HO without osteoarticular damage. In this type "the HO excision is a greater surgical demand than soft tissue contracture release."
- Grade 3. A contracture of soft tissue with or without HO is in association with the osteoarticular damage. The joint loss, the articular surface congruity, and the bone is distorted such as:
  a. malunions or nonunions of intra-articular fractures;
  b. chronic unreduced subluxation.

In this grade "the articular surface incongruity and surgical correction of the bone articular distortion are greater surgical demand than HO excision and soft tissue contracture release."

This classification provides some guidelines for the management of elbow stiffness in relation to the entity of the lesion and to the difficulty of the surgical treatment.

Evaluation

In patients presenting with a post-traumatic stiffness, the physician should gather:
- a precise history;
- a physical examination;
- imaging studies to determine the osteoarticular integrity of the joint and the presence of HO.

The non-operative treatment should be considered only if the imaging studies show the absence of the mechanical block caused by a distorted bone anatomy or the presence of HO with or without bone bars linking the joint.

The History

The cause of a contracture is usually explained by:
- the imaging studies after trauma and before any treatment;
- the duration of the clinical symptoms and their progression;
- the previous treatment, including duration of prolonged immobilization and fitness of physical therapy and manipulation under anesthesia, or surgery;
- the presence of the internal fixation device and the knowledge of any remote complications (infection, skin suffering) or periodical complications such as elbow inflammation or edema after physical therapy.

The Physical Evaluation

The physical evaluation includes gathering general information and performing a detailed evaluation of the elbow and the remaining joints in both upper limbs.
- The general information must include:
  - age;
  - dominant arm;
  - entity of the disability during daily living activities, manual work, and the recreative program;

- the skin of the involved limb around the elbow should be inspected to look for evidence of any previous surgical approach;
- the neurological state with special attention paid to the ulnar nerve;
- the patient's capacity to have normal motor strength and voluntary control of muscles;
- the functional evaluation of the elbow uses a simple and sensitive rating system that considers subjective and objective symptoms such as pain, motion, stability, and ability to perform daily activities.

Many authors have described [25-28] elbow functional assessment and rating schemes to evaluate the outcomes after prosthetic replacement. The system, called "the Mayo Elbow performance score (MEPS)" described by Morrey [29], well represents the residual function of the posttraumatic elbow and it also allows surgeons to compare outcomes after surgical treatment in the follow-up. Elbow post-traumatic stiffness is often painless but the presence of pain should be noted: intensity, location, radiation, and where it occurs in the arc of movement.

During passive forced elbow flexion or extension the presence of pain helps to localize the anterior or posterior block with impingement of the olecranon or the RH against an osteophyte or incongruity of articular surface of the trochlea. The range of the elbow movement can be measured through a goniometer in a reproducible way.

A loss of full extension is often the sign of an intra-articular ulno-humeral incongruity.

Morrey [30] asserted that most activities of daily living can be accomplished with an arc of motion from 30° to 130° of flexion and 50° of forearm pronation and supination.

In case of elbow stiffness the patient tolerates 50°-60° loss of extension. The use of the hand is limited to the space around the body. Otherwise the patient does not tolerate a 30°-40° of flexion because the use of the hand is very limited for the individual needs.

The axial bone alignment (varus and valgus deformity) and rotational stability of the elbow should be carefully tested.

In chronic unreduced subluxation the elbow becomes stiff in flexion-extension, preserving the prono-supination movements. Pain is always present (Fig. 5).

After RH malunion or nonunion, the forearm can present rotational stiffness and pain. In case of RH resection there may be associated distal radius-ulna dissociation (Essex-Lopresti lesion).

The wrist is limited in extension and the forearm becomes stiff in supination. The patient also feels

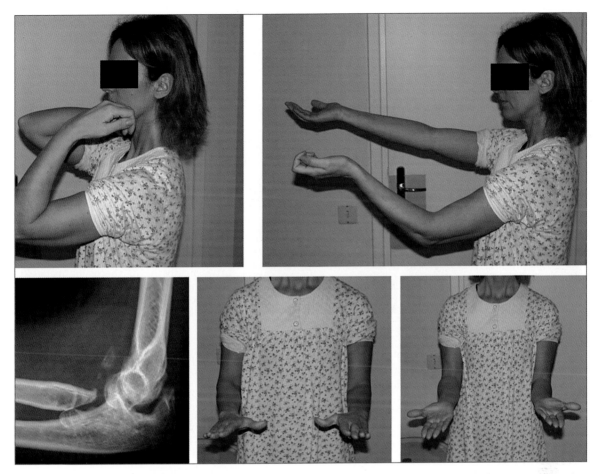

Fig. 5. In chronic unreduced subluxation, the elbow become stiff in flexion extension, preserving the prono-supination movements; pain is always present

pain at the distal radio-ulnar joint, and the end of the ulna is posteriorly subluxated. At the end of the elbow stiffness clinical evaluation, the neurological status, which is indicated by the motor strength of the muscle around the upper limb, should be carefully evaluated, and also any peripheral paresthesias and sensory deficit should be noted.

The Imaging Studies

Imaging studies should be performed before proceeding with treatment.

Routine lateral, oblique, and anteroposterior radiographs provide most of the information regarding the osteoarticular causes of elbow contracture and, in particular, they determine the integrity of the joint and the presence of para-articular HO.

Computer tomography (CT) scanning should be employed to evaluate the residual articular congruity and the precise localization and extension of HO around the elbow.

Magnetic resonance imaging (MRI) may be useful in identifying any associated loose bodies.

The lateral tomogram is the most helpful to define:

- the humeral-olecranon and the humeral-radius correct relationship and also it may be valuable to determine the normal articular surface contours.
- the presence of HO in the anterior or posterior aspect of the joint.

The anteroposterior radiograph is not particularly helpful if the elbow is contracted in flexion. In this case CT provides precise information regarding the state of the articular surface, the presence of fragment malunion or nonunion and the HO bone geometry. In order to reduce the risk of the recurrence of HO after surgery, their radiographic "maturity" must be taken into consideration. HO is defined as "mature" when linear trabeculation is present and the margin separating the HO from the surrounding soft tissues is distinct with cortical borders identical to the native bone (Figs. 6 a-d).

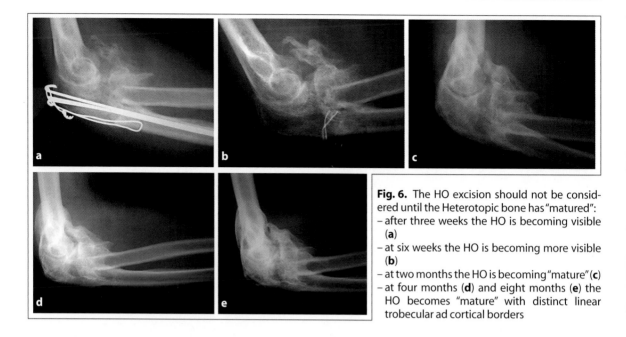

Fig. 6. The HO excision should not be considered until the Heterotopic bone has "matured":
– after three weeks the HO is becoming visible (**a**)
– at six weeks the HO is becoming more visible (**b**)
– at two months the HO is becoming "mature" (**c**)
– at four months (**d**) and eight months (**e**) the HO becomes "mature" with distinct linear trobecular ad cortical borders

The technetium bone scan is not predictable for assessing the maturity or biological activity of HO to minimize recurrence after surgical intervention [31, 32].

Treatment Options

The choice of the treatment of the elbow stiffness has to consider:
- nonsurgical management;
  - rehabilitation program;
  - manipulation under anesthesia;
- surgical management with:
  - arthroscopic capsular release;
  - open capsular release;
  - debridement arthroplasty;
  - distraction interposition arthroplasty;
  - elbow replacement.

A) Nonsurgical Management

Nonoperative treatment should be considered when:
- the articular bone anatomy is preserved;
- the contracture is mild and hasn't been present for more than 6 months;
- the absence of the HO bridge as Class II or Class III in Hastings and Graham Radiographic Classification [14].

The end point of the ROM is springy without firm block as bone impingement.

Nonsurgical treatment includes various strategies.

1. The Rehabilitation Program

Physical therapy with active and passive assisted elbow motion is often not sufficient to gain functional ROM. The passive assisted therapy has to avoid aggressive exercises that can increase elbow swelling and pain and the secondary risk of HO and stiffness development.

The active or passive exercises only, for a short time every day, will not be able to lengthen the contracted soft tissues. Continuous passive motion (CPM) is an important adjunct to achieving this goal.

In order to preserve the gained arc of motion, static adjustable splinting or dynamic splinting can be used after the active and passive exercises. The inflammatory and fibroplasia phase after the forced motion that stretches the periarticular soft tissue can be protected with the use of splints. The splints maintain the soft tissue at its maximal length (the static or serial static progressive splint).

During the rehabilitation program, static adjustable splinting can be useful. Most commercial hinged splints present adjustable blocks to the ROM and the mechanical possibility to increase passive ROM, and also they can be used as static splints. The guidelines for the use of the splints, their specific position, and their wearing time have been described by Morrey [33].

The typical splint program is:
1. remove the splint in the morning after having used it at night;
2. apply the splint in an opposite direction to the one used at night;

3. remove the splint for 1 h in the morning, 1 h in the afternoon, and 1 h in the evening;
4. use the elbow only when it is out of the splint;
5. if the elbow is inflamed, apply ice for 15 min and take an anti-inflammatory agent;
6. if the elbow is not inflamed but stiff, apply heat for 15 min and gently work the joint in flexion and extension;
7. at night, apply the splint in the most-needed direction. Analgesics are often required to tolerate the splint through the night.

2. Manipulation Under Anesthesia

Forced passive manipulation in the operating room is not generally advocated because of possible adverse early and late sequelae. During manipulation under anesthesia the physician has to avoid:
- periarticular fractures;
- ORIF mobilization;
- ulnar nerve injury.
  Otherwise, late sequelae could be:
- HO;
- elbow instability;
- increased risk of nonunion and secondary bone deformity.

B) Surgical Management

The choice of the surgical technique and the timing of the surgical intervention must take into consideration:
- the patient's needs and expectations and their involvement;
- the etiology and the clinical assessment of the elbow stiffness;
- the operative technique and skill of the surgeon.

1. Patient Involvement

The indications for surgical intervention are based on the patient's needs and expectations regarding improved elbow function without incurring a high risk of complications. Before the surgery the surgeon has to explain to the patient the real gain of the desired arc of motion and the risk of complications, which depend on the complexity of the lesions.

The patient should feel confident with the surgeon's ability to realize his needs.

The indication for surgery is correct when the loss of the functional arc of motion is inadequate for particular personal needs (such as occupational,

professional, or recreational activities) or when the conservative treatment has failed after 6-8 months.

Otherwise, in cases where the joint is damaged by osteoarticular deformity and incongruity without periarticular HO, the surgical treatment can be performed as soon as the soft tissue fibrous scar is organized. In these cases with osteoarticular deformity, a nonsurgical management (therapy, splinting CPM, or aggressive manipulation) is not able to gain the elbow motion but it increases pain and inflammatory reaction with degenerative arthrosis.

The nonoperative management is advised only when the state of articular bone is preserved.

2. Clinical Assessment

The knowledge of any clinical details about the traumatic lesion, the subsequent surgical treatment, and the imaging studies (X-rays or CT), allow us to determine the best surgical procedure.

Elbow stiffness following a soft tissue trauma with integrity of the joint (we classified it as grade 1 in the clinical presentation) indicates that the causes of the stiffness are the contractures of the capsule, of the ligaments, and of the periarticular muscle-tendon unit. These patients are the best candidates for soft tissue releases: arthroscopic or open surgical procedure. The contracture of soft tissue could be associated with HO (grade 2). Specific anatomic information which can be useful for the surgery is obtained from physical and radiographic examination. For instance, bone extrinsic impingement for HO in the olecranon fossa can be associated with anterior capsular contraction and the choice of surgical procedure has to consider the approach to the anterior and posterior aspect of the elbow.

When the articular surfaces are not violated and the cartilage is preserved in the open surgery, HO resection is a greater surgical priority than soft tissue contracture release.

A difficult surgical technique is needed when a contracture of soft tissue is associated with an articular surface incongruity with or without periarticular HO (grade 3 of our classification). The surgeon removes any articular adhesions, incongruities, or malunions.

In these cases, the surgeon's experience is essential in dealing with very complicated challenges during the surgical treatment.

3. The Surgical Technique

The general principles of the surgical technique are:

1. remove all the contracted structures and intra-articular deformities to obtain elbow motion;
2. maintain elbow stability by preserving the anterior band of MCL and the posterior band of the LCL;
3. avoid any damage to neurovascular structures.

In order to achieve this goal with open surgery three surgical approaches are always followed (see Chapter 4):

1. the posterior midline approach (the global approach);
2. the lateral approach;
   - limited "lateral column procedure";
   - extensive "Kocher approach";
3. the medial approach;
   - limited "medial column procedure";
   - extensile "over-the-top approach."

The surgeons choose the most appropriate surgical approaches after a clinical assessment that allows localization of all relevant abnormalities.

The decision about which operative techniques to use is made on the basis of the presence of elbow stiffness with:

- intact articular surface with preserved congruity;
- violated articular surface without congruity for malunion or nonunion.

Stiffness in Intact Articular Surfaces with Preserved Congruity

1. Arthroscopic Release

This procedure can be helpful in properly selected cases, but it is technically demanding and it requires experience to be performed safely [34].

In elbow stiffness the capsular volume is reduced from 25 ml to 6 ml [35] and the potential risk to neurovascular structures is high, especially for the ulnar nerve and the deep motor branch of the radial nerve.

The arthroscopic capsular release for "simple" elbow contracture can be performed with three possible options [36]:

- capsular detachment from the humerus with minimal risk;
- capsulotomy, with moderate risk;
- capsulectomy, dangerous but the most effective.

The capsular release is completed with synoviectomy and debridement of all olecranon and coronoid osteophytes, of the RH resection, and also of the olecranon fossa fenestration (Outerbridge-Kashiwagi procedure) [37].

Any further information about the indications, techniques, and outcomes of arthroscopic capsular release are discussed in Chapter 20.

2. Open Capsular Release

The isolated open capsulectomy is uncommon in our practice, often associated with HO resection. Consequently, the choice of the surgical approach depends on the type, on the location, and on the extension of HO.

The limited or extensile lateral approach is carried out when the contracture of the anterior or posterior capsule is associated with lateral HO with olecranon and coronoid osteophytes or RH malunion or nonunion.

Under general anesthesia we can perform the proximal half of Kocher's skin incision (the lateral column procedure) [38] and the main steps of the deep exposure, which are reported in the Chapter... on surgical exposures. If we need to expose the anterior and posterior aspect of the radio-capitellar joint and RH neck, the skin incision should be extended distally in the Kocker's interval (Fig. 7).

The LCL complex is identified and preserved, and in order to make the largest excision of the inferolateral capsule we have to identify the annular ligament and the LCL. The identification of the annular ligament without damage is done only before elevating the extensor carpi ulnaris very carefully. The relationship between both structures is very close. The LCL-sparing technique [39] can be useful to perform anterior and posterior capsulectomy without disturbing the extensor tendon insertion and the underlying LCL complex.

The deep surgical technique starts proximally; the brachialis is reflected anteriorly, exposing the anterior humerus in the same way as with the column procedure. The dissection is continued distally in a muscle splitting between the extensor carpi radialis longus (ECRL) and brevis. The surgeon can visualize the splitting area, distinguishing the extensor carpi radialis brevis (ECRB) tendon covered with a thin white fascia from the ECRL, which is predominantly muscular at this level. The advantage of this approach is that it reduces the risk of postoperative instability after release. The possible disadvantage is the risk of damage to the posterior interosseous nerve (PIN) and also the terminal motor branch to the ECRB, which arises from the lateral side of the PIN, proximally at the level of the radio-capitellar joint.

The Hohman retractor enables reflection of the brachialis and ECRL from the distal humerus and

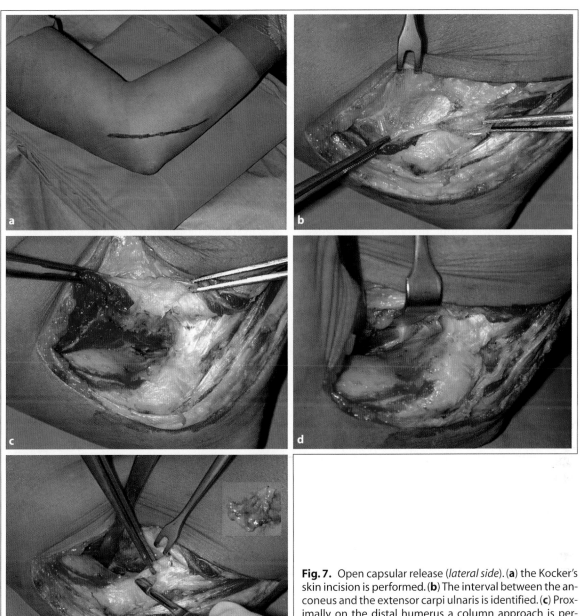

Fig. 7. Open capsular release (*lateral side*). (**a**) the Kocker's skin incision is performed. (**b**) The interval between the anconeus and the extensor carpi ulnaris is identified. (**c**) Proximally on the distal humerus a column approach is performed. (**d**) The anterior capsula is exposed with the lateral collateral ligament complex. (**e**) The anterior and posterior capsulectomy are performed, preserving the lateral collateral and annular ligaments

the capsule. The capsule is typically thickened and contracted and it often adheres to the underlying humerus.

The anterior capsule is excised from its points of insertion on the humerus, on the coronoid process, and on the RH, always respecting the annular ligament. Extensive capsulectomy rather than capsulotomy has been advised to reduce the risk of recurrent contracture. The lateral approach implies a greater difficulty in excising the medial half of the

anterior capsule without disturbing the anterior bundle of the MCL.

If elbow flexion is not achieved, Wada et al. [40] suggest that the thickened and scarred posterior oblique bundle of the MCL plays an important role in posttraumatic flexion contracture.

A small posteromedial skin incision after isolated ulnar nerve allows the excision of the posterior bundle of the MCL with the medial part of the posterior capsule. Elbow full flexion is achieved.

When the extension contracture is present, the triceps is elevated from the posterior and distal surface of the humerus, and the fibrotic tissue in the olecranon fossa should be completely excised.

The medial operative approach described by Hotchkiss [41] for the treatment of posttraumatic elbow contractures is indicated when we have ulnar neuropathy or posteromedial HO located over the posteromedial aspect of the elbow (Fig. 8). The medial extensive approach is also indicated when the severe capsule contracture is associated with posteromedial or anteromedial HO bone bars (class IIA, IIB, or III of Hastings and Graham classification) [14]. In these cases the ulnar nerve is often encased in HO, without clinical symptoms of nerve entrapment. The ulnar nerve should be carefully protected from any surgical injury when the operative bone excision and capsulectomy are performed. After ensuring nerve freedom, the anterior transposition is indicated in the subcutaneous or submuscular position.

The lateral or medial approach is generally the best choice to treat contracture of the soft tissue and isolated posterolateral or posteromedial HO.

We suggest the use of a midline posterior approach ("the global approach") when the elbow is ankylosed for multilocation or extensive HO. The postoperative management is essential to keep the arc of motion achieved in the operating room.

The post-operative protocol program is:

- leave one or two drains in the anterior and the posterior aspect of the joint and another one posteriorly in the subcutaneous tissue;
- keep the elbow in a full extension bandage; the arm should be elevated with the elbow above the shoulder for 24-36 h;
- after surgery, examine the nerve function, in particular the state of the ulnar nerve, before performing the continuous brachial plexus block anesthesia with axillary catheter;

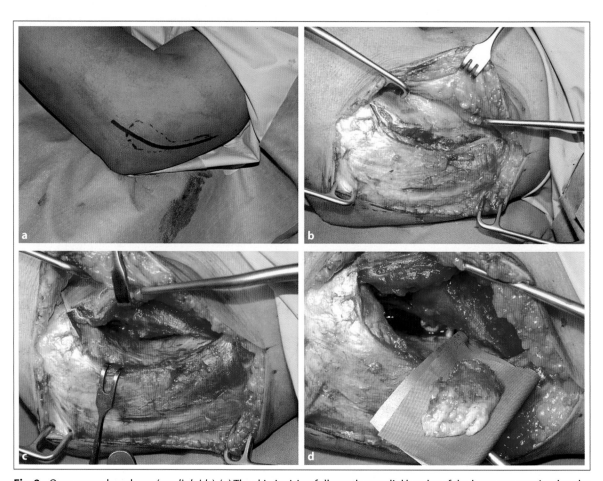

Fig. 8. Open capsular release (*medial side*). (**a**) The skin incision follows the medial border of the humerus proximal to the lateral epicondyle. (**b**) The ulnar nerve is identified and released if necessary. (**c**) The anterior muscles are lifted up from the anterior aspect of the humerus and a wide retractor allows the exposure of the anterior capsula. (**d**) The anterior capsulectomy is performed and the coronoid process is visualized

- on the same day, start the CPM machine through the full arc of motion. The maximum benefit of CPM occurs in the first 2-3 days when the movement reduces the early accumulation of fluid in the periarticular soft tissue;
- remove the bandage and maintain a simple elastic sleeve during the CPM exercises. It will prevent edema fluid and any stress to the skin and wound;
- stop the anesthesia block after 2-3 days;
- send the patient home with a CPM machine if there are no complications;
- help the patient to maintain the extreme position (full extension and full flexion) with adjusted static splint;
- prescribe indometacin as a prophylaxis against HO for 6 weeks post-operatively. The indometacin also helps to limit joint and soft tissue inflammation during the rehabilitation program.

Stiffness in Violated Articular Surfaces Without Osteoarticular Congruity

In the pre-operative clinical and radiographic assessment, the presence of significant articular deformity for fracture malalignment often creates a refashioning of the articular surface with painful elbow stiffness.

In planning the operative treatment several factors and several surgical options should be considered:
- the possibility of anatomically restoring the distorted articular surfaces (patients under 50 years old) in order to recover the appropriate alignment and osseous union with osteoarticular surgical corrections;
- the possibility of recognizing the articular surfaces if the limited loss of the articular cartilage is less than 50%: the best surgical option is the debridement arthroplasty;
- the presence of a distortion of joint surfaces and the lack of more than 50% of hyaline cartilage [42], in young patients with high physical demands, the distraction arthroplasty is performed. In recent literature, when the olecranon and radius articular surfaces are preserved, humerus hemiarthroplasty is advised as a salvage reconstruction [43];
- the impossibility of recovering any anatomical aspect of the articular surfaces for malunion, fixation failure, or nonunion or secondary osteoarthritis: in elder patients with low physical demands, the total elbow arthroplasty (TEA) is a salvage procedure.

The Osteoarticular Surgical Correction

In younger, active patients the anatomical restoration of the ulno-trochlear and radio-capitellar joints could be a good option to solve the problems of loss of motion and pain. Loss of motion of the elbow may be due to the articular deformity and the intra-articular or extra-articular adhesions, while pain is often due to intra-articular bone impingement and the presence of nonunion sites.

The first goal of surgical management is to restore the anatomical shape and size of the trochlea and capitellum so that they match the olecranon and RH during the flexion-extension movement.

The second goal is to achieve a secure internal fixation to allow early motion to attain a functional arc of motion.

In the intra-articular malunion the imaging studies (X-rays, CT) should help to define the real possibility of achieving the preoperative goals. In case of small osteopenic bone fragments the reconstruction may be difficult. The intra-articular osteotomy can be difficult to perform if there is a poor bone stock condylar element. In these cases TEA should be considered.

In distal humerus or proximal ulna and radius nonunions or malunions we have to distinguish the extra-articular pathology from the intra-articular [44].

The supracondylar distal humerus is the most frequent location of the extra-articular malunion or nonunion. The supracondylar malunion is usually "extension malunion," with retroversion of the articular condyles, as "the gun stock" deformity. The articular bone retroversion (if more than 10°-20°) changes the anatomical flexion-extension offset (the distance from longitudinal humeral axis to flexion-extension condylar axis): the elbow loses the over 90° flexion for coronoid impingement with anterior border of the distal humerus.

In the supracondylar malunion, the corrective osteotomy is performed with:
- posterior midline skin incision;
- neurolysis and transposition of the ulnar nerve into the subcutaneous tissue at the end of the surgery;
- the transtricipital or triceps sparing approach is adequate to have a good exposure;
- a biplanar osteotomy is performed in the sagittal plane and the articular surface is rotated anteriorly about 20°-30°.

We emphasize that we reach the 30° of the condylar antiversion when the anterior border of the distal humerus transects the midportion of the trochlea. In this way we have restored the normal anterior offset of the osteoarticular bone.

- Osteotomy stable fixation is obtained with two lateral precontoured plates;
- Soft tissue release is not often necessary.

The open reduction, instead of TEA option, could be considered in the treatment of the intra-articular humerus nonunion or malunion, especially in younger patients with higher physical demands and with good bone stock.

In 20 patients with intra-articular nonunion, Ackermann and Jupiter [19] reported the following outcomes: excellent and good function regained in 7 patients (45%), and fair and poor in 13 patients (55%), although the union was achieved in 95% of the patients.

Mitsunaga et al. [45] reported an osseous healing in only 20 patients out of 25 (80%) and only 2 patients were judged to have sufficient stability after fixation to allow early postoperative motion. In this study the authors emphasized this concept as "union first and motion second."

Recently, in a retrospective study, Helfet et al. [46] reported that 51 out of 52 patients had bad union after open reduction and internal fixation. These authors believe that in order to achieve union it is more important to release the elbow contractures at the time of surgery. The main advantage is the redistribution of the normal forces across the elbow during postsurgical early motion. This reduces the bending forces through the ORIF in the delayed unions or nonunion sites.

A failed identification of coronal shearing trochlear and capitellum fractures may lead to elbow stiffness in extension and in flexion as well as the reduction of the elbow intrinsic osteoarticular stability, provided by the trochlea-olecranon joint [47].

The malunion of anterior articular fragments requires surgical treatment to correct the articular incongruity.

The supracondylar osteotomy is recommended to restore the articular alignment, avoiding narrowing the trochlea. The surgeon should pay attention while recovering an appropriate contact between the medial trochlea and anteromedial facet of coronoid and also between the capitellum and RH.

The definitive fixation is made with a contoured lateral column plate if the size of the fragment is sufficient. If the fragment is too small, the fixation is provided by using only buried Herbert screws and/or small threaded K wires.

Recently we performed an internal fixation of the articular fragment with rigid reabsorbable wires in association with an external fixator which is applied to attain the joint distraction, and which avoids early motion stresses on the articular fragment.

The distal humerus malunion or nonunion osteoarticular surgical correction is an extreme procedure that requires careful preoperative planning and a surgeon experienced in elbow surgery in order to recover the complex anatomy of the distal end of the humerus.

The rigid internal fixation and immediate postoperative mobilization enable improvement of the arc of motion with a high rate of fragment union.

In olecranon fractures, an inadequate reconstruction can lead to elbow stiffness with or without elbow instability.

The nonunion or malunion of the olecranon trochlear notch is relatively unusual because the fracture often occurs in the "void zone," between the coronoid and olecranon contact area.

The malunion often occurs during the surgical stabilization of the comminuted fractures. The compressive force with screws or tension band wiring narrows the olecranon-coronoid distance. In these cases, the patient may lose full elbow extension (about 30°).

The nonunion of the proximal ulna is not common. The technical errors to reduce the bone fragment or inadequate rigid internal fixation are important causes of olecranon nonunion [48].

The coronoid process nonunion often leads to posterior olecranon subluxation. The elbow becomes stiff in extension for impingement with the anterior border of the trochlea.

The goals of the treatment options are:

1. In case of malunion:
   - restore congruity of the sigmoid notch and realign the proximal ulna with the trochlea;
   - coronoid nonunions often require autologous bone grafts from the iliac crest to recover anterior olecranon stability;
   - recover the ligamentous stability and to maintain the ligamentous stability
   - recover early motion after surgery.
2. In case of nonunion:
   - debridement of the nonunion site and realignment of the fracture;
   - placement of an autologous cancellous bone graft;
   - fixation with a contoured dorsal plate.

In elderly patients when the proximal olecranon nonunion is less than 50%, and it is associated with malalignment of the articular surface, the most reliable option is the excision of the proximal nonunited fragment and the triceps tendon reattachment at the articular level [49-50].

TEA is a viable option when the malunion or nonunion is associated with osteoporosis or degenerative osteoarthritis.

The Arthroplasty – With or Without Total Elbow Replacement

In the current literature the surgical management of stiff elbow with more or less significant articular involvement is not well defined.

In many articles, there is terminological confusion about the term elbow arthroplasty.

Many elbow surgeons advocate the use of this term only when the surgery is related to the total elbow prosthesis procedures.

In the same way, other authors use this term for different surgical conservative options (interposition arthroplasty, debridement arthroplasty, and also distraction, resurfacing, remodelling, or recontouring arthroplasty).

In our opinion, the elbow arthroplasty embraces different surgical reconstructive procedures whose goal is to preserve, change, or replace the joint articular surface in order to recover painless motion and stability.

As a consequence, there are two types of elbow arthroplasty:
- conservative arthroplasty;
- replacement arthroplasty (hemi- or total elbow arthroplasty).

The choice of the treatment depends mainly on the state of the joint surface and on the patients' age.

In the preoperative clinical and radiographic assessment the surgeon should define the presence and the type of the articular abnormalities, which are frequent after-effects of intra-articular fractures.

Conservative Arthroplasty – Historical Review

We distinguish different periods in the history of elbow conservative arthroplasty.

The first period was characterized by efforts to recover motion through extra-articular resection of the elbow. Park [51], Park and Moreau [52], and Ollier [53] in Europe, and Barton [54] in USA were the main pioneers of this surgical procedure in the nineteenth century.

The second era of elbow arthroplasty begins at the dawn of the twentieth century. Surgeons abandoned the extra-articular resection because it often caused serious unstable elbows; a new, more conservative concept was developing, the intra-articular resection, which implied the removal of any damaged articular surfaces, followed by the interposition of the fascia lata.

In the USA, Murphy [55,56] was the first surgeon to introduce elbow arthroplasty with fat interposition, a technique that he further changed by using muscular fascia.

Years later Lexer [57] and Albee [58] declared the fat and fascia lata to be better substances for arthroplasty interposition and exalted the value of autologous tissues.

In 1918 Baer [59] used an animal membrane (a pig's bladder) as the interposition muscular flap. Meanwhile,

Putti [60] spread the use of elbow arthroplasty in Europe: in 1921 he performed a high number of interventions which implied the interposition of aponeurotic flap, previously drawn from fascia lata and fixed through catgut suture. Putti always chose his patients carefully: his target constituted young and adult patients (older than 20 years, younger than 50) affected by posttraumatic arthritis.

In 1922 Campbell [61] proposed a transtricipital approach to the elbow, while the European School always preferred Kocher's approach: he carved the aponeurotic tricipital flap which he used as interposition tissue between resected articular surfaces, then he fixed this flap to the anterior portion of capsule [62]. According to Campbell's theory this surgical intervention should be proposed to patients affected by post-traumatic ankylosis and acute arthritis (by Staphylococcus, Pneumococcus, and Streptococcus), obviously after a careful evaluation of the degree of patient collaboration. Patients with tubercular infection, high muscular atrophy, and large cicatricial tissue were excluded.

In the meantime, Mc Ausland [63] from Boston and Henderson from Mayo Clinic [64] developed the fascia lata interposition.

In Italy, we have to keep in mind remarkable authors Giuntini [65], Agrifoglio [66], Cappelin [67], and also Knight and Van Zandt [68]. In 1952, Lars [69] played an outstanding role.

Many authors tried out new materials in arthroplasty interposition: Froimson in 1976 [70] tried abdomen skin, whereas in 1977 Kita tested the J-K membrane with good results [71]. Meanwhile, Smith employed a kind of spongy gel called gefoarm [72]; in 1983, he also used a silicon membrane in six hemophilic patients with elbow ankylosis.

Today, after this long period of surgical experience, two different conservative options can be performed: the debridement arthroplasty and the interposition distraction arthroplasty.

The Debridement Arthroplasty

Tsuge described the debridement arthroplasty for elbow advanced primary osteoarthritis [73,74]. The debridement arthroplasty is generally indicated when more than 50% of the articular cartilage is preserved, and the size and shape of the articular bone anatomy are recognizable.

In our experience we have performed this technique in 60 patients from 1989 to 2000. The patients were affected by elbow stiffness due to degenerative osteoarthritis such as a sequela of intra-articular fractures or fracture-dislocation.

We have achieved 91.2% patient satisfaction and we concluded our review observing that the debridement arthroplasty is indicated in young, non-manual worker patients, and that the pain after this surgical treatment increases with manual activities and is often correlated to joint instability.

The bone debridement is an essential aspect of the elbow release.

Articular surfaces undergo characteristic pathologic changes in case of primary or secondary posttraumatic osteoarthritis involving elbow stiffness.

The changes include:

- osteophytes are often present in the olecranon, and olecranon fossa, and in the coronoid and coronoid fossa;
- heterotopic bone between the ulna-olecranon and radio-capitellum joints;
- deformity and narrowing of the ulno-humeral joint space;
- bone stock deficiency or erosion often affect the capitellum and the corresponding surfaces of the RH;
- deformity of both olecranon and coronoid fossa;
- the intra-articular soft tissue adhesion and triceps retraction;
- the ulnar nerve adhesion in the cubital tunnel and the posterior band of the MCL retraction.

In the debridement arthroplasty it is necessary to remove all these pathologic changes, then to reshape the articular surfaces border and at last to release the soft tissues, with ulnar nerve subcutaneous transposition.

The debridement arthroplasty does not require soft tissue interposition when the articular cartilage of the ulno-humeral joint is well preserved. The tissue interposition is indicated when the shape and size of the trochlea are preserved although a large cartilage deficiency is present.

The tissue interposition prevents the pain that early motion triggers after articular debridement.

If the olecranon and coronoid fossa are narrowed by hypertrophic bone formation or by fracture malunion, the articular surface could be debrided and reshaped after removing the olecranon and coronoid tip.

We perform the olecranon fossa fenestration (Kashiwagi's procedure) during the debridement arthroplasty only if the elbow loses the anterior rotation of the articular condyles (supracondylar malunion) with consequent ulno-humeral impingement in extension.

Kashiwagi [75] and Morrey [76] described this technique for the osteoarthritis treatment of the elbow joint. Morrey called this technique "ulno-humeral arthroplasty" [76] and considered it very appropriate for the treatment of primary osteoarthritis which had already minimally or moderately restrained the elbow extension.

The goal of an elbow debridement is to gain a wide exposure for removal of all the pathoanatomic structures which cause elbow stiffness.

The basic steps of the surgical techniques of the intra-articular debridement that we perform is similar to Tsuge's description, but our technical approach to deep structures is different. Specifically, we avoid detaching the triceps olecranon insertion, so the ulnar nerve neurolysis is not associated at medial epicondylectomy. In our technique we release the LCL from the humerus insertion rather than perform the Z lengthening of the LCL as described by Tsuge

The surgical steps:

- The patient is supine: his arm is flexed over the chest.
- An extensile posterolateral or longitudinal posterior skin incision (global approach) (Fig. 9a) is used.
- Full thickness soft tissue flap may be raised on both sides of the elbow.
- Subcutaneous medial flaps are cleared to expose and release the ulnar nerve at the cubital tunnel, and if necessary the common flexor tendon insertion for deep medial approach (Fig. 9b).
- The starting point for deep approach is lateral in the Kocher's interval and along the lateral column (Fig. 9c).
- The humerus brachio-radialis and the ECRL are detached anteriorly, and reflected from the triceps and anconeus posteriorly. We have to be careful about the radial nerve in the case of a dissection that lies proximally more than 7-8 cm from the lateral epicondyle [77].
- The dissection proceeds distally to isolate and preserve the LCL complex. We can spare the LCL through:
  - Cohen and Hastings' LCL sparing technique [78];
  - the extensile lateral exposure in order to detach and elevate the common extensor aponeurosis from the LCL;
  - to detach the LCL from the humeral insertion (Fig. 9d).

The LCL sparing technique involves an anterior and distal dissection [78] which runs between the extensor radialis longus and brevis. The whole anterior joint capsule can be exposed without disturbing the extensor tendon origins of the humeral epicondyle. The underlying lateral ligament complex is also preserved. We usually place a retractor under the brachialis and under the triceps: the anterior and posterior aspects of the joint are recognizable.

- We perform the anterior and posterior capsulectomy, paying attention to preserve the MCL (Fig. 9e).
- After releasing both the anteroposterior capsular contracture and the brachialis and triceps scar adhesion, the bone debridement starts removing anteriorly the overgrown soft tissue, reshaping the coronoid tip and deepening the coronoid and radial fossa (Fig. 9f).

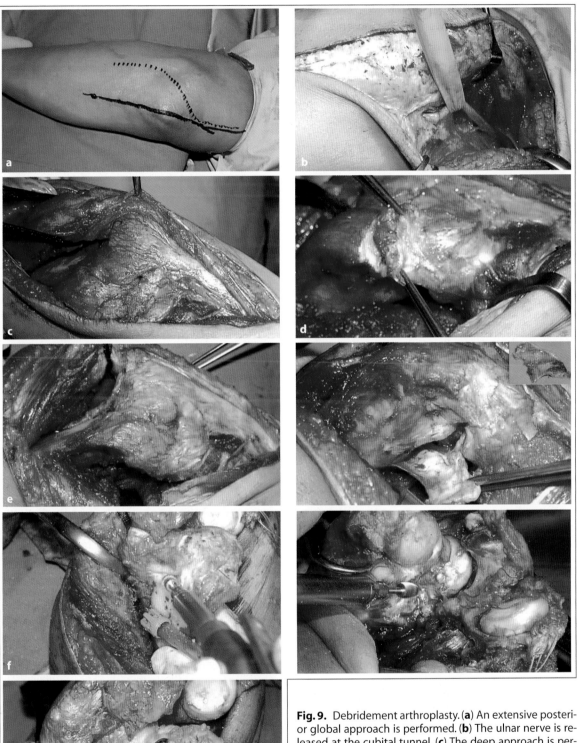

Fig. 9. Debridement arthroplasty. (**a**) An extensive posterior global approach is performed. (**b**) The ulnar nerve is released at the cubital tunnel. (**c**) The deep approach is performed laterally through the Kocher's interval and along the lateral column. (**d**) The LCL complex can also be detached from the humeral insertion, if necessary. (**e**) The anterior and posterior capsulectomy is performed. (**f**) The bone debridement is performed, restoring the coronoid tip and deepening the coronoid and radial fossa. (**g**) The posterior aspect of the trochlea is trimmed by removing all the osteophytes

- A trochlear notch recontouring osteotomy is often necessary to recover full flexion and to release the contracted posteromedial and transverse MCL band.
- After the excision of the posterior capsule, we smooth hypertrophic ridges around the olecranon fossa, which is deepened by rongeur and chisels.
- Osteophytes are usually recognizable on the tip of the olecranon as well as the bone deformity on medial and lateral edge. An oscillating saw is used at the olecranon border in order to avoid olecranon humerus impingement.
- The posterior aspect of the trochlea is trimmed by removing all the osteophytes and every articular incongruity (Fig. 9g).
- The debridement is complete after removing the HO which caused impingement.
- Lastly, we check the joint stability, flexo-extension movement, and forearm rotation.
- We use to make a plaster after surgery, in order to keep the elbow extended. The active and passive motion starts after 24 h. The splint may be often applied during the night.

The Interposition Arthroplasty

The interposition arthroplasty is a well-defined surgical procedure: it is useful in young and adult patients whose articular surfaces have been severely damaged (Figs. 10a-c).

The interposition arthroplasty is indicated if the articular anatomy cannot be recovered. In this case it is necessary to reshape the articular surfaces; therefore, autologous or omologous soft tissue interposition is useful to replace the cartilage absence.

Morrey et al. [79] proposed considering the interposition arthroplasty as the first option in case of a 50% cartilage loss and an incongruity due to articular fractures.

The interposition also is a viable surgical option for persistent dislocation or subluxation in younger patients (often involving bone and ligamentous structures with articular cartilage degeneration or articular bone loss).

Froimson and Morrey [80] described the use of Achilles' tendon allograft in order to cover the humerus and to reconstruct the lateral and medial collateral ligament.

The general concepts regarding elbow interposition arthroplasty are as follows:
- a wide surgical exposure is recommended in order to allow the management of the damaged extensive peri- and intra-articular tissue;

- the recontouring osteotomy and reshaping of the humerus and ulna surfaces: to recreate a new joint with a relative congruence, similar to anatomic articular bone;
- the fascial tissue interposition; (omologous or autologous);
- hinged elbow external fixator is applied.
The surgical steps:
- A posterior skin incision (the global posterior approach [81] or the posterolateral extensible Kocher's approach) allow the surgeon to obtain circumferential deep exposure of the elbow.
- The ulnar nerve is decompressed, released, and protected.
- The anterior capsule and the brachialis muscle are released from the anterior aspect of the humerus. The posterior capsule, the triceps, and anconeus muscles are released from the posterior cortex and the humerus lateral column in order to preserve the triceps tendon insertion on the olecranon.
- Any adhesions between the muscles and the humerus are removed.
- The anterior and posterior capsulectomy are performed (Fig. 11).
- The LCL complex is released from the humerus insertion, often linked to the common extensor tendon, detaching it from the humerus without dissection in order to preserve the complex tendon and the ligament unit. The muscular splitting is carried out between the ECRL and brevis. Otherwise, we detach the LCL complex separately from the common extensor muscles and the tendons, which are elevated in continuity with the ECRL.
- The LCM anterior band is preserved: the elbow is opened and dislocated with hypersupination and flexion manoeuvres are generally useful to associate the external rotation of the humerus.
- The joint is hinged at the medial side on the ulnar collateral ligament and the tendon flexor insertion.
- The distal humerus is contoured by cutting out osteophytes and malunited bone fragments and fibrous debris. After removing the outstanding amount of cartilage, the trochlea is deepened and widened without changing its smooth, round surface. The deepness of the humeral articular surface should be preserved. It is necessary to remove any bone irregularity that could disturb the movement. This way we keep the shape of the trochlea and consequently relative ulno-humeral bone stability. Besides, we debride and resect the RH only if necessary, in case of malunion or nonunion limiting the prono-supination movement. The RH presence improves medial lateral stability.

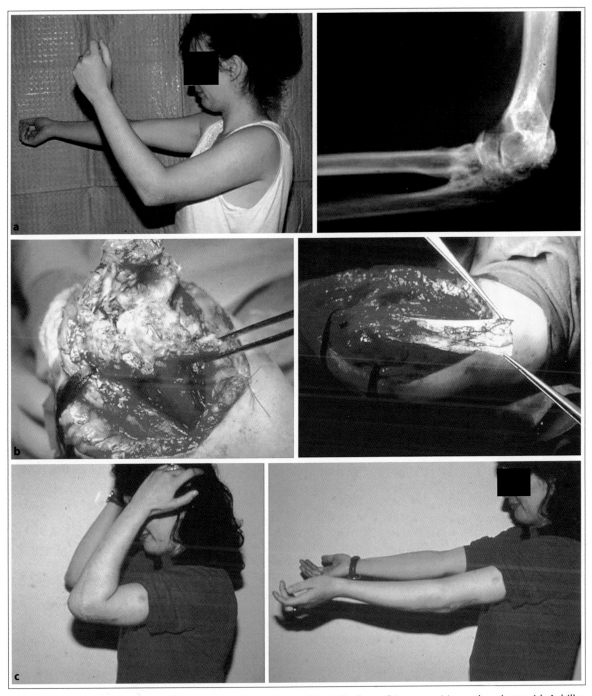

Fig. 10. (**a**) 35-year-old patient with posttraumatic ankylosis of her left elbow. (**b**) Interposition arthroplasty with Achilles tendon allograft (used for the ulno-humerus interposition and for the ligaments reconstruction). (**c**) Clinical evaluation at 8-year follow-up

There is general agreement about the tissue interposition, which can be:
- Autologous tissue:
  - Fascia lata graft harvest: the dissection is done from the lateral aspect of the thigh, measuring 8 cm by 20 cm, from proximal to distal direction.

- Cutis graft: according to Froimson's Technique [82] the skin graft is removed from the patients' lower abdomen, while for Morrey's Technique [79-80] strips of epidermis are sharply removed from an ellipse of skin taken from the groin region or bikini line.

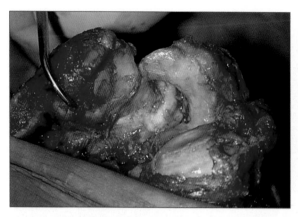

Fig. 11. The interposition orthroplasty. The anterior and posterior capsulectomy is performed, the LCL is released from the humerus and the elbow joint is exposed with hypersupinations and flection monoeurvres

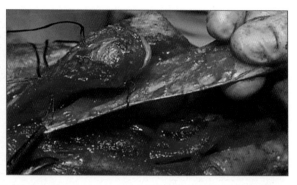

Fig. 12. The interposition orthroplasty. The Achilles tendon allograft is interposed to cover the humeral articular surface and to reconstruct the ligaments

- Omologous tissue:
  - Achilles tendon allograft (Morrey's technique) [83] is used to cover the humerus, and in case of ligament deficiency one or both ligaments can be reconstructed using the remaining parts of the tendon graft (Fig. 12). We have to be careful not to remove more trochlea and capitellum bone in order to avoid articular instability. It is important to remember that the maximum graft thickness could reduce the ulno-humeral bone congruity.
  - The surgeon transfers the graft to cover the humerus and, if necessary, the olecranon greater sigmoid notch; therefore, he sutures the interposed tissue with several small holes through the proximal condyles and along the medial and lateral epicondyle ridges. If the collateral ligaments are defective they could be reconstructed through lateral and medial strips of the Achilles' tendon graft used to cover the humerus.
  - At the end of the procedure the lateral ligament and tendon complex are reattached to the bone through drill holes placed in the lateral epicondyle. The hinged external fixator is always applied: the hinged fixation allows better joint stability until the soft tissues heal adequately during the postoperative free motion. It is also possible to distract the joint space (at least 3 mm through a full arc of motion) to protect the interposition material (Fig. 13).

The most critical step in the hinged fixation application is the correct placement of the axis pin in the center of the elbow axis of rotation [84].

The flexo-extension axis pin on the capitellum has to be generally located at the site of attachment of the lateral ligaments, while the axis pin has to ex-

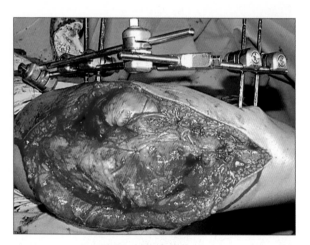

Fig. 13. The interposition orthroplasty. The external fixator is used to protect the ligaments and to distract the joint space

it medially at the anterior and inferior site of the medial epicondyle.

Different hinged elbow external fixators are available.

In our experience we consider the Mayo Device (Dynamic Joint Distractor II) simple to use and very comfortable for the patients (Fig. 14). On the contrary, the Orthofix Elbow Fixator is simple to apply but it is heavy and very uncomfortable. The Compass Universal Hinge is more difficult to apply: it is recommended only for single use. This device is very expensive.

The continuous brachial plexus block permits early postoperative mobilization of the elbow. After the interposition distraction arthroplasty a patient should use a CPM device for many hours each day (18-20 h).

Early active motion is recommended. We do not permit passive forced stretching by the therapist. After 4-5 weeks the hinged fixator is removed under anesthesia, and elbow motion and stability are

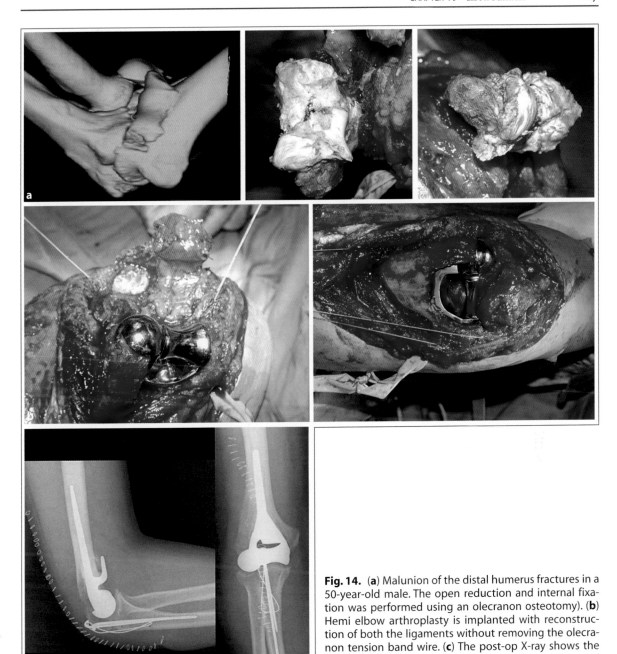

Fig. 14. (**a**) Malunion of the distal humerus fractures in a 50-year-old male. The open reduction and internal fixation was performed using an olecranon osteotomy). (**b**) Hemi elbow arthroplasty is implanted with reconstruction of both the ligaments without removing the olecranon tension band wire. (**c**) The post-op X-ray shows the congruency between the olecranon articular surface and the trochlea of the hemi-implant

examined. The elbow brace is applied to protect active and passive motion.

Replacement Arthroplasty (Total or Hemi Elbow Arthroplasty)

Total elbow arthroplasty (TEA) (both linked and unlinked prosthesis) are performed in extreme cases:
• if no salvage procedure is possible;

• if patients are aged, with low physical demands, and osteoporotic bone and a conservative treatment could imply complications [85-86].

Implant failure is the most common complication after TEA in younger patients.

The choice between the linked or unlinked device depends on the type and amount of the joint deformity. The linked semiconstrained designs play a predominant role in our institution: we usually implant the Conrad Morrey prosthesis. We consider the main indication for elbow replacement in the post-traumatic elbow stiffness in cronic unreduced subluxation or dislocationin aged patients or in case of intra-articular bone deformity for malunion or nonunion.

Distal humeral hemiarthroplasty could be appropriate in younger patients who need reconstruction of malunion, intra-articular avascular necrosis and unreduced shear fracture involving the capitellum and lateral trochlea (Figs. 14a-c) [43].

The Authors Preferred Classification and Management of The Post-traumatic Stiff Elbow

Various attempts have been made to relate treatment options to the types and extension of the anatomo-pathological lesions in the posttraumatic stiff elbow.

Similarly, the classification was defined on the basis of the schematic principle to localize the injury in to the articular and extra-articular area.

Most adverse outcomes in stiff elbow management are related to failure in the choice of treatment options.

The decision-making process regarding operative technique must be correlated with the surgeon's capacity to localize the relevant abnormalities in the periarticular or intra-articular tissue and to choose and perform an adequate surgical technique.

To make the task of the readers easier regarding a better scientific rationale in the management of the stiff elbow, we point out in a schematic summary the relationship between the main injury patterns and the management options (Table 1).

Table 1. The posttraumatic stiff elbow can be classified in three grades of progressive main injury patterns. Our schematic summary enables definition of the correct surgical choice for each grade of stiff elbow

Posttraumatic Elbow Stiffness	The Main Injury Patterns	Associated Lesions	Limited Motion	Management Options
Grade 1	Contracture of the periarticular soft tissue	• Capsule and ligament contracture • Muscle and tendon retraction	In FLEXION Contracture of: • Posterior Capsule • Posterior band of LCM In EXTENSION: Contracture of: • Anterior Capsule • Anterior band of the LCM In FLEXION-EXTENSION: Contracture of: • Anterior and Posterior Capsule • LCL ± Posterior band of LCM	• Rehabilitation program • Surgical release: – Arthroscopic – Open Limited approach
Grade 2	Hectopic Ossification • Limited areas – Medial – Lateral – Anterior – Posterior • Myositis ossificans • Bone bridge • Osseous ankylosis	• Contracture of the periarticular soft tissue	• FLEXION-EXTENSION (II-A)* • PRONO-SUPINATION (II-B) * • FLEXION-EXTENSION and PRONO-SUPINATION (II-C)* • ANKYLOSIS (III)* * Hastings and Graham classification (14)	OPEN SURGERY: – Limited approach: – Hectopic Ossification excision – Extensile approach: Hectopic bone brigde excision

Grade 3	The Articular Surface Incongrunity
	
	• LIMITED CARTILAGE EROSION
	– Less than 50%
	– Articular marginal bone deformity
	– Osteophytes
	  - Omero-radial
	  - Omero-olecranon
	
	• EXTENSIVE CARTILAGE EROSION
	– More than 50%
	– Bone distortion
	– Osteoarticular instability
		• Contracture of the periarticular soft tissue
		• Hectopic ossification
			SEVERE LOSS OF MOTION:
			• FLEXION-EXTENSION
			• PRONO-SUPINATION
				Limited debridment:
				– Arthroscopic
				– Ulno-Humeral (O.K. procedure)
				Extensile debridment:
				– Debridment arthroplasty (Tsuge technique)
				– Osteoarticular correction
				
				– Interposition arthroplasty (Morrey procedure)
				– Replacement arthroplasty

The stiff elbow was graduated in three progressive injury patterns:

- In the first grade, the greater surgical priority is the soft tissue release.
- In the second grade, the most important surgical priority is the excision of HO.
- In the third grade, surgical treatment of the articular surface incongruity is the greater priority than HO excision and soft tissue release.

References

1. Demling RH, Lalonde C (1989) Rehabilitation and wound remodelling. In: Burn trauma. Thieme, New York pp 209-213
2. Peterson SL, Mani MM, Crawford CM et al (1989) Post burn heterotopic ossification in sights for management decision making. J Trauma 29:365-369
3. Josefsson PO, Johnell O, Gentz CF (1984) Long-term sequalae of simple dislocation of the elbow. J Bone Joint Surg Am 66:927-930
4. Mehlhoff TL, Noble PL, Bennet JB et al (1988) Simple dislocation of the elbow in the adults. Results after closed treatment. J Bone Joint Surg Am 70:244-249
5. O'Driscoll SW, Morrey BF, Karinek S et al (1992) Elbow subluxation and dislocation: A spectrum of instability. Clin Orthop 74:1235-1241
6. Linscheid RL, Wheeler DK (1965) Elbow dislocation. JAMA 194:1171-1176
7. Joseffson PO, Gentz CF, Johnell O et al (1987) Surgical versus non surgical treatment of ligamentous injuries following dislocation of the elbow joint: A prospective randomized study. J Bone Joint Surg Am 69:605-608
8. Buring K (1975) On the origin of cells in heterotopic bone formation. Clin Orthop 110:293-302
9. Urist MR, De Longo RJ, Finerman S (1989) Bone cells differentiation and growth factors. Science 220:680
10. Thompson HC III, Garcia A (1967) Myositis ossificans: Aftermath of elbow injuries. Clin Orthop 50:129
11. Bromberg MA, Morrey BF (1973) Results of delayed excision of the radial head after fracture. J Bone Joint Surg Am 55:1629
12. Sazbon L, Najenson T et al (1981) Widespread periarticular new-bone formation in long term comatose patients. J Bone Joint Surg Br 63:120
13. Garland DE, Dowling V (1983) Forearm fractures in the head-injured adult. Clin Orthop 176:190-196
14. Hastings H II, Graham TJ (1994) The classification and treatment of heterotopic ossification about the elbow and forearm. Hand Clin 10:417-437
15. Garland DE, Blum C, Waters RL (1985) Periarticular heterotopic ossification in head injured adults: Incidence and location. J Bone Joint Surg Am 67:1261-1269
16. Jupiter JB (1994) Complex fractures of the distal part of the humerus and associated complications. J Bone Joint Surg Am 76:1252-1264
17. Jupiter JB, Goodmann LJ (1992) The management of complex distal humerus non unions in the elderly by elbow capsulotomy, triple platting and ulnar nerve neurolysis. J Shoulder Elbow Surg 1:37
18. Bryan RS, Bickel WH (1971) "T" condylar fractures of the distal humerus. J Trauma 11:830-835
19. Ackerman G, Jupiter JB (1988) Non union of fractures of the distal end of the humerus. J Bone Joint Surg Am 70:75-83
20. Kolenak A (1977) Ununited fracture of the lateral condyle of the humerus. A 50 years follow-up. Clin Orthop 124:181
21. Heldsworth BJ, Mossadmn (1984) Elbow function following tension band fixation of displaced fractures of the olecranon. Injury 16:182-187
22. Helm RH, Hornshy R, Miller SWM (1987) The complication of surgical treatment of displaced fractures of the olecranon. Injury 18:48-50
23. Kiviluoto O, Santavirta S (1978) Fractures of the olecranon. Acta Orthop Scand 49:28-31
24. Morrey BF (1990) Posttraumatic contracture of the elbow. J Bone Joint Surg Am 72:601-618
25. Ewald FC, Scheinberg RD, Poss R et al (1980) Capitello condylar total elbow arthroplasty: Two to five year follow up in rheumatoid arthritis. J Bone Joint Surg Am 62:1259
26. Inglis A, Pellicci PM (1980) Total elbow replacement. J Bone Joint Surg Am 62:1252-1258
27. Pritchard RW (1977) Total elbow arthroplasty in joint replacement in the upper limb. London Mechanical Engineering Publications, London, p 61
28. Broberg MA, Morrey BF (1987) Results of treatment of fracture dislocations of the elbow. Clin Orthop 216:109-119
29. Morrey BF (1993) Functional evaluation of the elbow In: Morrey BF (ed) The elbow and its disorders, 2nd edn. WB Saunders, Philadelphia
30. Morrey BF, Askew LJ, An K, Chao E (1981) A biomechanical study of normal functional elbow motion. J Bone Joint Surg Am 63:872-877
31. Garland DE, Blum C, Waters RL (1980) Periarticular heterotopic ossification in head injured adults: Incidence and location. J Bone Joint Surg Am 62:1143-1146
32. Stover SL, Hataway CJ, Zeiger HE (1975) Heterotopic ossification in spinal cord-injured patients. Arch Phys Med Rehab 56:199
33. Morrey BF (2000) Splints and bracing at the elbow. In: The elbow and its disorders. WB Saunders, Philadelphia, pp 150-155
34. O'Driscoll SW, Morrey BF (1992) Arthroscopy of the elbow: Diagnostic and therapeutic benefits and hazards. J Bone Joint Surg Am 74:84-94
35. Gallay SH, Richards RR, O'Driscoll SW (1993) Intra articular capacity and compliance of stiff and normal elbows. Arthroscopy 9:9-13
36. O'Driscoll SW (2004) Arthroscopic release. Instructional course: The assessment of management of elbow stiffness and arthritis. 71st Meeting of A.A.O.S., San Francisco
37. Kashiwagi D (1978) Articular changes of the osteoarthritic elbow especially about the fossa olecranon. J Jap Orthop Assoc 52:1367-1382
38. Mansat P, Morrey BF (1998) The column procedure: A limited lateral approach for extrinsic contracture of the elbow. J Bone Joint Surg Am 1603-1615
39. Cohen MS, Hastings H (1998) Post traumatic contracture of the elbow: Operative release using a lateral collateral sparing approach. J Bone Joint Surg Br 80:805-812
40. Wada T, Ishii S, Usui M et al (2000) The medial approach for operative release of post traumatic contracture of the elbow. J Bone Joint Surg Br 82:68-73

41. Hotchkiss RN (1999) Elbow contracture. In: Green DP, Hotchkiss RN, Pederson WC (eds) Green's operative hand surgery, 4th edn. Churchill Livingston, Philadelphia, pp 667-682

42. Morrey BF (1990) Post-traumatic contracture of the elbow. Operative treatment including distraction arthroplasty. J Bone Joint Surg Am 72:601-618

43. Parson M, O'Brien S, Hughes J (2005) Elbow hemiarthroplasty for acute and salvage reconstruction of intra articular distal humerus fractures. Tech Shoulder Elbow Surg 6:82-97

44. Sim FH, Morrey BF (2000) Non union and delayed union of distal humeral fractures. In: Morrey BF (ed) The elbow and its disorders, 3rd edn. WB Saunders, Philadelphia pp 331-340

45. Mitsunaga MM, Bryan RS, Linscheid RL (1982) Condylar non union of the elbow. J Trauma 22:787-791

46. Helfet D, Kloen P, Anand N, Rosen H (2003) Open reduction and internal fixation of delayed unions and non unions of fractures of the distal part of the humerus. J Bone Joint Surg Am 85:33-40

47. McKee MD, Jupiter JB, Bamberger HB (1996) Coronal shear fractures of the distal end of the humerus. J Bone Joint Surg Am 78:49-54

48. Papagelogoulos P, Morrey B (1994) Treatment of non union of olecranon fractures. J Bone Joint Surg Br 76:627-635

49. Gartsman GM, Sculo TP, Otis JC (1981) Operative treatment of olecranon fractures. J Bone Joint Surg Am 63:718

50. Dunn N (1939) Operative for fracture of the olecranon. Br Med 1:214

51. Park H (1783) An account of a new method of treating diseases of the joint of the knee or elbow, in a letter to Mr. Percivall Pott. Printed for J Johnson. HDM Collection, London

52. Park H, Moreau PF (1806) Cases of the excision of carious joints. HDM Collection, University Press, Glasgow

53. Ollier L (1885) Traite' des resections et des operations conservatrices qu'on peut pratiquer sur le systeme osseux. Tome Troiseme, Masson, Paris, pp 991-970

54. Barton JR (1827) On the treatment of ankylosis by the formation of artificial joints. North Am Med Surg J 3:279-400

55. Murphy JB (1904) Ankylosis: Arthroplasty-clinical and experimental. Trans Am Surg Assoc 22:215

56. Murphy JB (1905) Ankylosis: Arthroplasty of elbow. JAMA 44:1573

57. Lexer E (1917) Das beweglichmachen versteifter gelenke mit und ohne gewebszwischenlagerung. ZBL Chir 44:1

58. Albee F (1931) The principles of arthroplasty. J Am Med Ass 96:245-249

59. Baer WS (1918) Arthroplasty with the aid of animal membrane. Amer J Orth Surg 16:171-199

60. Putti V (1921) Arthroplasty. AM J Orthop Surg 3:421

61. Campbell WC (1922) Arthroplasty of the elbow. Ann Surg 76:615-623

62. Campbell WC (1924) Mobilization of the joints with bony ankylosis. JAMA 83:976-980

63. Mac Ausland WR (1947) Arthroplasty of the elbow. New Engl J Med 236:97

64. Henderson MS (1925) Artrhoplasty. Minnes Med 8:97

65. Giuntini L (1934) Sulla cura delle fratture di gomito e dei loro esiti. Archivio Ortopedico 50:291

66. Agrigoglio E, Marcacci G (1953) Emiresezione artroplastica nelle fratture comminute del gomito. Minerva Ortopedica, pp 134-138

67. Cappelin M (1952) L'artroplastica come trattamento precoce primario delle gravi fratture comminute del gomito e dell'adulto. Minerva Ortopedica, pp 186-194

68. Knight R, Van Zandt L (1952) Arthroplasty of the elbow. J Bone Joint Surg 34:610-618

69. Lars U (1965) Experience of arthroplasty of the elbow. Acta Orthop Scand 36:54-61

70. Froimson AI, Silva JE, Wayne G (1976) Cutis arthroplasty of the elbow joint. J Bone Joint Surg 58:863-865

71. Kita M (1977) Arthroplasty of the elbow using J-K membrane, analysis of 31 cases. Acta Orthop Scand 48:450-455

72. Smith M, Savidge G, Fountain E (1983) Interposition arthroplasty in the management of advanced haemophilic arthroplasty of the elbow. J Bone Joint Surg 65:436-440

73. Tsuge K, Murakami T, Yasumaga Y et al (1982) Arthroplasty of the elbow: Twenty years experience of a new approach. J Bone Joint Surg Br 69:116-120

74. Tsuge K, Mizusek T (1994) Debridement arthroplasty for advanced primary osteoarthritis of the elbow: Results of a new technique used for 29 elbows. J Bone Joint Surg Br 76:641-646

75. Kashiwagi D (1986) Outerbridge-Kashiwagi arthroplasty for osteoarthritis of the elbow in the elbow joint. In: Kashiwagi D (ed) Proceedings of the International Congress. Kobi Japan Excerpta Medica, Amsterdam

76. Morrey BF (1992) Primary arthritis of the elbow treated by ulnohumeral arthroplasty. J Bone Joint Surg Br 74:409-413

77. Guse TR, Ostrum RF (1995) The surgical anatomy of the radial nerve around the humerus. Clin Orthop 320:149-153

78. Cohen MS, Hastings H (1998) Post traumatic contracture of the elbow: Operative release using a lateral collateral ligament sparing approach. J Bone Joint Surg Br 80:805-812

79. Morrey BF (1990) Post traumatic contracture of the elbow operative treatment including distraction arthroplasty. J Bone Joint Surg Am 72:601-618

80. Froisom AI, Morrey BF (2002) Interposition arthroplasty of the elbow. In: Morrey BF (ed) The elbow master technique in orthopaedic surgery, 2nd edn. Lippincott, New York, pp 391 408

81. Patterson SD, Baw GI, Mhta SA (2000) Surgical approaches to the elbow. Clin Orthop 370:19-33

82. Froimson AI, Silva JE, Rickey D (1976) Cutis arthroplasty of the elbow joint. J Bone Joint Surg Am 58:863-865

83. Wrigt PE, Froimson AI, Morrey BF (2000) Interposition arthroplasty of the elbow. In: Morrey BF (ed) The elbow and its disorders. WB Saunders, Philadelphia, pp 718-730

84. Tan V, Saluiski A, Capo J, Hotchkiss R (2005) Hinged elbow external fixates: Indication and uses. J Am Acad Orthop Surg 13:503-514

85. Schneeberger AG, Adams R, Morrey BF (1992) Semiconstrained total elbow replacement for the treatment of post traumatic osteoarthrosis. J Bone Joint Surg Am 79:1211-1222

86. Moro JK, King GW (2000) Total elbow arthroplasty in the treatment of post traumatic conditions of the elbow. Clin Orthop 370:102-114

CHAPTER 20

The Arthroscopic Treatment of the Stiff Elbow

S.W. O'DRISCOLL

Introduction

Loss of elbow motion due to trauma or arthritis is common and significantly impairs function of the upper extremity. Morrey et al. [1] documented in 33 normal volunteers that the activities of daily living (ADLs) require a functional arc of approximately 100° of flexion and extension of the elbow (30°-130°).

The purpose of the elbow is to place the hand within the volume of a sphere that is centered about the shoulder. This is distinguished from the purpose of the shoulder, which places the hand on the surface of the same sphere. As the elbow permits the hand to move to and from the center of the sphere, it effectively determines the radius of the sphere of reach of the hand. The volume of the sphere is proportional to the cube of its radius, so that any loss of elbow motion can significantly diminish the volume of reach of the hand. Unfortunately, contractures of the elbow are common following trauma, but can also result from surgery, arthritis, and other conditions.

Assessment

To appreciate how much the loss of mobility compromises a patient's functional capabilities, questions are asked concerning ADLs. As many patients also have pain it is important to ask which is the higher priority-relief from pain or improvement in motion. Patients with congenital contractures and those acquired at a very young age typically feel less impaired than does a patient who acquired a similar degree of contracture as an adult or teen. Thus, management decisions are more appropriately made according to the degree of functional impairment rather than on the basis of the absolute loss of motion or joint contracture. It will be important to understand the details of the original injury as well as initial treatment. Associated conditions including infection, neurologic dysfunction, and ipsilateral limb injury will also influence management decisions.

Examination of the patient should include an assessment of the entire upper limb. Particular attention is given to the ulnar nerve in light of its all too common involvement in elbow trauma. Patients should be specifically asked whether or not they have pain in the region of the cubital tunnel with attempts to fully flex or extend the elbow. A positive response would suggest ulnar neuritis as a possible contributing factor to the contracture. In some instances, a patient may not appreciate subtle changes in the ulnar innervated muscles, due to greater focus on the difficulty associated with their elbow. Testing for evaluation of two-point discrimination, pinch strength, and intrinsic muscle function as well as electrophysiologic parameters can be important to document pre-operatively the status of the ulnar nerve.

With the widespread availability of high-quality 3-D CT scanning, particularly surface rendering, radiological assessment of the stiff elbow is now most complete by adding this imaging modality to the standard radiographs, especially when there are osteophytes, heterotopic ossification, or any other alteration in the bony or articular anatomy. CT scans with sagittal and coronal reconstructions along with 3-D surface rendering have completely replaced conventional tomograms.

In determining the optimal timing for removal of heterotopic ossification, there are two factors to be considered. The first is the maturity of the heterotopic bone, as indicated by a smooth well-demarcated cortical margin and defined trabecular markings. These are best appreciated by comparing sequential radiographs. The second factor is the time since onset. Usually bone is mature enough to be removed by 3-6 months following its appearance.

Arthroscopic Treatment Options

Surgical treatment can be performed using open or arthroscopic techniques, or by a combination of the two. This chapter will focus on arthroscopic release of an elbow contracture, a procedure that is clearly efficacious, though its safety is still being studied.

The indications and techniques for arthroscopic contracture release are rapidly evolving. It has become clear to those surgeons experienced in the technique that arthroscopy will indeed play a major role in the surgical treatment of elbow stiffness [2-11].

Indications for Arthroscopic Contracture Release

The indications for arthroscopic contracture release include impairment of function with limitation in the activities of daily living or other important activities that a patient may wish to pursue. In some patients, the loss of motion is painless, while in others the primary complaint is pain at the end-points of motion. Often due to impingement of fractured osteophytes or loose bodies, this is commonly seen in osteoarthritis. Traditionally, surgery has been offered only to patients with flexion contractures of at least 30° or who could not flex past about 120° or 130°. However, as arthroscopic contracture release evolves, the potential for restoring even more minor losses of motion with minimal complications appears more feasible. For some patients who require full or nearly full motion due to specific lifestyle demands, this is an important concern.

Simple vs Complex Contractures

In considering the arthroscopic management of elbow contractures, it is extremely helpful to distinguish those cases that require extensive surgical expertise in both arthroscopy and stiff elbow surgery, or have a high likelihood of complications, from those cases for which neither of these two concerns apply. In other words, one might wish to differentiate complex from simple cases. For the purpose of this discussion, the term "simple" in relation to elbow stiffness will be used to denote those contractures that meet all of the following criteria:
- mild to moderate contracture (ROM = 80° or less);
- no or minimal prior surgery;
- no prior ulnar nerve transposition;
- no or minimal internal fixation hardware in place;
- no or minimal heterotopic ossification;
- normal bony anatomy has been preserved.

It is likely that these criteria will be present in patients with contractures due to mild to moderate primary osteoarthritis or rheumatoid arthritis, as well as those adolescents with contractures related to osteochondritis dissecans of the capitellum. The majority of patients with post-traumatic stiffness fail to meet one or more of these criteria.

Patients with complex contractures (i.e. those who fail to meet all of the criteria for a "simple contracture") are probably best referred to a surgeon with special training and expertise in elbow surgery, both open and arthroscopic. For safety reasons, arthroscopic treatment, if it is a consideration in a patient with a complex contracture, should only be performed by a surgeon with a substantial volume of experience in arthroscopic techniques of contracture release.

Technique of Arthroscopic Contracture Release

Before describing the technique of performing an arthroscopic contracture release, it would be wise to consider the risks and difficulties. Gallay et al. [12] showed that capsular contracture leads to marked loss of intra-articular volume capacity to an average of just 6 ml in stiff elbows compared to 25 ml in normal elbows [13]. This limits the value of capsular distension in displacing the nerves away from operating instruments (Fig. 1). Timmerman et al. [14] found that access was so difficult in some cases of arthroscopic release as to prevent visualization altogether. Thus, it is essential that the operating surgeon be aware of special techniques developed for working in stiff elbows.

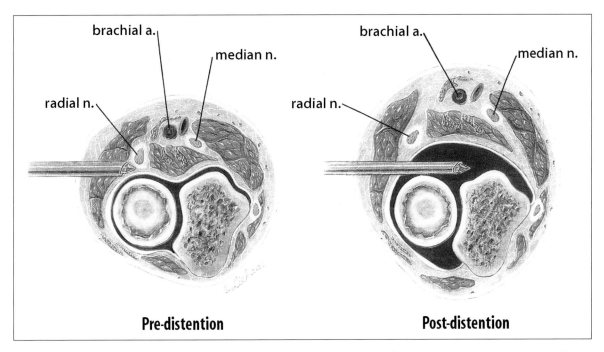

Fig. 1. Capsular distention, which in a normal elbow displaces the nerves away from the operating instruments, is of limited value in a stiff elbow due to decreased capsular compliance. Thus, it is important to retract the capsule away from the humerus, thereby creating a space within which to work. (Figure reproduced with permission from Chantal O'Driscoll)

In our experience, the most important technical factor that facilitates performing a capsular release is the use of retractors inside the joint [8]. In this regard, the use of retractors in the authors' experience is also the key determinant that permits more complex procedures to be performed safely, without nerve injury. Retractors, which are routinely used in open surgery, are required for proper visualization and to retract nerves away from motorized and cutting instruments. In addition, by retracting the capsule, pressurized distension is not needed and therefore swelling is less likely to become a serious impediment to progress. Therefore, one must be prepared to use multiple portals (one for the scope, one for the shaver/cutter, one or two for retractors). I am often asked whether one should start anteriorly or posteriorly. Apart from personal preference or how one was taught, several factors influence this decision. Included in this consideration are one's experience and confidence operating posteriorly *vs* anteriorly, familiarity and proficiency with the use of retractors, and nature and location of major pathology, as well as other factors. After trying both ways for a number of years, I have come to believe that it may be more effective to begin with the posterior capsule release and then procedure to the anterior release, which is what I now do routinely.

Posterior Capsular Release

The sequence of steps for arthroscopic posterior capsular release is as follows. The first objective is to *get in and establish a view*. With the scope in the posterolateral portal and the shaver in the posterior portal (or the scope in the direct midlateral or/and the shaver in the posterolateral portal), establish a view by debriding the olecranon fossa and 'create a space' within which to work. A radiofrequency ablation device can be helpful to remove dense scar tissue, but over heating the joint fluid can cause chondrolysis. Next, the capsule can be elevated from the distal humerus to further increase further the working space. This can be done with a shaver or periosteal elevator. A retractor placed in a proximal posterolateral portal is useful to maintain that space. The next step is to perform a synovectomy if there is synovitis. The capsule should be preserved until the synovectomy is complete. Doing so makes it easier and safer to perform the capsulectomy. At this stage, the osteophytes are removed. Loose bodies are removed as they are encountered. Once any abnormal bone or osteophytes have been removed, the posterior capsule is resected. This is performed with a shaver or radiofrequency ablation device, most easily through the posterolateral portal.

The posterolateral capsule is then resected. The posteromedial capsule must be released if there is a significant lack of flexion. If the elbow does not flex past about 90°-110°, the posterior band of the MCL will have to be released to regain that motion. Since this tissue represents the floor of the cubital tunnel, the ulnar nerve is at significant risk of injury (Fig. 2). The nerve is closer to the epicondyle than to the tip of the olecranon, so release of the capsule is safer along the olecranon. A retractor placed in the proximal posterolateral portal, or even a proximal posterior portal (sometimes two retractors), is invaluable in this step. The capsule should be kept on tension as it is divided. One should not perform posteromedial release without knowing where the nerve is or being capable of identifying it prior to resecting any tissue. One option is to identify the nerve through a small open incision in order to know exactly its location (Fig. 3) [8]. In many contractures open decompression of the ulnar nerve is performed to prevent delayed-onset ulnar neuropathy. Arthroscopic nerve exposure is a highly demanding procedure that should be performed only with a high level of experience and prior cadaveric training.

As stated in the section on clinical assessment, ulnar neuritis is implicated in the etiology of the contracture for some patients. A subcutaneous ulnar nerve transposition can be performed prior to the release, or as soon as it has been completed. In those patients with ulnar neuropathy, our preference is to fully expose the ulnar nerve, but not destabilize it, prior to performing the arthroscopic release. This permits fluid to exit the soft tissues posteromedially,

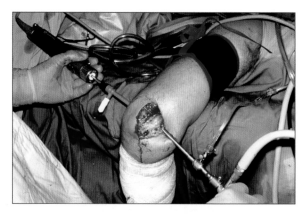

Fig. 3. Open decompression of the ulnar nerve just prior to arthroscopic contracture release can be performed for a number of indications. In some cases, such as this one, transposition is also indicated. (Figure reproduced with permission, Mayo Foundation)

and gentle retraction of the nerve provides the operator safer access to the posteromedial capsule, and the opportunity for direct visual feedback regarding where the shaver is in the vicinity of the (transposed) nerve. If the nerve is destabilized and/or transposed, it must be identified and protected each time an instrument is inserted or used in an anteromedial portal. The scope is move to visualize the lateral gutter. The posterolateral capsule is then resected.

Anterior Capsular Release

Anterior capsular release performed arthroscopically has evolved through three phases based on concern about the risk of nerve injury: capsular stripping from the humerus, capsulotomy, capsulectomy [15, 8]. Our experience would suggest that the efficacy of these three techniques might be proportional to the completeness of the capsular excision. Yet this presents a paradox, as the efficacy of the procedure might be inversely related to the risk of nerve injury. This is discussed further below under Complications.

Based on experience with over 300 capsulectomies, a technique and sequence have been developed for arthroscopic anterior capsulectomy. For reasons of safety and efficacy, yet at the risk of sounding elementary, I would like to emphasize a step-wise sequence in four steps: (1) get in and establish a view; (2) get ready; (3) bone and loose body removal; (4) capsulectomy. Step 1 is to get in and *establish a view*. Sometimes this is the most challenging part of the operation. I prefer to enter the joint with a pointed, but blunt-tipped, switching stick, then slide the scope sheath over the stick into the

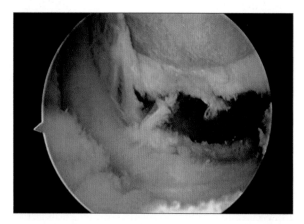

Fig. 2. The ulnar nerve is at risk during posteromedial capsular dissection as it lies immediately adjacent to the posterior bundle of the MCL, which forms the floor of the cubital tunnel. In this case, the nerve has been dissected out, the cubital tunnel retinaculum released, and the heterotopic ossification removed from the epicondyle. Currently, we would prefer to transpose the nerve. (Figure reproduced with permission, Mayo Foundation)

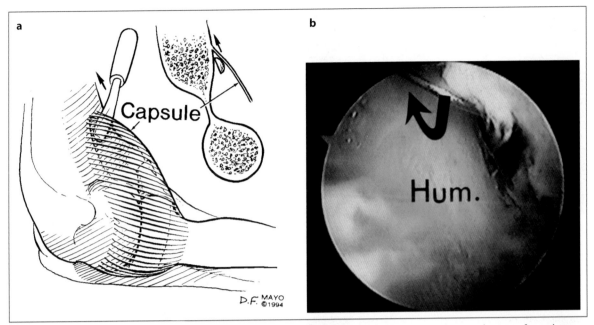

Fig. 4. (a, b) Steps 1 and 2 in anterior capsulectomy involve getting into the joint and getting ready to perform the capsulectomy, respectively. An important component of this initial phase is to establish a space within which to work by stripping the capsule and scar tissue off the humerus, permitting the tissues to be retracted anteriorly. (Figure reproduced with permission, Mayo Foundation)

joint. To do this one establishes three anterior portals and starting with the scope and shaver in the anterolateral and proximal anteromedial portals [16-19] and a retractor in the proximal anterolateral portal. A second retractor can be inserted if necessary (through the anteromedial portal). Step 2 is to *get ready*. To do this one must establish a space in which to work. After identifying sufficient normal articular anatomy to confirm location and orientation, one strip the capsule/scar off the humerus and supracondylar ridges to increase the space within which to work (Fig. 4). Although it is tempting to start removing the capsule, wisdom dictates that patience and attention to detail will yield better results and lower risks. Once these have been done, a synovectomy is performed as necessary and the capsule is superficially debrided in order to define it as a structure. This facilitates the actual capsulotomy/capsulectomy. Step 3 is *bone and loose body removal*. Loose bodies are generally removed as they are encountered. Numerous techniques have been described for removal of large loose bodies [16-19]. Bony recontouring (removal osteophytes, abnormal bone) is performed prior to removing the capsule. Step 4, *capsulectomy*, is best performed by first dividing the capsule from medial to lateral with a wide-mouthed duckling punch, as the plane of dissection between the capsule and the brachialis is more distinct on the medial side (Fig. 5). The capsulotomy is continued down to the level of the collat-

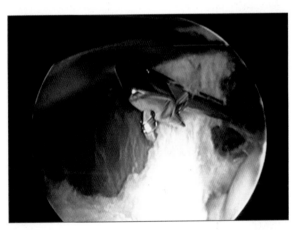

Fig. 5. Prior to capsulectomy, a capsulotomy is performed from medial to lateral. The final strip of capsule over the radial nerve is being released with a reverse-cutting punch biopsy. (Figure reproduced with permission, Mayo Foundation)

eral ligaments on each side. Finally, the capsule is excised, commencing on the medial side from proximal to distal (Fig. 6). Next the lateral capsule is excised proximally and distally. This is the most dangerous part of the anterior surgery, as the radial nerve is not protected behind the capsule. It is located just anterior to the radial head, between the brachialis and the ECRB (Fig. 7). The incremental risk of nerve injury in going from capsulotomy to capsulectomy must be emphasized. While we feel

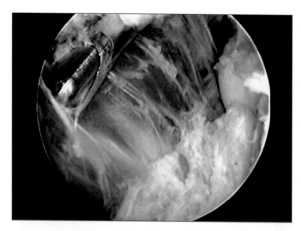

Fig. 6. The final step is capsulectomy. It is important that the brachialis be retracted anteriorly with a retractor and the shaver be kept rotated away from the anterior neurovascular structures. (Figure reproduced with permission, Mayo Foundation)

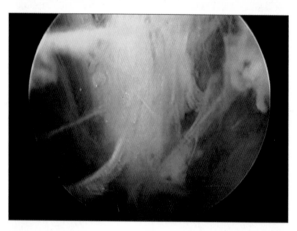

Fig. 7. The radial nerve is at risk at the lateral edge of the brachialis. A layer of thin fat tissue normally surrounds it. (Figure reproduced with permission, Mayo Foundation)

that the efficacy may also be greater with a complete capsulectomy, this remains to be proven by appropriate comparative or randomized studies.

At the completion of the procedure, two drains are placed – one through the proximal anterolateral portal and one posteriorly that is brought out through a separate exit wound. Portal wounds are closed with locked horizontal mattress sutures to minimize problems with prolonged drainage. If an incision was used to expose the ulnar nerve, it can be closed with staples.

Post-operative Care

Whether an open or arthroscopic release has been performed, the elbow is lightly wrapped in a bulky bandage with an anterior plaster slab from the shoulder to the hand, with the elbow in full extension. This maintains tension in the anterior soft tissues, and compression against the posterior soft tissues, such that bleeding and edema of the periarticular soft tissues are minimized in the immediate post-operative period [20, 21]. Once the neurologic status is confirmed to be intact, an indwelling axillary catheter can be placed for brachial plexus block anesthetic, or a single-shot injection performed (we now wait 36 hours, then perform a single-shot injection). Continuous passive motion (CPM) is commenced in hospital. The CPM must be from full flexion to full extension to be effective in preventing fluid accumulation around the elbow. It is the fluid accumulation that is responsible for loss of the motion gained at the time of surgery. As soon as the patient is ready to commence CPM, the splint and dressing must be entirely removed and exchanged for a thin elastic sleeve with absorbent gauze over the wounds. Constrictive or nonelastic dressings are contraindicated with CPM, as they cause shearing of the skin during motion. Optimally, the patient is treated in hospital for about 3 days. If the patient is able to maintain the range of motion without severe pain, he or she is discharged. If not, the block may need to be resumed for another day.

Home CPM is continued for an average of 3-4 weeks. Total hours of usage that are required each day vary with the pathology, the severity and duration of the contracture before release, and the nature of the surgery. Patient-adjusted static splints are helpful in maintaining the range of motion achieved in surgery and are routinely used by many surgeons [22, 23].

The post-operative administration of indomethacin is recommended for those at risk of developing ectopic ossification, although its efficacy in the prevention of recurrence is unknown. Meticulous surgical technique as well as copious irrigation during surgery is thought by some to decrease the likelihood of heterotopic ossification.

Results

Several studies have documented the efficacy of open [24-35] and arthroscopic [2-11, 14, 34, 36-40] contracture release. Based on early studies [41], it has commonly been said that patients can be expected to gain about half of the lost motion. However, a review of the literature over the past 15 years suggests that about 90% of patients gain motion

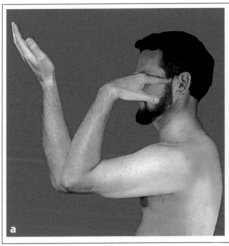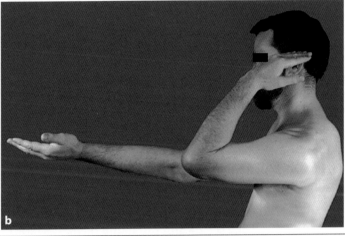

Fig. 8. (a, b) The efficacy of arthroscopic release in severe elbow contractures is exemplified in this male patient with a severe contracture despite two prior attempts at open contracture release. (**a**) Pre-operative photograph showing severe left elbow contracture (80°-110°). (**b**) Post-operative photograph showing excellent restoration of motion following arthroscopic contracture release and ulnar nerve transposition (20°-130°). (Figure reproduced with permission, Mayo Foundation)

(defined by at least a 10° increase in the arc of motion) and about 80% obtain a functional arc of motion (30° to 130°) as defined by Morrey et al. [1]. Another 5%-10% get to within 5°-10° at each end of this functional range. While some believe that the motion diminishes immediately after surgery and then gradually increases, this diminution may be prevented by the diligent use of CPM in the immediate post-operative period.

A valid comparison of arthroscopic *vs* open contracture release cannot be made from the literature, nor has a randomized study been reported comparing these two techniques. However, even in complex contractures, arthroscopic release appears efficacious (Fig. 8).

Complications

Complications of open contracture release are reported to be in the range of 10%-30%, depending on the nature of the underlying pathology and the treatment required [24-33]. Complications of orthoscopic contracture release include persistent drainage from portal sites, infection, wound healing complications such as hematoma if the ulnar nerve was transposed, heterotopic ossification and nerve injury. In addition, a recently recognized complication has caused us to rethink our approach to the management of the stiff elbow – delayed-onset ulnar neuropathy. A patient whose significant lack of flexion is restored acutely with

surgery and then maintained post-operatively is at risk of developing irritation or even loss of function of the ulnar nerve. This occurs due to compression under the cubital tunnel retinaculum. Normally this structure is tight only in terminal flexion [42]. However, in patients with loss of flexion, the retinaculum may shorten and become tight in lesser degrees of flexion. However, this can also occur after release of a flexion contracture release in patients with flexion to 130° or more pre-operatively. Patients with this complication may lose their ulnar nerve function in the first few days post-operatively, or may simply have too much pain to maintain their motion. The pain is localized to the cubital tunnel. Treatment is ulnar nerve transposition. This problem may be preventable by decompression of the ulnar nerve prophylactically or by a less intensive rehabilitation program post-operatively. Firm recommendations will not be possible until further data have been collected and verified.

Wound problems that occur with CPM should be managed by stopping the CPM, elevating and extending the elbow for 1-2 days, and re-evaluating it. Hematomas and seromas are washed out surgically, as they have a tendency to impede flexion and can become infected.

Complications of arthroscopic contracture release occur in the range of 10%-20% [3, 7, 8, 10, 14, 34, 36-40]. Of these, the most worrisome is nerve injury. Nerve injuries have been reported with both open [25, 41] and arthroscopic releases [18, 39, 43, 44]. The risk of nerve injury with arthroscopic release has anecdotally been considered to be higher than that with open release. That may or may not be the case, but is probably dependent on a number of factors including experience of the operator and not just the complexity of the surgery. Most reported nerve injuries occurred early during the development of arthroscopic release. Our experience with over 300 arthroscopic releases suggests that the risk of nerve injuries can be reduced by a number of safety measures. These include the use of retractors, avoiding the use of suction anywhere near a nerve (leave the shaver outlet open with no tube connected to it), using a shaver instead of a burr near a nerve to avoid the 'power takeoff' effect in which the burr wraps tissue and pulls the nerve into it, knowing where the nerves are or actually seeing and retracting them (if the operator has the expertise to identify them), and, most importantly of all, the surgeon knowing his or her own limits and also operating within them.

References

1. Morrey BF, Askew LJ, An KN, Chao EY (1981) A biomechanical study of normal elbow motion. J Bone Joint Surg Am 63:872-877
2. Savoie FH 3rd, Nunley PD, Field LD (1999) Arthroscopic management of the arthritic elbow: indications, technique, and results. J Shoulder Elbow Surg 8:214-9
3. Kim SJ, Shin SJ (2000) Arthroscopic treatment for limitation of motion of the elbow. Clin Orthop Relat Res 375:140-148
4. Norberg FB, Savoie FH 3rd , Field LD (2000) Arthroscopic treatment of arthritis of the elbow. Instr Course Lect 49:247-53
5. O'Driscoll S (2000) Elbow arthroscopy: loose bodies. In: Morrey B (ed) The Elbow and its Disorders. WB Saunders, Philadelphia, pp 510-514
6. O'Driscoll S (2000) Elbow arthroscopy: the Future. In: Morrey B (ed) The Elbow and its Disorders. WB Saunders, Philadelphia, p 522
7. Savoie FH 3rd, Field LD (2000) Arthroscopi capsular release. In: Morrey B (ed) The Elbow and its Disorders. WB Saunders, Philadelphia, pp 516-519
8. Kelly E, Morrey B, O'Driscoll S (2001) Complications of elbow arthroscopy. J Bone Joint Surg Am 83:25-34
9. Savoie FH 3rd, Field LD (2001) Arthrofibrosis and complications in arthroscopy of the elbow. Clin Sports Med 20:123-129
10. Ball CM, Meunier M, Galatz LM et al (2002) Arthroscopic treatment of post-traumatic elbow contracture. J Shoulder Elbow Surg 11:624-629
11. O'Driscoll SW, Savoie FH 3rd (2002)Arthroscopy of the elbow. In: Morrey BF (ed) Master Techniques in Orthopedic Surgery: the Elbow. Lippincott Williams & Wilkins, Philadelphia, pp 27-45
12. Gallay SH, Richards RR, O'Driscoll SW (1993) Intra-articular capacity and compliance of stiff and normal elbows. Arthroscopy 9:9-13
13. O'Driscoll SW, Morrey BF, An KN (1990) Intra-articular pressure and capacity of the elbow. Arthroscopy 6:100-103
14. Timmerman LA, Andrews JR (1994) Arthroscopic treatment of post-traumatic elbow pain and stiffness. Am J Sports Med 22:230-235
15. O'Driscoll SW (1995) Arthroscopic treatment for osteoarthritis of the elbow. Orthop Clin North Am 26:691-706
16. Lindenfeld TN (1990) Medial approach in elbow arthroscopy. Am J Sports Med 18:413-417
17. Marshall PD, Fairclough JA, Johnson SR, Evans EJ (1993) Avoiding nerve damage during elbow arthroscopy. J Bone Joint Surg Br 75:129-131
18. Miller C, Jobe C, Wright M (1995) Neuroanatomy in elbow arthroscopy. J Shoulder Elbow Surg 4:168-174
19. Lynch G, Meyers J, Whipple T, Caspari R (1986) Neurovascular anatomy and elbow arthroscopy: inherent risks. Arthroscopy 2:191-197
20. Bain GI, Mehta JA, Heptinstall RJ (1998) The dynamic elbow suspension splint. J Shoulder Elbow Surg 7:419-421
21. O'Driscoll S, Giori N (2000) Continuous passive motion (CPM): theory and principles of clinical application. J Rehabil Res Dev 37:179-188
22. Gelinas JJ, Faber KJ, Patterson SD, King GJ (2000) The effectiveness of turnbuckle splinting for elbow contractures. J Bone Joint Surg Br 82:74-78
23. Bonutti PM, Windau JE, Ables BA, Miller BG (1994) Static progressive stretch to reestablish elbow range of motion. Clin Orthop Relat Res 303:128-134
24. Mansat P, Morrey BF (1998) The column procedure: A limited lateral approach for extrinsic contracture of the elbow. J Bone Joint Surg Am 80:1603-15
25. Mansat P, Morrey BF, Hotchkiss RN (2000) Extrinsic contracture: the column procedure. Lateral and medial capsular releases. WB Saunders, Philadelphia, pp 447-456
26. Morrey BF (2000) Surgical treatment of extra-articular elbow contracture. Clin Orthop Relat Res 370:57-64
27. Morrey B (1993) Post-traumatic stiffness: distraction orthoplasty. In: Morrey B (ed) The Elbow and its Disorders. WB Saunders, Philadelphia, pp 476-491
28. Morrey BF (1990) Post-traumatic contracture of the elbow. Operative treatment, including distraction arthroplasty. J Bone Joint Surg Am 72:601-618
29. Gates HS, Sullivan FL, Urbaniak JR (1992) Anterior capsulotomy and continuous passive motion in the treatment of post-traumatic flexion contracture of the elbow. A prospective study. J Bone Joint Surg 74:1229-1234
30. Husband JB, Hastings H (1990) The lateral approach for operative release of post-traumatic contracture of the elbow. J Bone Joint Surg Am 72:1353-1358
31. Mih AD, Wolf FG (1994) Surgical release of elbow-capsular contracture in pediatric patients. J Pediatric Orthop 14:458-461
32. Viola RW, Hanel DP (1999) Early "simple" release of post-traumatic elbow contracture associated with heterotopic ossification. J Hand Surg Am 24:370-380
33. Moritomo H, Tada K, Yoshida T (2001) Early, wide excision of heterotopic ossification in the medial elbow. J Shoulder Elbow Surg 10:164-168
34. Cohen AP, Redden JF, Stanley D (2000) Treatment of osteoarthritis of the elbow: a comparison of open and arthroscopic debridement. Arthroscopy 16:701-706
35. King GJ, Faber KJ (2000) Post-traumatic elbow stiffness. Orthop Clin North Am 31:129-143

36. Phillips BB, Strasburger S (1998) Arthroscopic treatment of arthrofibrosis of the elbow joint. Arthroscopy 14:38-44
37. Kim SJ, Kim HK, Lee JW (1995) Arthroscopy for limitation of motion of the elbow. Arthroscopy 11:680-683
38. Redden JF, Stanley D (1993) Arthroscopic fenestration of the olecranon fossa in the treatment of osteoarthritis of the elbow. Arthroscopy 9:14-16
39. Jones GS, Savoie FH III (1993) Arthroscopic capsular release of flexion contractures (arthrofibrosis) of the elbow. Arthroscopy 9:277-283
40. Nowicki KD, Shall LM (1992) Arthroscopic release of a posttraumatic flexion contracture in the elbow: a case report and review of the literature. Arthroscopy 8:544-547
41. Urbaniak JR, Hansen PE, Beissinger SF, Aitken MS (1985) Correction of post-traumatic flexion contracture of the elbow by anterior capsulotomy. J Bone Joint Surg Am 67:1160-1164
42. O'Driscoll SW, Horii E, Morrey BF, Carmichael SW (1991) The cubital tunnel and ulnar neuropathy. J Bone Joint Surg Br 73:613-617
43. Haapaniemi T, Berggren M, Adolfsson L (1999) Complete transection of the median and radial nerves during arthroscopic release of post-traumatic elbow contracture. Arthroscopy 15:784-787
44. Papilion J, Neff R, Shall L (1988) Compression neuropathy of the radial nerve as a complication of elbow arthroscopy: a case report and review of the literature. Arthroscopy 4:284-286

CHAPTER 21

The Surgery of Neglected Distal Humerus Fractures in Children and Adults

L.P. Müller, M. Hansen, B.F. Morrey, K.J. Prommersberger, P.M. Rommens

Introduction

The restoration of function after a neglected distal humerus fracture presents a formidable challenge to the surgeon because of both the complexity of the regional anatomy and the proximity of numerous neurovascular structures. Inadequate or unstable fixation, a failure to reposition the articular fragments anatomically, prolonged post-operative immobilization, or the development of soft-tissue complications will result in substantial disability for the patient. Complications after injuries affecting a child's elbow are common due to understimating the severity of the injury on the native X-rays where the growth plates and cartilage structures can not be seen.

The technically demanding reconstruction procedures of neglected fractures of the distal humerus include osteotomy for malunion or debridement for nonunion, realignment with stable fixation and autogenous bone grafts, anterior and posterior capsulectomy and ulnar neurolysis, which are discussed in this chapter.

The primary goal is to restore the intrinsic anatomy of the elbow. The surgical tactic for this demanding goal is highlighted. Excising the peri-articular fibrosis is a critical feature when treating neglected distal humerus fractures – poor overall functional outcome will result if treatment is only focused on gaining union alone.

The definition of "to neglect" includes the "lack of attention, failing to do something and to leave something undone". In other words to neglect in general is something bad and negative. Sometimes though a fracture can be "skillfully-neglected": this in order to emphasize the fact, that in some cases where an isolated neglected humerus fracture presents late with a pseudarthrosis, no surgery is needed due to a surprisingly good clinical result, in contrast to the X-ray findings. The following "neglected situations" are discussed here in:
- non union and delayed union;
- angular deformity (esp. pediatric deformities);
- stiffness and instability combined with a neglected fracture of the distal humerus.

Evaluation

The evaluation of neglected distal humeral fractures often lead to difficult treatment problems that require a great deal of judgement. Each case has its own characteristics, and the treatment of each case must be individualized. Evaluation requires a careful assessment of the patient's age, functional demands, functional status of the soft tissues, and presence of infection. The evaluation of the X-ray appearance must be related closely with the clinical evaluation: Smith [1] reported an 84-year follow-up of a lateral condylar nonunion in an individual with a near-painless extremity who pursued a 35-year career as a professional musician as a possibly good or better result than could have been produced by surgery. Sim and

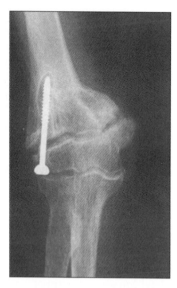

Fig. 1. A 75-year-old female sustained a nonunion after inadequate fixation of a low transcondylar fracture. The patient tolerated the nonunion without pain, requiring no additional surgery ("skillfull neglect")

Morrey [2] made similar observations (Fig. 1). Hence, not all nonunions are dysfunctional or require intervention.

The status of the elbow joint itself is a very important consideration – the post-traumatic arthritis, the state of function of the ulnar nerve, and the extent of joint stiffness in the specific context of the anticipated functional demands must be carefully evaluated. Pain is the most consistent problem, followed by instability [2], up to 75% of patients have motion loss [3].

Delayed Union and Nonunion

An excellent surgical result is only achieved with reduction and restoration of an axis of rotation that passes through the center of the arcs formed by the capitellum and the trochlear sulcus. Early mobilization is important for a good functional outcome. However, in underdeveloped countries, not all of these fractures are seen primarily by the orthopedic surgeons. Various forms of management ranging from splints to massage are attempted prior to presentation at specialized centers, making our task more complicated and treatment options limited.

Overall the literature suggests non union rates in 0%-7% of distal humerus fractures [4, 5]. When a "real" nonunion without fibrous binding of the fragments and instability ocurs, there is a

significant disability because of pain, peri-articular fibrosis, and ulnar nerve symptoms. Fortunately nonunion is rare. Predisposing factors are infection, comminution, inappropriate initial treatment, multiple associated injuries, and excessive damage of soft tissues. Loosening or breakage of implants occurs when the initial open reduction and internal fixation (ORIF) is not anatomic and fixation insecure. In addition, the degree of comminution and the surgical exposure itself further compromise the blood supply to the fracture fragments [2].

Selection of the approach should be largely based on the area of scarring of the soft tissues from trauma or previous surgery and the dissection needed for exposure of the distal humerus. As exposure for low intra-articular neglected fracture situations a transolecranon approach seems reasonable; for extra-articular lesions medial or lateral reflection of the triceps may be an optimal approach, although the senior author (B.F. Morrey) uses the Mayo or modified Kocher exposure for both proximal and distal types of nonunions [6].

Leaving a painless pseudarthrosis alone is appropriate if reasonable motion and stability are present (Figs. 1, 2). The excision of a primary neglected fractured fragment in Milch type I injuries does not significantly affect the stability of the elbow joint. In a report by Nagi [7], a primary neglected totally intra-articular fragment was excised through an approach which involved distal reflection of the medial ligament of the elbow along with a bony chip. This was subsequently

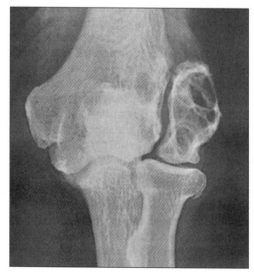

Fig. 2. A 40-year follow-up of a lateral Milch I nonunion. The patient is without significant symptoms and has a motion from 15° to 140° ("skillfull neglect")

reattached by a screw after the fractured fragment was excised. No instability developed.

Still, resection arthroplasty offers little and should be avoided – the effectiveness of stable ORIF is emerging as the desired solution. Inadequate fixation techniques (Fig. 3) should be interpreted as a neglected fracture situaton and addressed surgically as soon as the soft tissue situation allows a secure surgical exposure of the involved lesions. Double plate osteosynthesis, refixation of intra-articular fragments with Herbert screws or Ethipins, bone grafting including interpositional bicortical grafting of the trochlea to restore the width (Fig. 4) are to be considered. Jupiter [8] reported using triple plating of complex distal humerus nonunions in six elderly patients, radiographic follow-up re-

vealed only one case with a focal area of avascular necrosis involving a previously ununited intra-articular fracture of the trochlea. He emphasized the importance of elbow capsulectomy and ulnar nerve neurolysis to regain ulnar nerve function and a good arc of motion. The surgical technique for elbow release before stabilizing the nonunion is described below in the section titled "Stiffness and Instability Combined with a Neglected Fracture of the Distal Humerus".

Reconstruction of intra-articular malunion and nonunion of the distal humerus is technically challenging, but can improve function by restoring the intrinsic anatomy of the elbow (Fig. 5). As incongruence of the joint surface is predisposing to later arthrosis, restoration of the intrinsic anatomy is nearly always indicated.

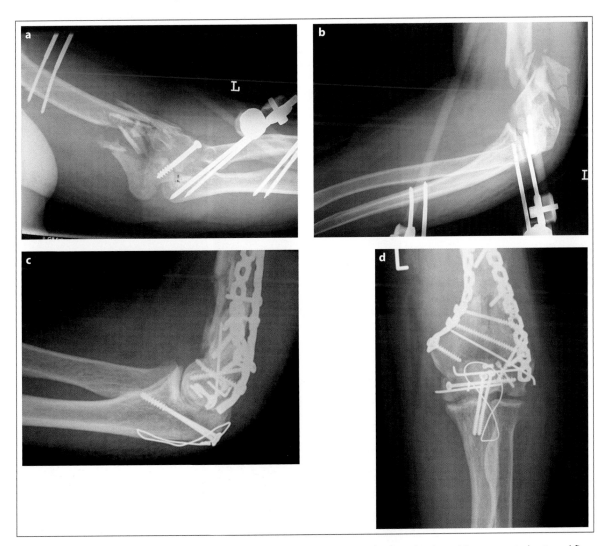

Fig. 3. (**a, b**) Provisional primary fixation of a C-fracture, in an attempt to obtain reduction with a screw and external fixateur. After soft tissues conditioning correction was performed. (**c, d**) Double plate osteosynthesis, refixation of intra-articular fragments with Herbert screws/K-wires of the case illustrated in (**a, b**)

Fig. 4. Malunion of condylar elements treated with osteotomy and interpositional bicortical grafting. (Figure reproduced with permission, Mayo Foundation)

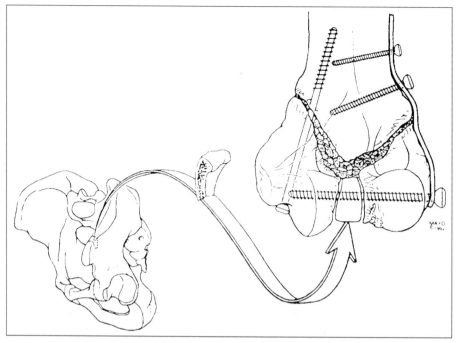

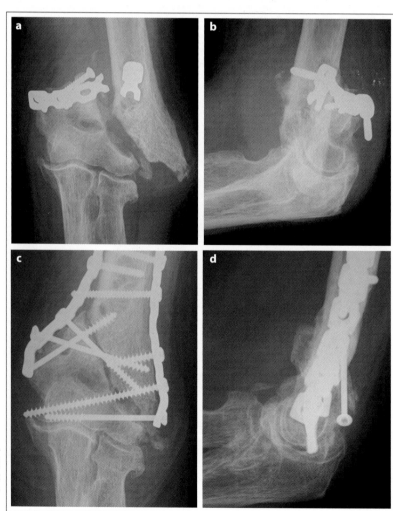

Fig. 5 a-d. Reconstruction of intra-articular nonunion of the distal humerus after failed osteosynthesis: double plate osteosynthesis plus anterior and posterior bone grafting

Total elbow prosthesis is a further valuable option for the treatment of neglected distal humerus fractures (Fig. 6) when due to comminuted low intra-articular fracture fragment; and when due to poor bone quality, stable and anatomical reduction of the width and angle of the trochlea and the capitellum is impossible to achieve and the loss of range of motion as a consequence of surgery itself are expected problems. Even if stable anatomic fixation is achieved by ORIF, joint stiffness or instability, nerve lesions, and heterotopic bone formation might spoil the result. Technically the operative procedure of TER is relatively simple in the neglected low fracture situation compared to reconstruction by open reduction and internal fix-

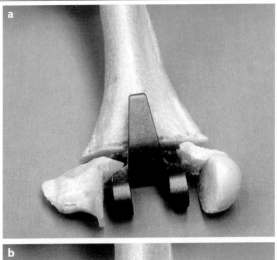

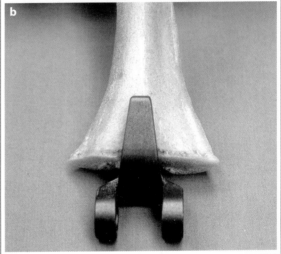

Fig. 7 a, b. Model of the distal humerus showing the normal axis of rotation. The axis of rotation is replicated by the Mayo-modified Coonrad-Morrey implant with the condyles intact. If the condyles are removed, the axis is maintained at the anatomic location. (Figures reproduced with permission, Mayo Foundation)

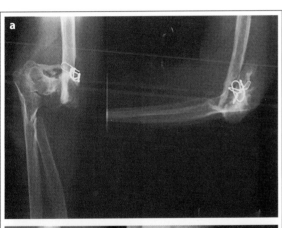

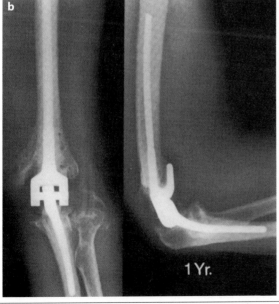

Fig. 6. (a) A 71-year-old female with ununited comminuted T-condylar fracture at 5 months after surgery. (b) Total elbow arthroplasty allowed 20° to 130° of flexion and no pain

ation. Even in the absence of humeral condyles (Fig. 7) the Coonrad-Morrey TER® (Zimmer) as a linked device with 7° valgus/varus laxity provides stability; excision of bone fragments of the distal humerus allows access to the humeral canal, releasing only 25% to 50% of attachment of the triceps muscle (Fig. 8). In the absence of the distal humerus, coupling of the ulnar and humeral prostheses components is easy.

We have no experience and do not perform treatment of non unions of distal humerus fractures with electrical stimulation or BMP products. We find that the elbow tolerates the necessary duration of immobilization poorly.

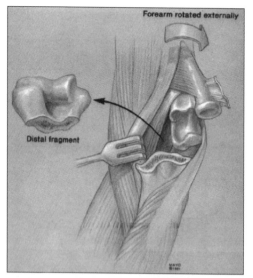

Fig. 8. Excision of bone fragments of the distal humerus leaving the triceps attachment intact. (Figure reproduced with permission, Mayo Foundation)

Angular Deformity

The most common significant adverse sequela of neglected or underestimated distal humerus fractures in children is angular deformity. Disturbances of growth plates include avascular necrosis and physeal injuries, or the position of the fracture has healed leads to deformities that need corrective procedures. Deformity may occur in any single plane or in a combination of planes, and remodelling can only be expected of sagittal plane deformity.

A common problem after distal humerus fractures in children is the estimation of the extent of the fracture: due to large cartilage fragments which can not be seen on native X-rays the extent of the fracture can be underestimated; an MRI scan – though very seldom indicated – might be helpful in questionable cases (Fig. 9). Valgus deformaty after conservative treatment of distal humerus fractures can be treated by correction osteotomy using a external fixateur (Fig. 10).

Neglected capitellum fractures, predispose arthrosis and angular deformities and should always be realigned securely (Fig. 11).

In battered child syndrome cases, neglected elbow dislocation plus malunited distal humerus fracture might be found, and especially in the very young patient an MRI (or ultrasound) helps to demonstrate the extent of the injury, for example, a complete epiphysiolysis (Fig. 12).

After osteosyntheses of distal humerus fractures in children with k-wires and repetitive postoperative falls, immediate X-ray controls should be performed.

Otherwise due to secondary dislocation and hardware breakage, deformation might develop and correction osteotomies must be carried out (Fig. 13).

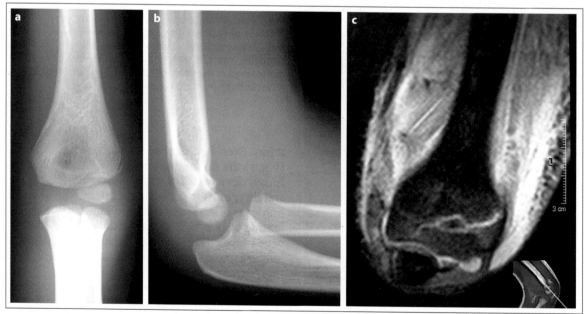

Fig. 9 a-c. Underestimated distal humerus fracture due to large cartilage fragment which can not be seen on native X-rays (9-year-old child): only in the anteroposterior view a slight incongruency (ulna-sided) can be seen – MRI demonstrated the extent of the injury. Treatment was performed conservatively with a cast for 3 weeks in 90° of flexion

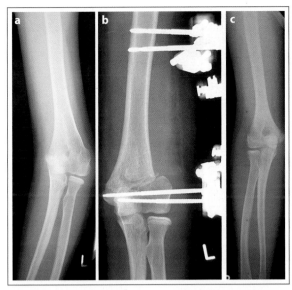

Fig. 10. (**a**) Misinterpretation of severity of fracture extent in a 15-year-old child: 18 months after distal humerus fracture after conservative treatment with cast development of a valgus deformaty. (**b**) Correction osteotomy using a external fixateur was performed. (**c**) Good realignment of axis after hard ware removal 3 months post-OR

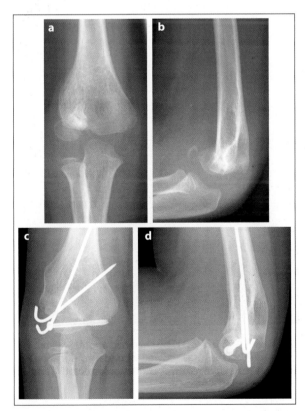

Fig. 11. (**a-b**) A 6-month neglected capitellum fracture in an 11-year-old child leaving a flexion deficit of 30°. Joint incongruence predisposes arthrosis. (**c, d**) Correction osteotomy and osteosyntheses with two smooth k-wires and a cannulated 3.5 mm screw

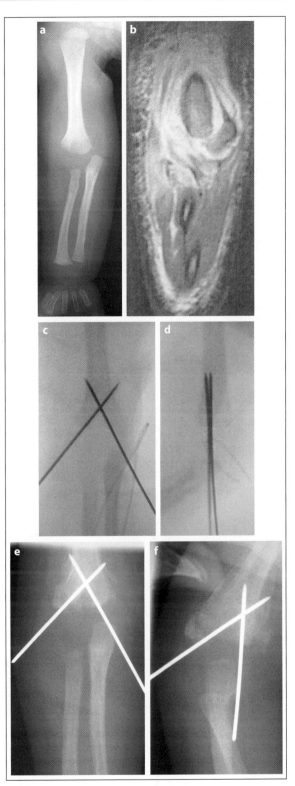

Fig. 12. (**a**) Battered child syndrome case (1-year-old child): Neglected elbow dislocation plus malunited distal humerus fracture. (**b**) MRI demonstrates cartilage of dislocated and malunited trochlea. (**c, d**) Open arthrolysis, osteotomy with correction of malunited trochlea, fixation with two smooth k-wires. (**e, f**) Follow-up 3 months post-OR

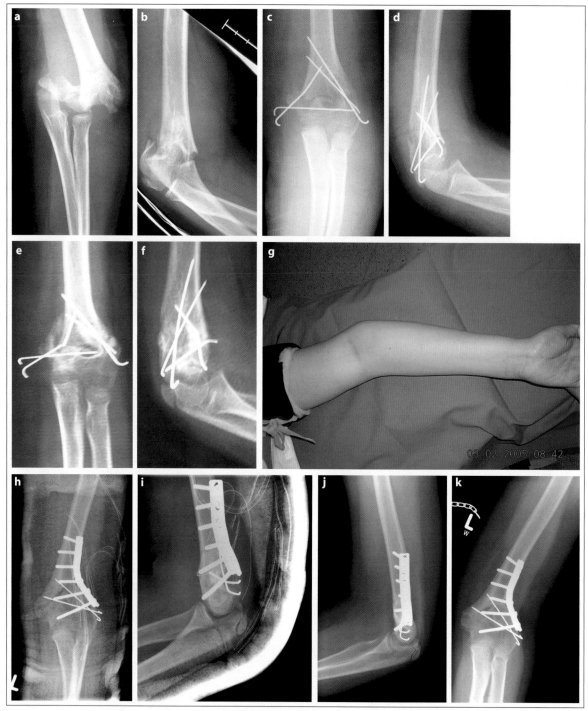

Fig. 13. (**a-d**) Distal humerus fracture in a 12-year-old child treated with k-wires. (**e, f**) The child had another fall but primary no X-ray investigation was performed. Three weeks after the second fall the X-ray showed secondary dislocation and hard ware breakage. (**g**) Clinically varus deformation developed. (**h, i**) Hard ware removal, correction osteotomy, and osteosynthesis using a 1/3 tubular plate was performed. (**j, k**) Follow-up 3 months post-OR

Stiffness and Instability Combined with a Neglected Fracture of the Distal Humerus

Due to extensive peri-articular fibrosis when treating neglected fractures of the distal humerus, in most adult cases a release of the elbow joint must be performed – in order to improve motion and to attain access to the involved non united fragments. The distal fragments will commonly be found to be flexed, and intra-operatively a bone hook will help stretch the anterior capsular fibrosis, facilitating its excision. This will allow mobilization of the distal fragment for reduction of the nonunion. Most patients have coincident significant scarring of the ulnar nerve, and the results of ulnar nerve neurolysis are rewarding. The difficult dissection of the nerve should preferably be done under surgical magnification and microsurgical instrumentation.

In cases of distal humerus nonunions combined with stiffness we perform a step by step procedure [9, 11].

1. Dorsal "global" incision.
2. A lateral deep triceps reflecting approach is first performed in cases of radial-sided nonunions. A primary medial deep approach is used for localized ulnar-sided nonunions, pre-operative signs of ulnaris irritation, or documented medial-sided heterotopic ossifications.
3. If an extension deficit is encountered, excision of anterior capsule from lateral deep approach is performed.
4. If the extension deficit persists after anterior capsule excision controll of impingement in olecranon fossa and debridement.
5. If the extension deficit persists, resection of tip of olecranon /osteophytes.
6. If a flexion deficit is present, primary resection of posterior capsule; for a persistent flexion deficit, resection of anterior capsule and revision of fossa coronoidea as well as the tip of the coronoid.
7. Potentially additional resection of the dorsal bundle of the medial collateral ligament in order to achieve full flexion.
8. Potentially lengthening of the triceps tendon in order to achieve full flexion.
9. Transposition of the ulnar nerve if signs of traction stress when testing full range of motion.
10. A combined anterior and posterior capsulectomy must be performed in most cases.
11. Potential hardware removal, debridement, and decortication of the bony fragments.
12. Bony contouring of distorted skeletal anatomy.
13. Reduction and provisional K-wire fixation, determination of the geometry of the skeletal columns (templates).
14. Double plating ulnar and radial.
15. Bone grafting both anteriorly and posteriorly.
16. If after ORIF of the nonunited fragments instability occurs due to ligamentous laxity, we apply a dynamic external fixateur for early beginning of motion post-OR (Fig. 14).

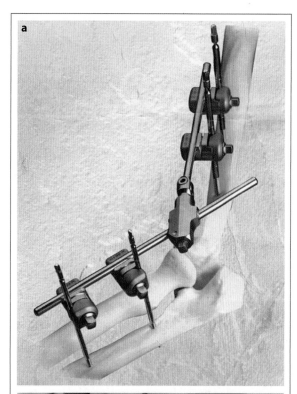

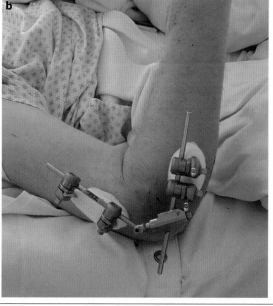

Fig. 14 a, b. Dynamic external fixateur (DJD II). In an situation of instability after release or secondary ORIF due to ligamentous laxity, a dynamic external fixateur for early beginning of motion post-OR is applied

However union, rather than motion, remains the priority, because motion can be restored reliably by subsequent contracture release, if necessary, as long as the fracture heals. For fractures that are judged intra-operatively not to be stable enough to commence early motion, the implementation of as hort period of immobilization followed by early soft tissue release will avoid exposing the patient to the risk of nonunion, and result in a more predictable functional outcome.

Discussion

The dilemma faced in the management of neglected distal humerus fractures is the tissue dissection needed to attain good exposure and reduction in cases presenting late, which may lead to further avascularity of the involved fragments and end up in poor results. Therefore apart from the X-ray finding a good evaluation of the patients status and expectations as well as an exact clinical investigation of the elbow are essential for a successful individual treatment protocol. We would like to emphasize the evaluation of the state of the soft tissues and the ulnar nerve before performing surgery and planning the procedure from incision to closure. A neglected fracture is not to be scheduled as an emergency procedure.

In young patients early anatomic restoration is to be achieved – possible complications include transient or permanent nerve lesions, especially to the ulnar (and radial) nerve. A persistent nonunion is uncommon but occurs with a frequency of about 5%.

When a neglected fracture has already existed for a long time, secondary arthritis may preclude correction and ORIF. Depending on the patients biological age it is probably best to consider arthroplasty in this situation.

The choice of the surgical approach for a stiff elbow should be based on the potential to meet unforeseen circumstances and the capability for providing adequate visualization to define and correct the underlying pathology [12].

If the achieved arc of motion intra-operatively after release of the involved structures is not sufficient, further dissection might be needed, stabilizing the elbow joint thereafter with an external fixator.

Neglected fractures of the distal humerus in adults and in most cases in children need ORIF (open reduction internal fixation) to allow functional recovery. In pre-operative planning and decision making for neglected distal humerus fractures, the following factors play a major role:
– soft tissue condition;
– stability of the elbow joint;
– joint congruence;
– arc of motion;
– neuropathy and pain (NB: ulnar nerve symptoms).

The X-ray findings play a minor role for the indication for an operative procedure of late/neglected cases. A CT scan can help to determine joint (in)congruence and the state of fracture healing and therefore should be performed when questionable native X-ray findings are obtained. In some cases of neglected distal humerus fractures ORIF may lead to a stiff and painful elbow, whereas the difficult decision to "skilfullyneglect" a non- or delayed union can result in a suprisingly good clinical result.

References

1. Smith FM (1973) An 84-year follow-up on a patient with ununited fracture of the lateral condyle of the humerus. J Bone Joint Surg Am 55:378-382
2. Sim FH, Morrey BF (2000) Nonunion and delayed union of distal humerus fractures. In: The elbow and its disorders. WB Saunders Co, Philadelphia, pp 331-341
3. Ackermann G, Jupiter JB (1988) Nonunion of fractures of the distal end of the humerus. J Bone Joint Surg Am 70:75-81
4. Bryan RS, Bickel WH (1971) "T" condylar fractures of the distal humerus. J Trauma 11:830-839
5. Solheim K, Daagev F (1973) Delayed union and nonunion of fractures: clinical experience with ASIF method. J Trauma 13:121-132
6. Morrey BF (ed) (2000) In the elbow and its disorders. WB Saunders Co, Philadelphia, pp 43-60
7. Nagi ON, Dhillon MS, Aggarwal A, Gill SS (2000) Fractures of the Medial Humeral Condyle in Adults. Singapore Med J 41:347-351
8. Jupiter JB, Goodman LJ (1992) The management of complex distal humerus nonunion in the elderly by elbow capsulectomy, triple plating, and ulnar nerve neurolysis. J Shoulder Elbow Surg 1:37-45
9. Dowdy PA, Bain GI, King GJW, Patterson SD (1995) The Midline Posterior Elbow Incision. J Bone Joint Surg Br 77:696-699
10. King JW, Faber KJ (2000) Post-traumatic elbow stiffness. Ortho Clin North Am 31:129-143
11. Morrey BF (2000) Surgical treatment of extra-articular elbow contracture. Clin Orthop 370:57-64
12. Morrey BF (2000) Surgical exposures of the elbow. In: Morrey BF (ed) The elbow and its disorders. WB Saunders Co, Philadelphia, pp 109-135

CHAPTER 22

Total Elbow Replacement for Rheumatoid Arthritis

B.F. MORREY

Introduction

Management of patients with rheumatoid arthritis of the elbow has changed significantly over the last several years. The reliability of both coupled and uncoupled elbow joint replacements have emerged as reliable interventions for this diagnosis. Mayo's experience with 78 procedures with rheumatoid arthritis undergoing total elbow arthroplasty has revealed a satisfactory outcome of approximately 92% at 12 years. The complication rate is approximately 15%, consisting primarily of delayed avulsions or deficiency of the triceps tendon (2%), deep infection (2%), and ulnar nerve irritation (3%).

Elbow Replacement

In recent years, improved outcomes after joint replacement have been documented, and joint replacement is the recommended treatment of most with advanced disease. In general, the indications for replacement follow the radiographic features as well as the clinical characteristics (Fig. 1, Table 1).

There are two distinct design philosophies applied to prosthetic elbow implant designs.

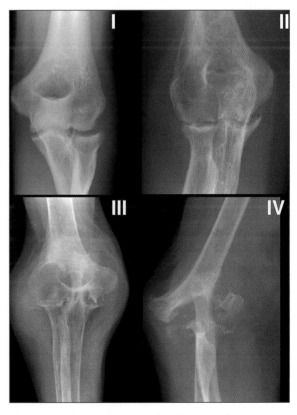

Fig. 1. Mayo Radiographic Classification of rheumatoid arthritis [1]. The Type V was recently added by Connor and Morrey to count for ankylosis

Table 1. Treatment options based on radiographic extent of disease

	Radiographic Appearance	Treatment
Type I:	Synovitis with a normal appearing joint	Synovectomy
Type II:	Loss of joint space	Synovectomy
	Maintenance of subchondral architecture	TEA: Resurfacing/Semiconstrained
Type IIIA:	Alteration of the subchondral architecture	TEA: Resurfacing/Semiconstrained
Type IIIB:	Alteration of the architecture with deformity	TEA: Semiconstrained
Type IV:	Gross deformity	TEA: Semiconstrained
Type V:	Ankylosis [1]	TEA: Semiconstrained

TEA, Total Elbowv Arthroplasty

Unlinked Arthroplasty

Unlinked arthroplasty emerged as a helpful solution to the disappointing outcomes from early failed linked highly constrained implants. The philosophy was and is prompted by an interest in performing more anatomic replacements, particularly at the knee and to some extent at the hip. Thus, the elbow design philosophy of uncoupled devices parallels that of hip resurfacing and knee condylar designs.

Indications

The pre-requisites for these designs are adequate humeral and ulnar bone and ligament integrity. Thus, the indications for an unlinked implant are primarily limited to dysfunction from rheumatoid or inflammatory arthritis, especially in the early stages of the disease.

Contraindications of Unlinked Implant Designs

Inadequate bone stock and insufficient ligamentous support are accepted as relative contraindications to the use of uncoupled devices.

The precise indications and contraindications are somewhat dependent on other design considerations. A persistent incidence of instability and distal humeral component migration has resulted in all currently available resurfacing implants having humeral and ulnar stems for supplemental fixation. The size and design of these stems determine the suitability for use in those with altered bone stock. Theoretically a radial head component continues to have value regarding stability and function. However, to date with the current implants it has not been demonstrated to be of long-term benefit. While uncoupled implants may be more physiologic, some are highly constrained, imparting considerable forces to the articulation

to the stem or interface fixation. Hence, the resurfacing implants are far from being homogenous in concept, application, or clinical results.

Linked Arthroplasty

Today the linked devices are designed and are termed semiconstrained implants. This term is used to refer to a captive articulation with some "laxity" or "play" at the articulation.

Indications

The indications for the linked semiconstrained implant in general terms constitute the full spectrum of elbow pathology. Hence, patients with rheumatoid arthritis can usually be managed regardless of the degree of bone or soft tissue present or destroyed. The precise design defines the extent of the pathology that can be reliably addressed by the system.

Contraindications

There are no unique contraindications to the linked devices. In the rheumatoid patient, a longer stemmed (15 cm) device is contraindicated in most, as concern exists of a possible future need of a shoulder replacement.

Results

Unlinked Devices

The results of several different unlinked designs from recent reports in the literature are summarized in Table 2. In general these data reveal an approxi-

Table 2. Results reported in last decade of resurfacing replacement: N=550. Nine authors, 4 implants

Author	Implant	No.	With R/A, %	Follow-up (yr)	Ext/ Flex, %	P/S, %	Pain Relief, %	Comp., %	Unstable, %	Loose, %	Revised, %	Satisfied, %
Ewald, 1993 [10]	Capitello-condylar	202	100	5.6	30/135	64/72	87	18	3	2	7	85
Kudo, 1994 [19]	Kudo	32	100	3.1	41/131	46/61	85	25	–	–	16	80
Verstreken, 1998 [8]	Kudo	16	100	3	37/140	–	100	17	12	0	6	83
Lyall, 1994 [3]	Souter	19	100	3.5	42/135	70/74	90	32	15	10	10	90
Ljung, 1995 [12]	Souter	50	100	3	–	–	100	38	2	0	16	–
Sjoden, 1995 [7]	Souter	19	100	5	41/136	65/75	75	50	5	20	15	80
Andreassen, 1997 [6]	Souter	30	97	5.0				50	6	6	20	74
Trail, 1999 [5]	Souter	186	100	12	–	–	–	–	–	13	13	≈85
Allieu, 1998 [20]	Roper/Tuke	12	100	9.5	40/140	61/62	67	33	8	16	16	50

mate 90% likelihood of a satisfactory outcome at 5 years in patients with rheumatoid arthritis. The arc of motion approximates the functional range but a variable degree of extension is lost.

Souter-Strathclyde. In the United Kingdom and parts of Europe, the Souter-Strathyclyde design

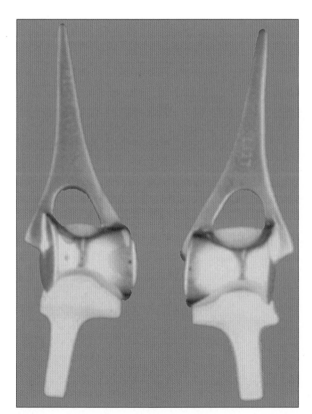

Fig. 2. The Souter-Strathclyde resurfacing implant is quite constrained at the articulation and employs the osseous integrity of the medial and lateral supracondylar columns for humeral stability

has been the most frequently employed implant, and outcome data continue to emerge (Fig. 2) [2-4]. One study from the Netherlands reviewed 31 of 34 implants with at least 2 years outcome information [4]. Of these three were revised because of dislocation, one because of loosening and one from infection. In those 26 patients who were not revised, with a mean follow-up of 4 years, function had improved and pain was dramatically reduced. Using the same implant, a more recent study from Hong Kong of 20 implants with a mean follow-up of 3.5 years documented 16 of the 20 with minimal or no pain [2]. They reported one instability (5%) among the 20 cases and an average of 7° of extension loss with this device. One loose implant required revision. It should be noted that both these reports are limited to patients with rheumatoid arthritis.

The most extensive experience regarding survival of the device is that of Trail et al. [5], who reported that 87% of 186 implants remained in place up to 12 years after implantation. However, if radiographic loosening is considered, the survival decreases to 80% at 12 years [5]. More recent experiences from Norway and Sweden reveal a higher complication rate of radiographic loosening of up to 30% [7] and as many as 20% requiring revision at 5 years [6]. The definitive report for this implant has not appeared but a complication rate of 32% [3], a loosening rate of 30% [7], and a revision rate of 20% [6] are worrisome as these problems increase with prolonged surveillance.

Kudo. The Kudo implant was designed in Japan but has been used in Europe as well (Fig. 3). A Belgian experience with 16 implants revealed success in 13 (81%) at 2.5 years [8]. More recently Kudo has shown that the implant was successfully

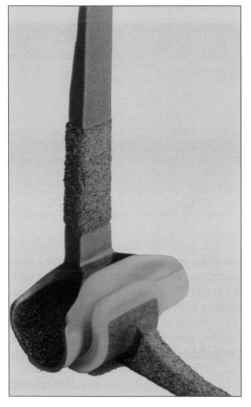

Fig. 3. The Kudo implant from Japan is designed with a saddle concept allowing the forces of the elbow to seat or stabilize the articulation

used in six patients with severe Type IV rheumatoid arthritis [9]. This is the first experience suggesting the possible value of an unlinked device in a grossly deformed joint. Of interest is that this is one of the least constrained of the unlinked device designs.

Capitellocondylar™. In the United States the Capitellocondylar™ has been the most commonly used resurfacing implant (Fig. 4). Ewald et al. [10] provided what to date is the definitive long-term documentation of the results with this device. Over a 13 year period from 1974 to 1987, 202 implants were inserted for rheumatoid arthritis with surveillance averaging 5.7 years. The mean post-operative rating score was 91, reflecting markedly improved function and less pain. Some flexion but little extension improvement was documented. Few revisions were required, 1.5% each for instability, loosening and sepsis. While X-rays showed loosening around eight humeral and 19 ulnar components, most did not appear progressive. The authors concluded that is an effective design for the rheumatoid patients if the surgical procedure is carefully executed. Not all can claim such results [11]. Ljung et al. [12] reported an experience from Sweden in which eight of 50 required reoperation, seven for instability. At final assessment most were pleased with their outcome.

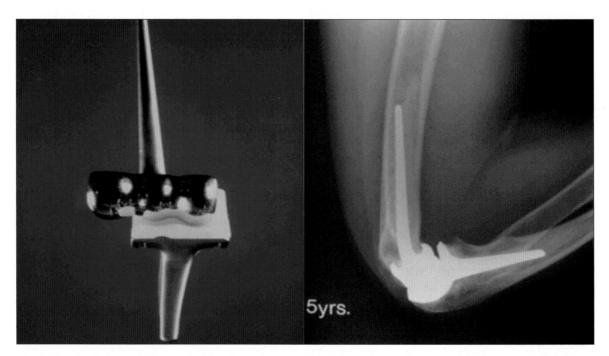

Fig. 4. The Capitellocondylar™ implant has been the most popular resurfacing devices in the United States. It is a two-piece minimally constrained implant, but is now no longer available

Current Generation "Convertable" Implants

In the last several years there have been several additional unlinked implant designs appearing on the market, especially in the United States. One interesting feature of several of these newer devices is the ability to convert the uncoupled to a coupled implant at the time of surgery if circumstances so dictate. There are no data on these devices as yet in the peer-reviewed literature.

Linked Joint Replacement

Several linked semi-constrained implants have been used in the United States and Europe over the last decade (Fig. 5). The characteristics are summarized in Table 3.

Triaxial™. There is limited information about this device. A number of reports have emanated from the designers, the most comprehensive being that of Kraay et al. [13]. This snap-fit design was used in 113 cases: 86 for rheumatoid arthritis and 27 traumatic or "other" etiologies. The outcome varied greatly in the two groups with variable surveillance, the maximum of which was 99 months. Six percent incidence of infection was reported. Loosening was less common in the rheumatoid (2%), compared to the post-traumatic group (22%). The survival at 3 years for rheumatoid and traumatic patients was 92% and 73% respectively. Over time the outcome deteriorated for the post-

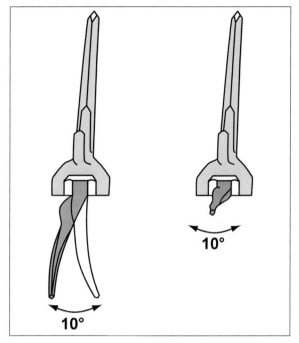

Fig. 5. The concept of a semiconstrained implant is one that allows some motion or laxity at the ulnohumeral articulation but yet is constrained with regard to separation of the components, usually by a pin

trauma group. At 5 years the survival was 90% and 53% for the two groups respectively.

The GSB™. This Swiss implant is most popular in Europe (Fig. 6). Possibly the best insight as to its effectiveness is gleaned from a review article on complications of elbow replacement by Gschwend et al.

Table 3. Semiconstrained elbow replacement for rheumatoid arthritis: N=843. Twelve reports, 6 implants

Author	Implant	No.	With Rheumatoid Arthritis, %	Follow-up, (year)	Extension Flexion, %	Pronation Supination, %	Pain Relief, %	Comp., %	Revised loose, %	Satisfied, %
Figgie, 1988 [21]	Triaxial	44	64	3.5	–	–	89	36	2	–
Pritchard, 1981 [22]	Pritchard II	92	60	2.5	–	–	98	15	2	85
Bayley, 1981 [23]	Stanmore	30	90	3.5	107 arc	107 arc	67	67	–	7
Rosenfeld, 1982 [24]	Pritchard I and II	14	100	2.6	–	–	100	53	–	94
Gschwend, 1988 [25]	GSB III	71	72	4	29-140	69-64	93	27	–	91
Leber, 1988 [26]	Triaxial	11	100	4 (est)	30-132	75-75	91	36	–	91
Morrey, 1989 [27]	Pritchard II	47	48	>5	30-135	60-65	90	32	4	80
Morrey, 1989 [27]	Coonrad-Morrey	237	40	>5	29-132	64-62	92	15	2	88
Madsen, 1989 [28]	Pritchard II	25	100	3	28-130	65-62	100	8	1	92
Kraay, 1994 [13]	Triaxial	86	100	5					3	92
Risung, 1997 [29]	Norway	118	100	4.3	–	–	–	–	4	–
Gill, 1998 [16]	Coonrad-Morrey	78	100	12.5	31-136	61-62	92	24	1	93
TOTAL		**853**		**5**	**29-133**	**65/63**	**91**	**26**	**2%**	**89**

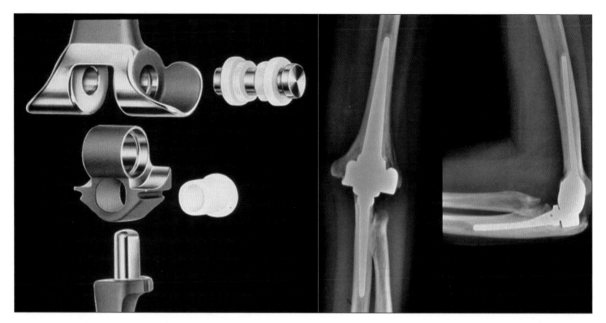

Fig. 6. The GSB-III is one of the more popular semiconstrained implants employed in Europe and for which there is considerable clinical experience

[14]. In this paper 133 procedures are discussed. Of 48 with severe rheumatoid disease, four (8%) were radiographically loose at 10-15 years. The Authors reported an overall rate of revision for loosening in the rheumatoid patients of 2.8% and of the post-trauma patients of 6.5%. As this is a snap-fit articulation, a far more common problem is that of articular disassembly occurring in 3.5% rheumatoid and 15.6% post-trauma patients. The Authors concluded that elbow replacement in selected patients performed by experienced surgeons approaches the success of hip or knee replacement.

Mayo Experience

Coonrad-Morrey. The device is characterized with a flange to resist posterior forces and a "loose hinge" to absorb transmitted forces (Fig. 7). Since 1982, our personal experience has been limited to this semiconstrained implant using the Mayo Elbow Performance Score to document outcome [15]. In 1998 Gill presented the 10-15 year outcome of 78 elbows undergoing the Coonrad-Morrey semiconstrained total elbow arthroplasty [16]. At latest follow-up averaging 12.5 years, 97% were not painful or only mildly so (Fig. 8). The mean arc of flexion was 28°-131°. Pronation averaged 68° and supination 62°. Of the 76 with long-term radiographic evaluation there were two loose ulnar components, one was associated with an infection.

The other did not require revision at the time of follow-up. However, five had worn bushings, none of which required revision at that time (7%). Subsequently, we have documented 4 of 450 patients with sufficient wear to require revision of the articular bushings [17].

Complications were documented in 11 of the 78 elbows (14%), and were serious enough to require a reoperation in 10 (13%). Delayed complications include avulsion of the triceps in three, two deep infections, two ulnar fractures, and fracture of an ulnar component in one. Two elbows were revised for aseptic loosening. The overall 12 year survival rate of this implant was 92.4% with 86% good or excellent according to the Mayo Elbow Performance Score [15] and 91% subjective satisfactory results (Fig. 9). Importantly, Whaley et al. [18] recently assessed a group of 16 patients with Coonrad/Morrey replacements after prior radial head resection and synovectomy. The study group had similar outcomes to the control group. Hence, if a prior synovectomy has been performed, a semiconstrained device can be implanted with confidence.

Conclusions

The current prosthetic elbow replacement options available to manage the patient with rheumatoid arthritis provide increasingly predictable out-

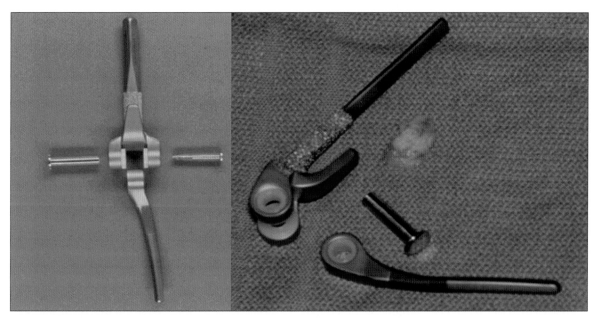

Fig. 7. The Coonrad-Morrey implant employs a loose hinge articulation (1978) and a flange (1981) to resist posterior and torsional stresses at the humerus

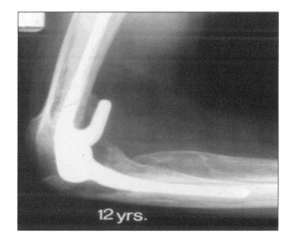

Fig. 8. Twelve year result in a patient with rheumatoid arthritis

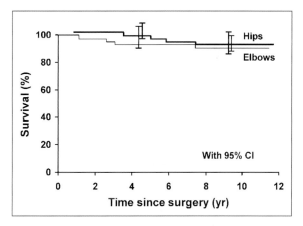

Fig. 9. The Coonrad-Morrey Kaplan Meier Survival Curve for revision at 10-15 years is similar to that of THA for rheumatoid arthritis

comes. Joint replacement with either linked or un-linked implants can be reliably employed but outcomes are enhanced in those with greater experience. The complication rate is higher than that of hip or knee replacement.

References

1. Connor PM, Morrey BF (1998) Total elbow arthroplasty in patients who have juvenile rheumatoid arthritis. J Bone Joint Surg 80:678-688
2. Chiu KY, Luk KDK, Pun WK (1996) Souter-Strathclyde el-bow replacement for severe rheumatoid arthritis. J Orthop Rheum 9:194-199
3. Lyall HA, Cohen B, Clatworthy M, Constant CR (1994) Results of the Souter-Strathclyde total elbow arthroplasty in patients with rheumatoid arthritis. A preliminary report. J Arthroplasty 9:279-284
4. Pöll RG, Rozing PM (1991) Use of the Souter-Strathclyde total elbow prosthesis in patients who have rheumatoid arthritis. J Bone Joint Surg Am 73:1227-1232
5. Trail IA, Nuttall D, Stanley JK (1999) Survivorship and radiological analysis of the standard Souter-Strathclyde total elbow arthroplasty. J Bone Joint Surg Br 81:80-84
6. Andreassen G, Solheim LF (1997) Follow-up of Souter elbow prostheses. Tidsskrift for Den Norske Laegeforening 117:940-942

7. Sjoden GO, Lundberg A, Blomgren GA (1995) Late results of the Souter-Strathclyde total elbow prosthesis in rheumatoid arthritis. 6/19 implants loose after 5 years. Acta Orthop Scand 66:391-394

8. Verstreken F, De Smet L, Westhovens R, Fabry G (1998) Results of the Kudo elbow prosthesis in patients with rheumatoid arthritis: a preliminary report. Clin Rheum 17:325-328

9. Kudo H (1998) Non-constrained elbow arthroplasty for mutilans deformity in rheumatoid arthritis: a report of six cases. J Bone Joint Surg Br 80:234-239

10. Ewald FC, Simons ED, Sullivan JA et al (1993) Capitellocondylar total elbow replacement in rheumatoid arthritis: Long-term results. J Bone Joint Surg Am 75:498-507

11. Dennis DA, Clayton MI, Ferlic DC et al (1990) Capitellocondylar total elbow arthroplasty for rheumatoid arthritis. J Arthroplasty 5[Suppl]:S83-S88

12. Ljung P, Jonsson K, Rydholm U (1995) Short-term complications of a lateral approach for non-constrained elbow replacement. Follow-up of 50 rheumatoid elbows. J Bone Joint Surg Br 77:937-942

13. Kraay MJ, Figgie MP, Inglis AE et al (1994) Primary semiconstrained total elbow arthroplasty. Survival analysis of 113 consecutive cases. J Bone Joint Surg Br 76:636-640

14. Gschwend N, Simmen BR, Matejovsky Z (1996) Late complications in elbow arthroplasty. J Shoulder Elbow Surg 5:86-96

15. Morrey BF, Adams RA (1992) Semiconstrained Arthroplasty for the Treatment of Rheumatoid Arthritis of the Elbow. J Bone Joint Surg Am 74:479-490

16. Gill DRJ, Morrey BF (1998) The Coonrad-Morrey total elbow arthroplasty in patients who have rheumatoid arthritis. A 10 to 15 year follow-up study. J Bone Joint Surg Am 80:1327-1335

17. Lee BP, Adams RA, Morrey BF (2004) Polyethylene wear in total elbow arthroplasty. J Bone Joint Surg Am (*in press*)

18. Whaley A, Morrey BF, Adams RA (2004) Total elbow arthroplasty following previous synovectomy and radial head resection of the elbow. J Bone Joint Surg Br (*in press*)

19. Kudo H, Iwano K, Nishino J (1994) Cementless or hybrid total elbow arthroplasty with titanium alloy implants. J Arthroplasty 9:269-278

20. Allieu Y, Meyer ZU, Reckendorf G, Daude O (1998) Long-term results of unconstrained Roper-Tuke total elbow arthroplasty in patients with rheumatoid arthritis. J Shoulder Elbow Surg 7:560-564

21. Figgie MP, Inglis AE, Mow CS, Figgie HE III (1988) Salvage of nonunion of supracondylar fracture of the humerus by total elbow arthroplasty. J Bone Joint Surg 3:235

22. Pritchard RW (1981) Long-term follow-up study: semiconstrained elbow prosthesis. Orthopaedics 4:151

23. Bayley JIL (1981) Elbow replacement in rheumatoid arthritis. Recon Surg Traumat 18:70

24. Rosenfeld SR, Ansel SH (1982) Evaluation of the Pritchard total elbow arthroplasty. Orthopedics 5:713

25. Gschwend N, Loehr J, Ivosevic-Radovanovic D et al (1988) Semiconstrained elbow prosthesis with special reference to the GSB III prosthesis. Clin Orthop 232:104

26. Leber C, Melone CP Jr (1988) Total elbow replacement. Orthop Rev 17:85

27. Morrey BF (1991) The Elbow: Semiconstrained Devices. In: Morrey BF (ed) Joint Replacement Arthroplasty. Churchill Livingstone, Philadelphia

28. Madsen F, Gudmundson GH, Søjbjerg JO, Sneppen O (1989) Pritchard Mark II elbow prosthesis in rheumatoid arthritis. Acta Orthop Scand 60:249-253

29. Risung F (1997) The Norway elbow replacement. Design, technique and results after nine years. J Bone Joint Surg Br 79:394-402

CHAPTER 23

Total Elbow Arthroplasty in Acute Fracture

A. CELLI

Introduction

The intra-articular fractures of the distal humerus are uncommon and difficult to treat with potentially disabling consequences. These fractures comprise about 1% of the adult fractures and about 10% of the humeral fractures; most of them are usually displaced and comminuted [1].

As the aging population is increasing, there is an increasing need to investigate the role of the surgical treatments of such fractures and in particular to define when the elbow replacement or the open reduction and stable fixation can be advised.

The epidemiologic studies have indicated that the incidence of the distal humeral fractures in women older than 60 years will have increased three times by 2030 [2].

The treatment of these lesions using the rigid osteosynthesis is well accepted, but in recent review of 846 procedures from 13 reports, in which were performed an open reduction and internal fixation for intra-articular fractures, 20% of the patients were described to have unsatisfactory outcomes [3].

It is often difficult to achieve stable fixation in elderly patients with poor bone quality associated with articular comminution. Helfet et al. [4] reported fair to poor outcomes in 25% of patients treated with open reduction and internal fixation for distal humeral fractures. The same result was also reported by John et al. [5]; they described 20% of fair and poor results in 49 elderly patients aged 75 to 90 years old. The open reduction and stable internal fixation can be difficult or sometimes impossible in elderly patients with marked intra-articular comminution and with an osteopenic bone that reduces the possibility to obtain a stable fixation [6-8].

The common sequale as joint stiffness, loss of the reduction, and early post-traumatic osteoarthritis are not rare in the treatment in these types of elbow fractures and in particular in older age groups [9-15].

The indications for total elbow arthroplasty (TEA) have expanded over the last decades, and the principle goals of the elbow replacement in these traumatic conditions is to provide a stable, painless range of motion during daily living activities [3, 7, 16, 17].

We have also to consider that patients older than 65 years of age with complex elbow fractures treated with TEA had better outcomes than those converted to TEA after the primary open reduction and internal fixation failed [18].

The linked semiconstrained implants are used in the majority of the series reported in the literature, and in particular the Coonrad-Morrey prosthesis for its design is able to be used in these acute conditions recovering the articular movements that allows most of the daily living activities in this age group [19].

The present chapter wants to define, with reference to the literature, the indications, the surgical technique and the outcomes of the TEA used in the acute elbow fractures.

Indications

The types C2 and C3 (comminuted intra-articular of the distal humerus fractures) of the AO classification are not uncommon in the older age group and typically occur as a result of a minor fall (Fig. 1) [18, 20].

The indication for the elbow replacement in these acute fractures are limited to a restricted number of patients older than 65 years with extensively comminuted fractures for which it is not possible to obtain a stable fixation that allows an early motion [16, 21, 22].

Usually these patients have a severe comminution with multiple small articular fragments associated with severe osteopenic bone and in some cases the pre-existing joint damage such as rheuma-

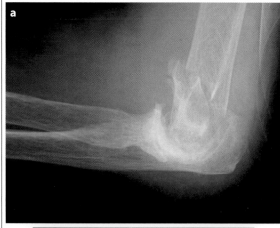

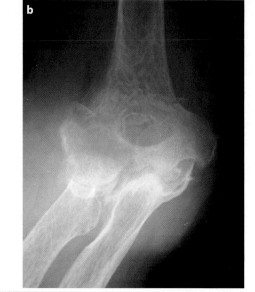

Fig. 2 a, b. Distal humeral fracture in patient with pre-existing rheumatoid arthritis

toid arthritis or other inflammatory joint diseases (Fig. 2) [18, 23].

The two most important aspects of the open reduction and internal fixation that allow satisfactory results are to recover the articular congruency and to stabilize the reduction with rigid fixation; when in elderly patients these can not be achieved, the elbow replacement must be considered as the correct choice [24-28].

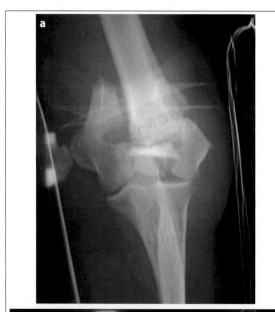

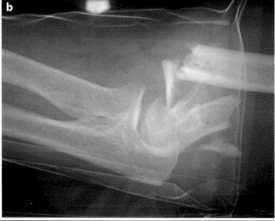

Fig. 1 a, b. C3 comminuted intra-articular fracture in older patient

Surgical Technique

The patient is in a supine position or in a lateral side position. The posterior midline skin incision is performed just medially or laterally to the tip of the olecranon (Fig. 3); the ulnar nerve is identified and mobilized distally to the first motor branch of the flexor carpi ulnaris and then proximally to be transposed into an anterior subcutaneous pocket without placing the nerve under tension (the anterior border of the intermuscular septum is resected to avoid a nerve impingement).

Different management of the extensor mechanism has been described in the literature. In the Bryan and Morrey approach [29], the triceps is reflected laterally from the olecranon in continuity with the ulnar periosteum and the fascia of the forearm, including the anconeus (Fig. 4).

At the end of the procedure the triceps is reattached to the olecranon through drill holes with a heavy nonabsorbable suture.

The advantage of this approach is that the triceps tendon is in continuity with the anconeus muscle and with the fascio-ulnar complex and this prevents the proximal migration of the extensor mechanism.

The disadvantages are the possible subluxation of the triceps tendon laterally and the difficulty of maintaining the continuity of the fascio-ulnar complex in the rheumatoid patient, or in case of previous surgical approaches which involved the extensor mechanism.

The second option is the paratricipital or bilaterotricipital approach [30, 31], which consists of leaving the triceps insertion intact (Fig. 5).

The joint is exposed through both medial and lateral fascia insertions by releasing the common flexor-pronator muscles from the medial epicondyle and the extensor supinator muscles from the lateral epicondyle.

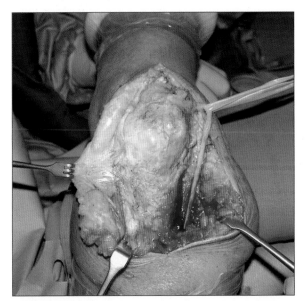

Fig. 3. The posterior midline skin incision with open medial and lateral cutaneous flaps and isolated ulnar nerve

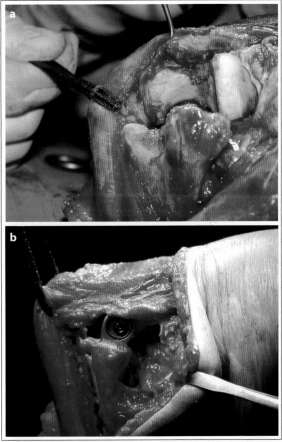

Fig. 5 a, b. The paratricipital approach consists of leaving the triceps tendon attached; the prosthesis is performed from the medial and lateral side

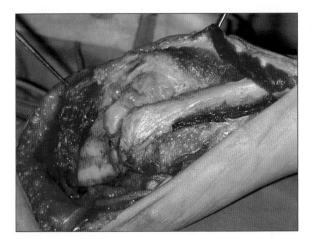

Fig. 4. In the Bryan and Morrey approach, the triceps is reflected laterally in continuity with the anconeus

The advantages are that the extensor mechanism remains intact from the olecranon insertion, and no post-operative protection is needed.

The disadvantages are the limited exposure of the articular surface and the difficulty in obtaining a visualization of the ulnar component to assess the correct version and rotation of the implant.

Another option is the triceps approach described by Stanley [32], in which he describes the medial edge of the triceps reflecting only 25%, leaving intact the other 75% of triceps insertion.

The advantage of this approach is that the triceps is still intact and allows a better visualization of the ulnar component during its implant than the paratricipital or bilaterotricipital approach.

Another possibility is the triceps splint [33, 34], which can be used in the implant of the prosthesis in acute trauma (Fig. 6).

The joint is exposed through a subperiosteal dissection of the triceps in continuity with the common extensor and flexor origins and the forearm fascia; some Authors reflect the two flaps with a piece of olecranon bone to obtain a better reinsertion at the end of the procedure.

The advantage of this technique is that it maintains a centralized extensor mechanism; the disadvantage is greater soft tissue disruption.

The modified approach (Tongue approach) consists of an incision along the border of the musculo-tendinous expansions of the triceps, leaving intact the muscle fibers; then it is reflected, leaving its insertion on the olecranon (Fig. 7).

Using this technique, the medial head of the triceps and the anconeus muscle are reflected in continuity, preserving the blood and nerve supply of the anconeus (Figs. 8, 9).

The dissection of the olecranon fat pad is made and reflected in continuity with the medial triceps flap and thus should prevent the post-operative adhesion between the triceps and the humerus.

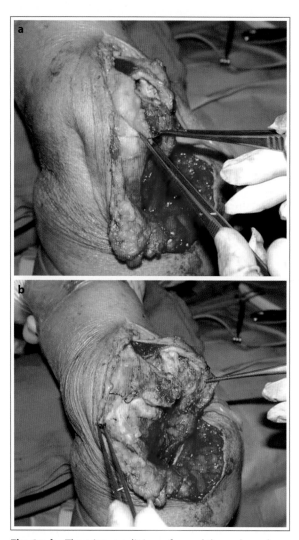

Fig. 6 a, b. The triceps split is performed through a subperiosteal dissection of the triceps

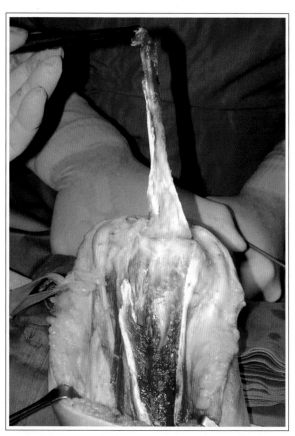

Fig. 7. The tongue approach consists of an incision along the border of the musculo-tendinous expansion of the triceps

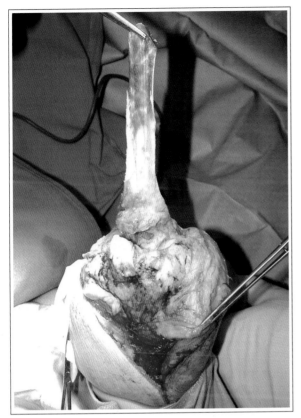

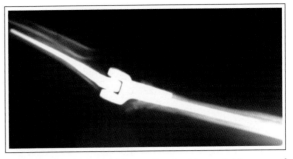

Fig. 10. The Coonrad-Morrey implant is useful in case of significant humeral bone loss

Fig. 8. The medial muscle part of the triceps and the anconeus are reflecting in continuity with the olecranon fat pad

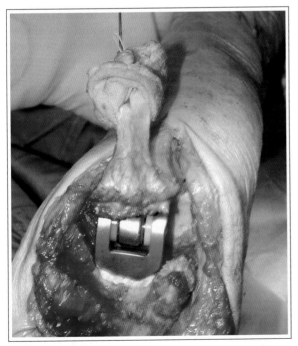

Fig. 9. The linked semiconstrain performed through the tongue approach

Once the distal humerus is exposed, the fracture fragments are excised; loss of one or both condyles makes it difficult to assess the correct rotatory alignment and the proper height.

The linked, semiconstrained implant such as the Coonrad-Morrey is preferred by several Authors in these traumatic conditions because it can be used also in case of significant bone loss with lack of one or both epicondyles (Fig. 10). It requires only the humeral diaphysis to obtain secure fixation and it does not need to have an internal fixation of the condyles [17,19].

The modularity of this implant allows better adaptation to the different traumatic conditions, and the long anterior flange reduces the risk of shortening of the humerus [3,17,19].

The intramedullary guide is seated in the humeral canal and it assists in the varus-valgus alignment. The humeral anterior flange helps align rotation because it fits with the bone graft and the anterior humeral cortex.

The ulnar preparation starts by removing the tip of the olecranon. Once the ulna intramedullary canal is entered, the trial rasp is used in the proper orientation.

The trial implants are inserted in both ulnar and humeral medullar canals; the elbow is put through a full range of motion to assess for impingement or capsular contractures.

The final components can be inserted using cement with antibiotic and placing the graft between the anterior humeral flange and the humerus cortex. Each component can be inserted separately starting with the ulna and then the locking central pin is placed.

The radial head resection is performed if it impinges on the anterior flange during the flexion.

The medial and lateral condyles can be reattached to the humerus using K wires and nonabsorbable sutures. This is useful to improve the stability of the implant (Fig. 11).

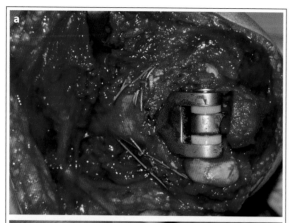

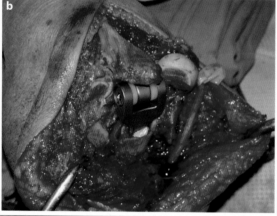

Fig. 11 a, b. The medial and lateral condyles are fixed to the humerus with K wires and sutures to improve the implant stability

The fixation of the extensor mechanism depends on which approach was used to reduce the risk of the triceps insufficiency. It must be securely fixed to the olecranon with heavy nonabsorbable N. 5 bone sutures (Fig. 12) [35].

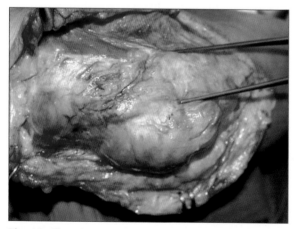

Fig. 12. The triceps is detached from the olecranon and moves laterally

Results

In 1997 Cobb and Morrey [7] reported their result of TEA used as primary treatment of distal humerus acute fracture in elderly patients.

Twenty patients (21 elbows) whose ages ranged from 48 to 92 years were treated using the TEA. The indications were an extensively comminuted fracture or an association with rheumatoid arthritis. They were followed patients were lost from the follow-up, the remaining were followed from a minimum of 2 years. According to the Mayo Elbow Performance Score (MEPS), 15 elbows had excellent results and five had good results. The mean arc of flexion-extension was 130°-25°. There were no fair or poor results.

In 1999 Frankle et al. [18] described their retrospective evaluation of the intra-articular distal humeral fractures in females older than 65 years, comparing the results of the patients treated with the open reduction and internal fixation (ORIF) with a second group in which was implanted TEA. Twelve patients were treated with primary TEA and according to the MEPS they obtained excellent results in 11 patients and one good result; no fair or poor outcomes were observed.

In this series better outcomes were obtained in the TEA group compared to the ORIF patients. The group that converted from ORIF to TEA had significantly worse outcomes.

In 2000 Ray et al. [36] reported their experience on seven patients treated with primary TEA and follow-up for 2-4 years. According to the MEPS five elbows obtained excellent results and two elbows rated a good result; six patients had no pain and one had mild pain. The mean arc of flexion-extension was 130°-20°.

In 2001, Gambirasio et al. [23] evaluated the outcome of 10 older patients (mean age of 85 years) treated with primary TEA for comminuted intra-articular distal humeral fractures.

According to the MEPS, eight patients rated an excellent result and two had good result at mean follow-up of one year. The mean arc of flexion-extension was 125.5°-23.5°.

In 2002, Garcia et al. [22] reported the results at 3 years of mean follow-up of 16 patients treated with primary TEA. Fifteen patients were satisfied with their outcome and the mean MEPS was 93 points; the mean arc of motion in flexion-extension was 24°-125°.

In 2004, Kaminemi [16] described the recent Mayo experience of 49 acute fractures in 48 patients treated using the TEA as primary option; the mean age was 67. In 43 fractures the mean follow-up was at least 2 years.

According to the MEPS, 93 points were obtained as a mean score and 32 elbows (65%) had neither complications nor any further surgery from the time of the implant to the most recent follow-up evaluation. The mean arc of flexion-extension recovered was 24°-131°.

Our Experience

We have used TEA for the treatment of the intra-articular comminuted distal humeral fractures in 18 patients. All of these patients had distal comminuted intra-articular fractures with associated poor bone stock for osteoporotic or prolonged therapy with cortisone. Two patients were also associated with a rheumatoid pathology and their elbows were painful before the trauma. All these elbows were replaced using the linked semiconstraint Coonrad-Morrey prosthesis. The average age of our group of patients was 73 years (range from 64 to 88 years). The mean follow-up was 38 months (range from 12 to 121 months).

According to the MEPS, 92 points were obtained as a mean score; one elbow underwent a revision of the prosthesis for septic loosening one year after the implant.

The other 17 elbows did not have any complications nor any further surgery from the time of the implant to the most recent follow-up evaluation. The mean arc of flexion-extension recovered was 20°-135°.

Discussion

Open reduction and internal fixation with early motion is the treatment of choice in distal humeral fractures. Problems arise due to osteopenia and comminution of the articular fractures that are correlated to inadequate internal fixation, and result in prolonged immobilization with a high rate of complications and poor results.

Recent literature has shown that open reduction and internal fixation of the distal humeral fractures in patients over the age of 60 years with comminuted fracture may not achieve acceptable outcomes [36, 37].

Pajarinen et al. [38] reviewed their results of internal fixation and they observed that patients younger than 40 years of age had a higher incidence of excellent and good post-operative results than patients over 50 years of age.

This result is influenced by a period of immobilization that is correlated to the rigid fixation of the synthesis and by bone quality; in their report they observed that younger patients had, on average, a shorter period of immobilization compared to those patients over the age of 50. They concluded that poor results in older patients were caused by the longer period of post-operative immobilization and subsequent elbow stiffness. The poor bone quality and comminution of the fractures provided an explanation for the prolonged immobilization.

Caja et al. [37] reported the same phenomenon in their series. They observed that patients over 40 years of age had a lower final range of motion compared to those younger than 40 years.

Morrey et al. [7, 19] have suggested TEA as a reliable option when adequate fixation of a fracture in an elderly patient is difficult due to comminution and poor bone quality.

Robison et al. [20] reported the same results with regard to the difficulty in obtaining stable fixation that can be correlated with higher risk for union complications in type C distal humeral fractures and they proposed the TEA as primary treatment for these types of fractures in elderly patients.

Cobb and Morrey [7] were the first to review retrospectively the results (21 patients) of a series of acute fractures treated with TEA.

The indications of the elbow replacement in this series were the comminution of the articular surface and in ten patients were associated to the destruction of the articular surface secondary to rheumatoid arthritis. The Authors reported that the presence of rheumatoid arthritis had a direct influence on their decision to treat these patients with TEA.

The results obtained in the Morrey's series prompted Frankle to re-examine osteosynthesis as the primary treatment for older women who may have bone loss related to osteoporosis [18].

At the end of the Frankle report [18], he described a decision-making algorithm for the treatment of the articular surface fractures in patients over the age of 65. Two factors are important to be considered in the decision-making process: bone quality and comorbidities such as osteoporosis, rheumatoid arthritis, diabetes, chronic steroid use, age of the patient, gender, etc., (the comorbidities factors are present in 69% of their patients) [16, 17].

Following this algorithm they concluded in their report that they treat preferentially comminuted and displaced intra-articular fractures of the distal humerus in older women with associated comorbidities with primary TEA. In older women with adequate bone stock and without associated comorbidities, the open reduction and internal fixation is the treatment of choice.

This study [18] is the only one that has compared osteosynthesis and TEA for the treatment of acute fractures in patients over 65 years of age. Although this study concerns selected fractures, better outcomes were obtained in the elbow replacement group in terms of range of motion and personal satisfaction.

A similar experience was described in the recent series from the Mayo Clinic in which they achieved satisfactory outcomes in 93% of their patients [16,17].

After a systematic review of recently published English-language literature, Little et al. [39] looked at 6 different papers, where in 79 TEAs were performed for acute distal humeral fractures. The Authors concluded that the clinical results (excellent and good results were obtained in 99% of the patients) reports for acute fracture were very good, although both the number of the procedures and the duration of the follow-ups were comparatively small.

In the literature [16, 40, 41], the majority of the elbow fractures were replaced using a linked semiconstrained Coonrad-Morrey implant. The design of this prosthesis is particular useful in the treatment of the acute comminuted fracture with poor bone stock. This implant allows 8° of varus/valgus through arc of motion closely simulating the normal axis of rotation of the elbow. The anterior flange allows good fixation to the anterior cortex of the humeral and avoids a shortening of the humeral in case of comminution of the distal part (Fig. 13).

McKee et al. [42] examined the effect of the condylar resection in the setting of TEA; they compared two groups of patients: the condyles resection and the condyles retained group. They concluded that condylar resection did not have a negative effect on patient functional strength. However, they did not examine the influence of the condylar

resection on the survival of the prosthesis in terms of aseptic loosening and bushing wear.

The aim of TEA is to allow the restoration of the functional arc of motion of the elbow without pain and post-operative immobilization. The correct choice of patients is an important factor to be considered in the preoperative plan for reducing the risk of complications.

In preparation for a surgical case, it is recommended that equipment for a primary TEA and for open reduction and internal fixation should be in the operation room. The decision must be made intra-operatively on the basis of the possibility of performing a stable internal fixation according to the type of the fracture and on the bone quality. For this reason, it is important to choose the appropriate approach.

The olecranon osteotomy allows a wide exposure of the articular surface but should be avoided in case we change intra-operatively the indication from the internal fixation to TEA.

The idea to perform an hemi-elbow replacement for the primary treatment of the acute fractures is relatively new (Figs. 14, 15). There is no long-term follow-up study or large group of patients; however, some Authors are working on the idea to replace only the humeral side in acute distal humeral fracture.

The results in acute fractures looks very interesting and they also advise the use of hemi-arthroplasty in case of revision (malunion or nonunion of distal humeral fractures) but the number of cases and the short time of the follow-up did not indicate if it is a real advantage in terms of reducing the number of complications and in the restoration of the functional range of motion without pain.

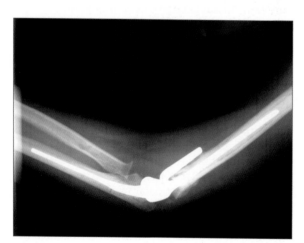

Fig. 13. The long flange allows good fixation on the anterior cortex and avoids shortening of the humerus

Conclusions

TEA does have a role in primary fracture fixation in selected patients. Many patients over the age of 60 years with distal humeral fractures can be well treated with open reduction and internal fixation. When patients have poor bone quality associated with comminuted distal humeral fractures, the TEA should be considered, especially for those patients with pre-existing joint disease from inflammatory arthropathy, poor mechanical bone quality, and extensive fracture comminution such as the AO C3 type.

The results of TEA in those cases are often better than internal fixation and are also better with the primary TEA rather than attempting to salvage a failed reconstruction. In the largest series pub-

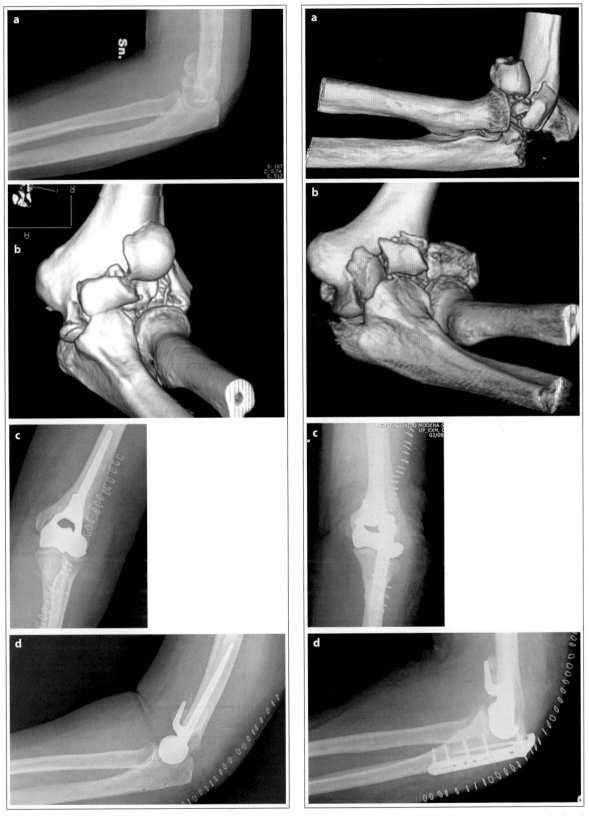

Fig. 14 a-d. X-ray and TC (3D) of comminuted distal humeral fracture in 67-year-old female treated with hemiarthroplasty and ligaments repaired

Fig. 15 a-d. X-ray and TC (3D) of comminuted distal humeral fracture with olecranon fracture in 70-year-old female treated with hemi-arthroplasty and olecranon plate

lished satisfactory results were obtained in 93% of the patients [16].

The Coonrad-Morrey linked semi-constrained implant is the most successful arthroplasty in acute fractures; it is designed to provide a good stability also in case of condilary resetion for particular comminution [43].

The hemiarthroplasty is being investigated as another solution for the treatment of these complex distal humeral fractures in older patients.

We believe that TEA is an option in the treatment of distal humeral fractures in properly selected patients and it is able to achieve satisfactory results in a high percentage of patients.

The intra-articular elbow fractures can be treated using different devices (plate osteosynthesis, total elbow arthroplasty, hemi-arthoplasty), all of which are able to obtain good results when the correct choice is taken on the basis of:
– the type of the elbow fracture;
– the presence of comorbidities;
– the patient's age;
– the patient's activities.

At the end of this chapter, we propose the following algorithm that can be useful in the decision-making process in case of intra-articular distal humerus fractures (Fig. 16).

References

1. Watson-Jones R (1960) Fractures and joint injuries. 4th edn. Vol. 2. Williams and Wilkins, Baltimore
2. Palvanen M, Kannus P, Niemi S, Parkkari J (1998) Secular trends in the osteoporotic fractures of the distal humerus. Eur J Epidemol 14:N2
3. Jupiter J, Morrey BF (1993) Fractures of the distal humerus in adult. In: Morrey BF (ed) The elbow and its disorders. WB Saunders, Philadelphia
4. Helfet DL, Schmerling GJ (1993) Bicondylar intra-articular fractures of the distal humerus in adults. Clin Orthop 26:292
5. John H, Rosso R, Meff V (1994) Operative treatment of the distal humerus fractures in the elderly. J Bone Joint Surg Br 74:793-796
6. Huang TL, Chiu FY, Chuang TY, Chen TH (2005) The results of open reduction and internal fixation in elderly patients with severe fractures of the distal humerus: a critical analysis of the results. J Trauma 58:62-69

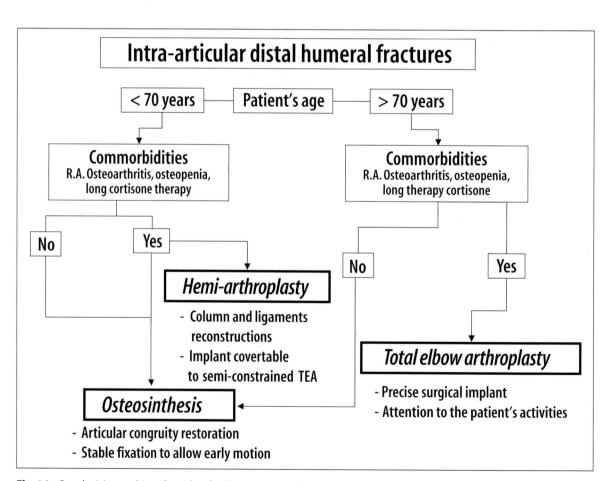

Fig. 16. Our decision making algorithm for the treatment of the distal humeral fractures

7. Cobb TK, Morrey BF (1997) Total elbow arthroplasty as primary treatment for distal humeral fractures in elderly patients. J Bone Joint Surg Am 79:826-832

8. Korner J, Lill H, Muller LP et al (2005) Distal humerus fractures in elderly patients: results after open reduction and internal fixation. Osteoporos Int 2:S73-S79. Epub 2004 Oct 29

9. Dubberley JH, Faber KJ, Macdermid JC et al (2006) Outcome after open reduction and internal fixation of capitellar and trochlear fractures. J Bone Joint Surg Am 88:46-54

10. McKee MD, Wilson TL, Winston L et al (2000) Functional outcome following surgical treatment of intra-articular distal humeral fractures through a posterior approach. J Bone Joint Surg Am 82:1701-1707

11. Aslam N, Willett K (2004) Functional outcome following internal fixation of intra-articular fractures of the distal humerus (AO type C). Acta Orthop Belg 70:118-122

12. Ring D, Jupiter JB, Gulotta L (2003) Articular fractures of the distal part of the humerus. J Bone Joint Surg Am 85:232-238

13. Soon JL, Chan BK, Low CO (2004) Surgical fixation of intra-articular fractures of the distal humerus in adults. Injury 35:954

14. Gofton WT, Macdermid JC, Patterson SD et al (2003) Functional outcome of AO type C distal humeral fractures. J Hand Surg Am 28:294-308

15. Tyllianakis M, Panagopoulos A, Papadopoulos AX et al (2004) Functional evaluation of comminuted intra-articular fractures of the distal humerus (AO type C). Long term results in twenty-six patients. Acta Orthop Belg 70:123-130

16. Kamineni S, Morrey BF (2004) Distal humeral fractures treated with noncustom total elbow replacement. J Bone Joint Surg Am 86:940-947

17. Kamineni S, Morrey BF (2005) Distal humeral fractures treated with noncustom total elbow replacement. Surgical technique. J Bone Joint Surg Am 87:41-50

18. Frankle MA, Herscovici D Jr, Di Pasquale TG et al (2003) A comparison of open reduction and internal fixation and primary total elbow arthroplasty in the treatment of intra-articular distal humerus fractures in women older than age 65. J Orthop Trauma 17:473-480

19. Morrey BF (2000) Fractures of the distal humerus: role of the elbow replacement. Orthop N Am 31:145-154

20. Robinson LM, Hill RN, Jacobs N et al (2003) Adult distal humeral metaphyseal fractures: epidemiology and result of the treatment. J Orthop Trauma 17:38-47

21. Muller LP, Kamineni S, Rommens PM, Morrey BF (2005) Primary total elbow replacement for fractures of the distal humerus. Oper Orthop Traumatol 17:119-142

22. Garcia JA, Mykula R, Stanley D (2002) Complex fractures of the distal humerus in the elderly. The role of total elbow replacement as primary treatment. J Bone Joint Surg Br 84:812-816

23. Gambirasio R, Riand N, Stern R, Hoffmeyer P (2001) Total elbow replacement for complex fractures of the distal humerus. An option for the elderly patient. J Bone Joint Surg Br 83:974-978

24. Srinivasan K, Agarwal M, Matthews SJ, Giannoudis PV (2005) Fractures of the distal humerus in the elderly: is internal fixation the treatment of choice? Clin Orthop Relat Res 434:222-230

25. Pereles TR, Koval KJ, Gallagher M, Rosen H (1997) Open reduction and internal fixation of the distal humerus: functional outcome in the elderly. J Trauma 43:578-584

26. Korner J, Lill H, Muller LP et al (2005) Distal humerus fractures in elderly patients: results after open reduction and internal fixation. Osteoporos Int 16:S73-S79. Epub 2004 Oct 29

27. Huang TL, Chiu FY, Chuang TY, Chen TH (2005) The results of open reduction and internal fixation in elderly patients with severe fractures of the distal humerus: a critical analysis of the results. J Trauma 58:62-69

28. Letsch R, Schmit-Neuerburg KP, Sturmer KM, Walz M (1989) Intraarticular fractures of the distal humerus. Surgical treatment and results. Clin Orthop Relat Res 241:238-244

29. Bryan R (1982) Extensive posterior exposure of the elbow: a triceps-sparing approach. Clinic Orthop 166:188-192

30. Alonso-Liames M (1972) Bilaterotricipital approach to the elbow. Its application in the osteosynthesis of the supracondylar fractures of the humerus in children. Acta Orthop Scand 43:479-490

31. Schildhauer T, Nork S (2003) Extensor mechanism-sparing paratricipital posterior approach to the distal humerus. J Orthop Trauma 17:374-378

32. Stanley D, Shahani SA (1999) A posterior approach to the elbow joint, J Bone Joint Surg Br 81:1020-1022

33. Frankle M (2002) Triceps split technique for total elbow arthroplasty. Tech Shoulder Elbow Surg 3:23-27

34. Gschwend N (1981) Our operative approach to the elbow joint. Arch Orthop Trauma Surg 98:143-146

35. Celli A, Arash A, Adams R (2005) Triceps insufficiency following total elbow arthroplasty. J Bone Joint Surg Am 87:1957-1964

36. Kay PS, Kakarlapudi K, Rajsekhar C, Bhamra MS (2000) Total elbow arthroplasty as primary treatment for distal humeral fractures in elderly patients. Injury 31:687-692

37. Caja VL, Moroni A, Vendemia V et al (1994) Surgical treatment of bicondylar fractures of the distal humerus. Injury 25:433-438

38. Pajarinem J, Bjorkemhein JM (2002) Operative treatment of type C intercondylar fractures of the distal humerus: result after a mean follow-up of 2 years in a series of 18 patients. J Shoulder Elbow Surg 11:48-52

39. Little C (2005) Total elbow arthroplasty; a systematic review of the literature in the English language until he end of 2003. J Bone Joint Surg Br 87:437-444

40. Hildebrand KA, Patterson SD, Regan WD et al (2000) Functional outcome of semiconstrained total elbow arthroplasty. J Bone Joint Surg Am 82:1379-1386

41. Armstrong AD, Yamaguchi K (2004) Total elbow arthroplasty and distal humerus elbow fractures. Hand Clin 20:475-483

42. McKee MD, Pugh DM, Richards RR et al (2003) Effect of humeral condylar resection on strength and functional outcome after semiconstrained total elbow arthroplasty. J Bone Joint Surg Am 85:802-807

43. Moro J (2000) Total elbow arthroplasty in the treatment of post-traumatic condition of the elbow. Clinic Orthopaedic N 370:102-114

CHAPTER 24

Latitude Convertible Total Elbow Prosthesis

G.J.W. KING, K. YAMAGUCHI, S.W. O'DRISCOLL

Introduction

Severe arthritis of the elbow was historically managed with resection or interposition arthroplasty. Dee was the first to report the use of total elbow arthroplasty in the English literature [1]. The fixed-hinge design was fully constrained and transferred stress directly to the prosthetic interface resulting in high rates of aseptic loosening and early failures. A greater understanding of elbow anatomy and kinematics has led to advances in prosthetic design and surgical technique.

Unlinked, resurfacing prostheses were subsequently designed in an attempt to address this problem of loosening. These prostheses had variable amounts of intrinsic constraint and relied primarily on the soft tissue envelope for stability. While often successful, a significant incidence of post-operative instability was reported and felt to be secondary to surgical inexperience and deficiencies in component instrumentation and design [2-6]. Advances in unlinked prosthetic design have favored a more anatomic ulnohumeral articulation that when properly positioned can restore near-normal kinematics of the elbow [8-12]. Some implants have been employed with greater articular constraint, which, while increasing stability, has

led to problems with loosening [9-13]. The option of a radial head prosthesis may theoretically improve elbow stability and lower forces at the ulno-humeral articulation by balancing the load distribution across the elbow joint. Radial head replacement has been reported to be an important factor for stability in some unlinked prostheses [8,12,14].

Newer designs of linked prostheses have a "loose-hinge" mechanical linkage that can accurately replicate the semi-constrained kinematics of the native elbow. Ideally, the rotational and varus/valgus forces that occur during normal flexion and extension should be dissipated through the soft tissues rather than through the mechanical articulation. It has been demonstrated that if the soft tissue envelope is balanced and the components are correctly positioned, the motion pathways of the implant will not reach the structural laxity of the hinge [7]. This should lead to a reduction in the incidence of polyethylene bushing wear, osteolysis, and aseptic loosening. An anterior flange has also been added to the humeral component of some linked designs to resist the posterior and rotational displacement forces thought to contribute to early prosthetic loosening.

Both linked and unlinked total elbow arthroplasty designs have been shown to be reliable for the treatment of patients with end-stage rheumatoid arthritis. Satisfaction and long-term, revision-free survival now approaches that of hip and knee arthroplasty in this population [15-17]. Mechanical failures have been higher with the use of elbow arthroplasty in a higher demand patient population. The unmet need to provide a reliable elbow arthroplasty for the younger rheumatoid patient and those with osteoarthritis has resulted in an increasing interest in the development of a more flexible, high performance total elbow system.

Restoration of the anatomical axis of flexion-extension and careful soft tissue balance is paramount in recreating normal elbow kinematics, in an effort to reduce mechanical failures and increase prosthetic survival. Modular implants and precision instrumentation should make determination and recreation of the flexion-extension axis more reliable and reproducible. A convertible implant allows the surgeon the versatility to choose to perform a hemiarthroplasty or an unlinked or linked total elbow arthroplasty with assurance that later revision can be performed without the need to remove well-fixed stems. Conversion from an un-linked to a linked prosthesis can be performed at the time of the initial implantation or post-operatively in a minimally invasive fashion if instability is a problem.

The Latitude (Tornier, Stafford, TX) total elbow system currently offers these options (Fig. 1). Alignment jigs and modular components assist in recreating an accurate center of rotation and soft tissue balance required for proper component tracking. The ability to repair the collateral ligaments through the prosthesis improves stability in the post-operative period. The Latitude system can also accommodate retention or replacement

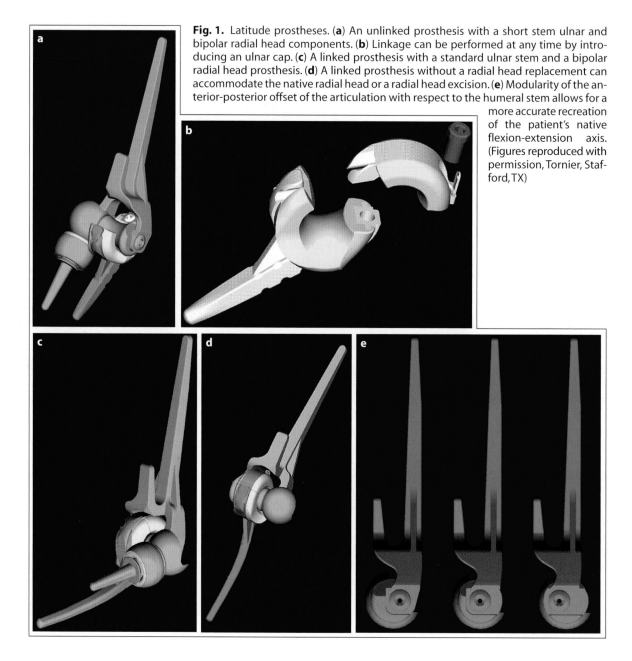

Fig. 1. Latitude prostheses. (**a**) An unlinked prosthesis with a short stem ulnar and bipolar radial head components. (**b**) Linkage can be performed at any time by introducing an ulnar cap. (**c**) A linked prosthesis with a standard ulnar stem and a bipolar radial head prosthesis. (**d**) A linked prosthesis without a radial head replacement can accommodate the native radial head or a radial head excision. (**e**) Modularity of the anterior-posterior offset of the articulation with respect to the humeral stem allows for a more accurate recreation of the patient's native flexion-extension axis. (Figures reproduced with permission, Tornier, Stafford, TX)

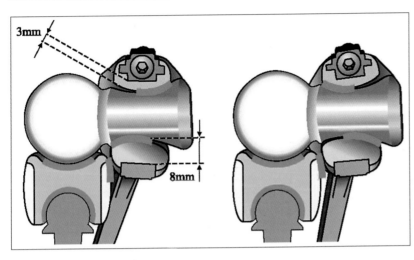

Fig. 2. Articular design. The humeral component has a concave barrel-shaped trochlea to maintain linear contact with the ulnar component throughout the 7° degrees of varus/valgus laxity of the articulation. The polyethylene of the ulnar component is thickest anteriorly (8 mm) in the area of maximal loading. The addition of a bipolar radial head component articulating with the prosthetic capitellum further dissipates loading across the elbow. (Figure reproduced with permission, Tornier, Stafford, TX)

of the radial head and has a thicker polyethylene articulation with a greater contact area to decrease wear (Fig. 2). An anatomic hemiarthroplasty of the distal humerus is also possible with modular components for the reconstruction of osteopenic, comminuted fractures of the distal humerus in elderly patients (Fig. 3).

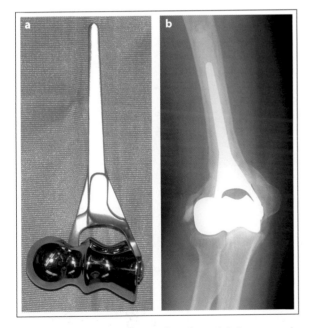

Fig. 3. Distal humeral hemiarthroplasty. (**a**) An anatomic distal humeral spool can accommodate the native olecranon and radial head. Later conversion to total elbow arthroplasty can be performed without the removal of the well-fixed humeral stem by replacing the anatomic spool with an arthroplasty spool and placement of an ulnar component. (**b**) An anatomic humeral hemiarthroplasty performed for a distal humerus fracture

Indications and Contraindications

Total elbow arthroplasty, whether linked or unlinked, is the most definitive functional procedure for end-stage elbow arthritis. Painful rheumatoid arthritis remains the most common indication for total elbow arthroplasty. Patients with complex nonunion, dysfunctional instability, periarticular tumors, and both primary and post-traumatic osteoarthritis have also been successfully managed with total elbow arthroplasty. More recently, complex acute intra-articular fractures of the distal humerus in elderly patients with osteopenia and comminution have become more frequent indications for total elbow arthroplasty [18, 19]. End stage arthritis with disabling pain, stiffness, or instability that continues despite conservative treatment is the primary indication for a total elbow orthoplasty. Major contraindications include active sepsis, an inadequate soft tissue envelope, and a neuropathic elbow joint.

Linked, prostheses are indicated in most primary situations as well as when significant osseous or ligamentous deficiency exists. Aseptic loosening and bearing wear are primary causes of failure, especially in the younger patient population. Unlinked arthroplasty requires adequate bone stock and collateral ligaments. The maintenance of bone stock and the potential for decreased polyethylene wear and aseptic loosening have made the unlinked design a favorable alternative for younger patients who are likely to require future revision. Patients with insufficient bone stock, advanced osseous deformity, gross instability or capsuloligamentous insufficiency are poor candidates for unlinked arthroplasty.

The decision to incorporate a radial head replacement or keep the native radial head is based on the intra-operative assessment of radiocapitellar and proximal radio-ulnar alignment. Proximal radial anatomy is complex and difficult to recreate with current prostheses [20, 21]. A bipolar radial head is one approach that can be used to accurately maintain the radiocapitellar and lesser sigmoid notch relationships.

If intra-operative or late instability is recognized with unlinked arthroplasty, ligamentous reconstruction or conversion to a linked articulation is indicated. The routine use of a convertible implant for patients undergoing unlinked arthroplasty simplifies the revision to a linked articulation without the need to remove well-fixed stems.

Surgical Technique

Under general or regional anesthesia, the patient is positioned supine with the arm across the chest. A sterile tourniquet is employed to allow more prox-

imal exposure if necessary. Prophylactic antibiotics are administered prior to tourniquet inflation. A straight posterior incision is made just medial to the tip of the olecranon and full thickness flaps are developed on the deep fascia (Fig. 4). The ulnar nerve is transposed anteriorly into a subcutaneous pouch.

The management of the triceps tendon varies with surgeon preference. A triceps-on approach will spare the insertion from the risk of rupture and post-operative weakness but sacrifices visualization when bone loss is minimal or the joint is contracted. The triceps can be elevated from medial to lateral, as in the Bryan-Morrey approach, or from lateral to medial, as in the extended Kocher approach [22-24]. The triceps-splitting approach divides the muscle-tendon unit centrally and the tendon is reflected medially and laterally, maintaining continuity with the flexor carpi ulnaris and anconeus, respectively. The medial and lateral collateral ligaments and their corresponding muscle attachments are sharply released from the epicondyles and tagged

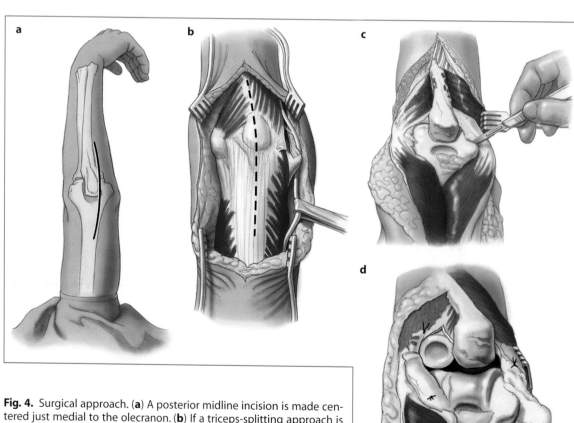

Fig. 4. Surgical approach. (**a**) A posterior midline incision is made centered just medial to the olecranon. (**b**) If a triceps-splitting approach is used the tendon is elevated subperiosteally medially and laterally off the olecranon. (**c**) The medial and lateral collateral ligaments are sharply divided off their humeral insertions and tagged to assist in later repair. (**d**) The elbow is dislocated to allow access for insertion of the arthroplasty. (Figures reproduced with permission, Tornier, Stafford, TX)

for later repair. The joint can then be dislocated to facilitate insertion of the prosthesis.

Four articular sizes are available (small, medium, large, and large-plus). The width of the anatomical spool is compared to that of the trochlea and capitellum of the distal humerus. The spool should also be placed into the trochlear notch of the ulna to assess fit (Fig. 5). The capitellum should align precisely with the radial head. When falling in between sizes, the smaller spool is preferred.

All subsequent surgical steps are based on accurately reproducing the flexion-extension axis of the elbow. The lateral point of isometry is the center of the capitellar arc, when visualized from a lateral viewpoint (Fig. 6). Medially, the anterior and inferior base of the medial epicondyle represents the location of the flexion/extension axis [25]. The central portion of the distal humerus is resected to the level of the proximal olecranon fossa prior to axis pin placement to verify that the axis pin is placed in the center of the capitellum and trochlea. The cut surfaces of the trochlea and capitellum are flat and round and may make confirmation of central pin placement easier. The axis drill guide is used to precisely place the axis pin. While an acceptable margin for error is not exactly known, the axis pin should probably be redrilled if a second hole is required to correct the axis (2-3 mm).

The humeral medullary canal is opened with a burr and the diaphyseal reamer. Distal humeral offset of the articulation with respect to the humeral stem in the sagittal plane is determined by measur-

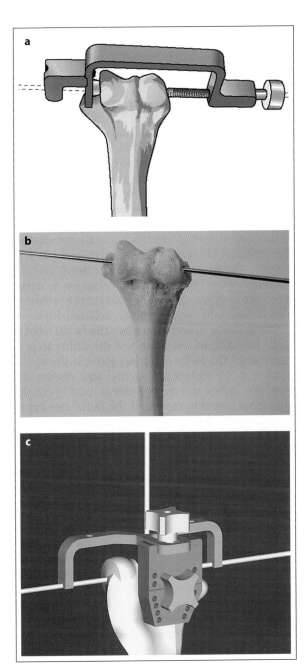

Fig. 6. Determination of the flexion/extension axis. (**a**) An axis drill guide is used to precisely place the flexion/extension axis. (**b**) The axis pin is drilled through the flexion axis from the center of the capitellum laterally to the antero-inferior base of the medial epicondyle. (**c**) A cutting block is used to make precise distal humeral cuts based on the both intramedullary and flexion/extension axis. (Figure reproduced with permission, Tornier, Stafford, TX)

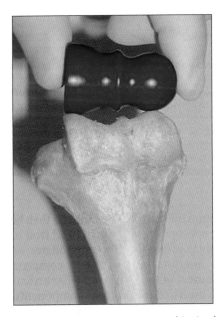

Fig. 5. Implant sizing. The anatomic spool is sized against the native distal humerus and then placed into the trochlear notch of the olecranon to assess fit. The radial head must align precisely with the capitellum. When the anatomy falls between sizes, the smaller spool size is preferred. (Figure reproduced with permission, Tornier, Stafford, TX)

ing the distance between the medullary alignment rod and the axis pin. Cutting blocks are then used to make precise distal humeral cuts based on the both intramedullary and flexion/extension axis. The humeral canal is then broached to the size previously determined by the anatomic spool. The broach is one size larger than the implant to ensure an optimal cement mantle. If the appropriate broach cannot be safely impacted but the previous smaller size broach was placed without difficulty, the appropriate final implant size can still be safely inserted. Alternatively, flexible reamers can be used to enlarge the canal. The humeral trial is inserted to seat the articulation flush with the bone cuts.

Radio-ulnar preparation is facilitated with a cutting guide also based on the flexion/extension axis. The anatomical spool and the ulnar diaphyseal axis are used to align the guide. The anatomical spool is placed in the trochlear groove and carefully aligned with the radial head (Fig. 7). The alignment of the radio-capitellar joint ensures accurate rotation of the proximal ulnar cut. The forearm axis pin sets the varus/valgus cut of the trochlear notch and the obliquity of the radial neck cut. Attention to detail is required while securing the guide to the proximal ulna to maintain these important relationships.

The decision to keep or replace the radial head is made based on its condition and the ability to precisely align the radio-capitellar joint. If the radial head is to be replaced, a sagittal saw resects the proximal radius and the bell saw is used to cut the ulna from lateral to medial. If the radial head is to be preserved, the ulnar cutting guide is reversed and the ulnar cut is made from medial to lateral. The bell saw should be continuously irrigated to prevent thermal injury to the bone. A triceps-on jig is available for radio-ulnar preparation when the triceps has not been released.

The ulnar canal is opened with a burr and broached to the desired size. The posterior flat spot on the proximal ulna is used to guide the axial rotation of the ulnar broach. Flexible reamers are used to prepare the ulnar canal if a standard length stem is desired. The decision to use a short or standard stem is based on the pathoanatomy of the diseased elbow and surgeon preference. A short stem may be preferred in a primary unlinked arthroplasty in a younger patient to preserve bone stock. A standard stem should probably be used in patients with poor bone quality, when linking the prosthesis and in revision situations. The appropriate ulnar trial is seated flush with the ulnar cut. Rotational malpositioning can be caused by not respecting the radial bow of the ulna during broaching or impinging bone in the olecranon. Repeat broaching or burring of the trochlear notch cut, respectively, should allow for

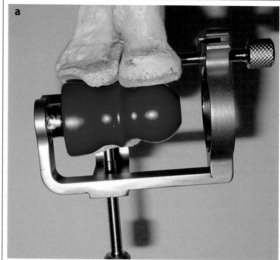

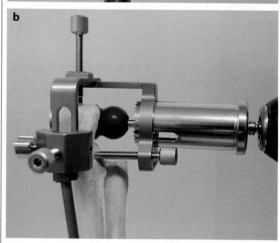

Fig. 7. Preparation of the radius and ulna. (**a**) The anatomic spool is used to align the ulnar cutting jig. The anatomic spool is placed into the trochlear notch and carefully aligned with the radial head to ensure proper rotation of the ulnar cut. (**b**) The jig is securely mounted to the ulnar diaphysis ensuring precise radial neck and ulnar cuts. If the radial head is to be preserved, the ulnar cutting guide is reversed and the ulnar cut is made with the bell saw from medial to lateral. (Figures reproduced with permission, Tornier, Stafford, TX)

proper implant seating. The radius is then broached and the appropriate size radial head trial is placed. The bipolar radial head accommodates +/- 10° of angular motion but will not compensate for malalignment of the radio-capitellar articulation.

After insertion of the trial components, the elbow is evaluated for alignment, stability, range of motion, and component tracking. A decision to proceed with unlinked or linked insertion is made based on patient factors and the pathoanatomy and stability of the elbow. If a linkage is required or desired, the trial ulnar cap is placed and an assessment of stability is repeated. If the radial prosthesis is malaligned with the capitellum and this cannot be corrected by component repositioning, a radial head replacement should not be performed.

Preparation for final implantation requires assembly of the modular humeral component, attaching the appropriate articular surface to the stem using a cannulated screw. Cement restrictors are employed and pulsatile irrigation is used to clear the intramedullary canals of blood and debris. Antibiotic-laden cement is inserted retrograde under pressure into the humerus, ulna, and radius and the components are inserted. Care is taken to ensure cement extrusion does not impede the functioning of the bipolar radial head. After the cement has cured, autologous cancellous bone from the resected distal humerus is placed under the anterior humeral flange. If the prosthesis is to be linked, the ulnar screw is removed after the cement has hardened and the ulnar cap is placed and secured using a torque-limiting screwdriver.

A locking stitch is used to repair the collateral ligaments and muscular origins (Fig. 8). Free suture ends from the collateral ligaments are passed through the cannulated humeral bolt for a secure isometric repair. A suture can also be passed through the cannulated humeral bolt and through the ulna as further protection against post-operative instability. If detached, the triceps are repaired with heavy braided nonabsorbable suture through drill holes in the ulna. The tourniquet is released prior to closure to achieve hemostasis. Drains are placed and a sterile dressing applied. The elbow is placed in a well-padded splint in near full extension and elevated for 3 days.

Rehabilitation

Post-operative rehabilitation should focus on early motion as the wound allows. If the wound appears dusky, splinting should be continued in less flexion until the wound declares itself. Active flexion and gravity-assisted passive extension exercises are instituted after splint removal. Active extension can be performed immediately when a triceps-on approach has been used. An anterior night extension splint is used to optimize terminal extension.

In triceps-reflecting approaches active extension can be instituted at 6 weeks but light strengthening

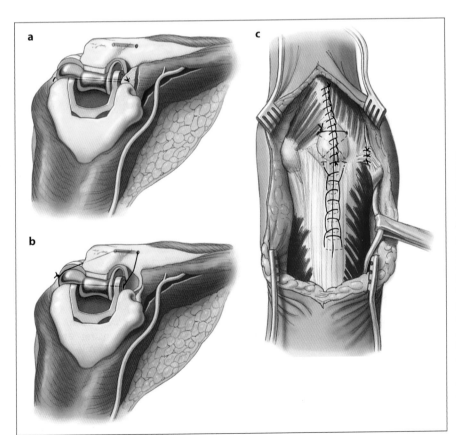

Fig. 8. Use of sutures. (**a**) Locking nonabsorbable sutures are placed in the medial and lateral collateral ligaments and passed through the cannulated humeral screw for a secure isometric repair. (**b**) A suture can also be passed through the cannulated humeral screw and through the ulna to serve as a temporary artificial ligament as further protection against post-operative instability. (**c**) The triceps are repaired if detached using locking nonabsorbable sutures and drill holes placed through the olecranon. (Figures reproduced with permission, Tornier, Stafford, TX)

should not be instituted until at least 10 weeks. Return to full activity can be recommended after 12 weeks although permanent restrictions should be emphasized. Repetitive lifting greater than 1 kg is not recommended and lifting greater than 5 kg should be strongly discouraged. It is important that the patient understand these long-term restrictions prior to surgical intervention to avoid early implant failure.

Results

The initial experience with the Latitude arthroplasty has been encouraging. The implant has been able to deal with a wide range of pathologies and patient profiles. Patients with relatively well-preserved bone stock and adequate ligaments have been managed with an unlinked arthroplasty (Fig. 9)

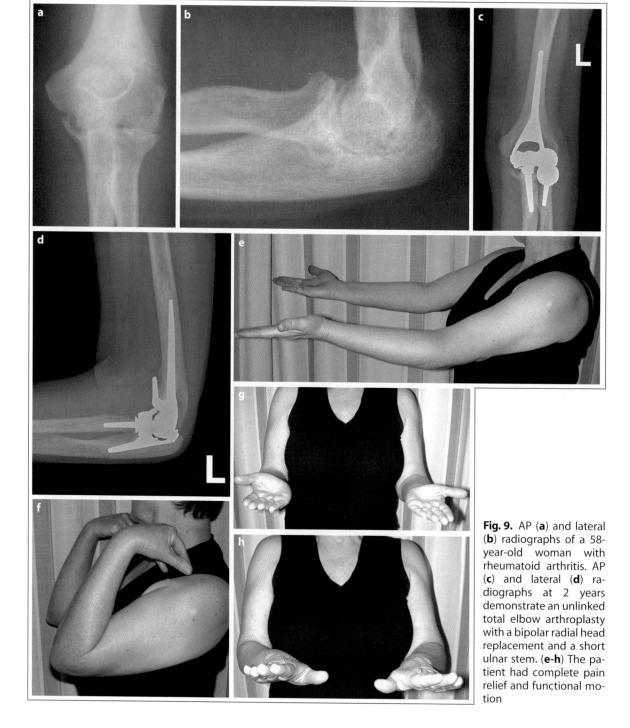

Fig. 9. AP (**a**) and lateral (**b**) radiographs of a 58-year-old woman with rheumatoid arthritis. AP (**c**) and lateral (**d**) radiographs at 2 years demonstrate an unlinked total elbow arthroplasty with a bipolar radial head replacement and a short ulnar stem. (**e-h**) The patient had complete pain relief and functional motion

while those with bone loss or ligament insufficiency have been treated with a linked arthroplasty (Fig. 10 and 11). The option to replace the radial head and the ability to place sutures through the axis of the implant has provided improved initial stability relative to the Authors' previous experience with other unlinked arthroplasty designs. As our experience with the prosthesis increases, a greater number of the implants are being inserted in the unlinked mode. This is due to our confidence

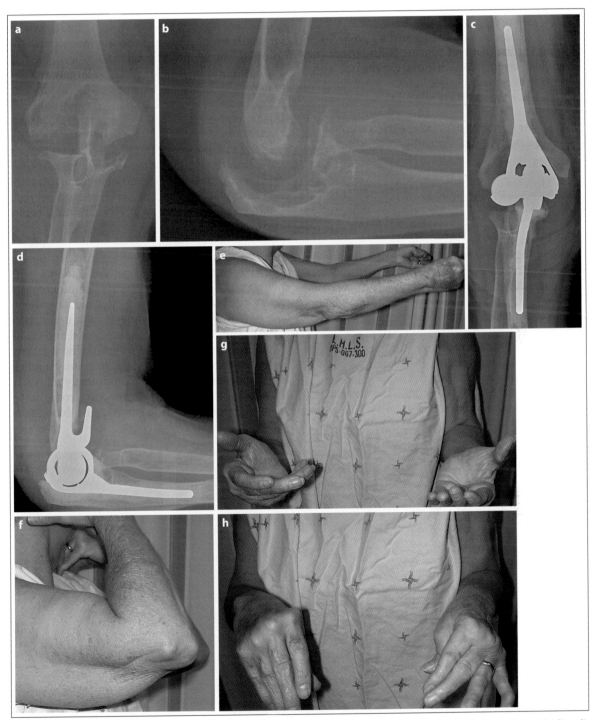

Fig. 10. AP (**a**) and lateral (**b**) radiographs of a 75-year-old woman with rheumatoid arthritis. AP (**c**) and lateral (**d**) radiographs at 1 year demonstrate a linked total elbow arthroplasty with a standard length ulnar stem. (**e-h**) The patient had an excellent functional outcome

in the initial ligament repair strength and the ability to easily convert the implant to a linked prosthesis through a minimal incision should instability occur. The more precise replication of the flexion/extension axis using the anatomically based modular component design and instrumentation should allow for improved implant biomechanics and therefore increased longevity. The increased polyethylene thickness and bearing surface area should decrease the incidence of bearing failure over time. As would be expected in an initial experience with a new implant system, loosening has been uncommon and to date has been related to technical factors. While our initial results have been encouraging, long-term follow-up of these patients will be required to determine the durability of this implant.

Complications

The success of any procedure is largely dependent on providing a sustained relief of symptoms and on the avoidance of complications. Elbow arthroplasty has historically been plagued by a high rate of complications [17]. While some complications, such as wound breakdown, deep sepsis, triceps insufficiency, and ulnar neuropathy are inherent in any elbow arthroplasty procedure, other complications are specific to implant design. Linked arthroplasty is more frequently associated with aseptic loosening and mechanical failure while unlinked resurfacing designs are more prone to instability. The more

"constrained" unlinked designs are susceptible to the problems of both, in proportion to their level of ulno-humeral articular constraint. Complications associated with radial head replacement are inherent to designs that can accommodate the radio-capitellar articulation. Osteolysis is a complication that is usually related to polyethylene wear and the design of the articulation. It also occurred with a polymethylmethacrylene precoat ulnar stem of the Coonrad-Morrey prosthesis [26].

Wound healing problems can be largely avoided by meticulous surgical technique and hemostasis. Patient factors should be addressed medically prior to intervention and prior surgical incisions respected when possible. Drains and post-operative splinting can minimize hematoma and tension on the wound during the critical early stages of healing. Full thickness flaps should be elevated from the deep fascial layers. Early signs of wound necrosis should be evaluated for flap reconstruction before deep sepsis ensues.

Patient-related factors and the tenuous soft tissue envelope make total elbow arthroplasty particularly susceptible to deep sepsis. Patients with rheumatoid disease are often immunocompromised by their medical treatment while patients who have undergone previous reconstruction may present with avascular bone, scar tissue, and occult infection. In large reported series of elbow arthroplasty for rheumatoid arthritis, deep infection has been reported to occur in approximately 2%-5% of elbows [16, 17, 27-29]. Deep infection complicates 5%-11% of post-traumatic elbows, most having un-

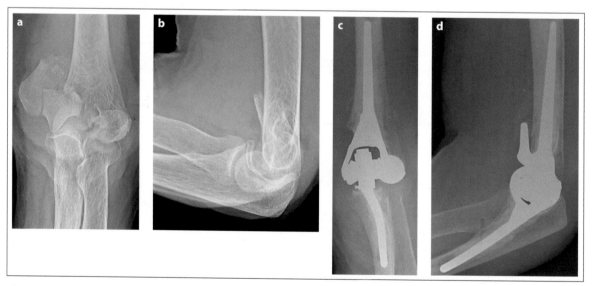

Fig. 11. AP (**a**) and lateral (**b**) radiographs of a 92-year-old woman with a comminuted distal humeral fracture. She was in good health and living independently. AP (**c**) and lateral (**d**) radiographs following a linked total elbow arthroplasty performed using a triceps on approach. The patient was able to return to her home and had no pain and a functional arc of motion

dergone previous surgery [31, 32]. Prosthetic retention is possible but multiple debridements and/or resection arthroplasty can be the unfortunate consequence of infection after TEA [32].

Triceps insufficiency or avulsion occurs in up to 11% of patients [16, 26, 33]. Methods of careful release and secure fixation may decrease this complication. The meticulous release of Sharpey's fibers from the proximal ulna should prevent excessive button-holing of the triceps whether the triceps is split or reflected as a sleeve. Refraining from active extension for at least 6 weeks should allow for early tendon healing to occur. A triceps-on approach, though more technically challenging, could decrease the rate of these complications [34, 35].

Ulnar neuropathies are not uncommon in patients with elbow arthritis presenting for arthroplasty [8, 33, 36, 37]. Osteophytes, pannus invasion, and scar tissue can produce varying degrees of neuropraxia. Resolution is unreliable after arthroplasty surgery with early ulnar nerve neuropraxia reported in up to 26% of elbows and up to 10% suffering permanent dysfunction [17, 27-29, 31, 33, 38, 39]. Post-operative ulnar nerve dysfunction can be exacerbated by devascularization of the transposed nerve segment, persistent proximal or distal tethering, or prolonged intra-operative dislocation when the nerve is inadequately released [42].

Intra-operative fractures of the humeral and ulnar shafts can occur [9, 26]. Excessive diaphyseal bowing, osteopenic bone and the use of longer stems are important risk factors for this complication. Unrecognized posterior cortical penetration of the humerus can lead to cement extravasation and thermal injury to the radial nerve [41]. Intra-operative condylar fractures are particularly important with unlinked designs and require secure fixation.

Aseptic loosening is primarily a complication of activity level, implant constraint, and imbalance across the elbow. The developments of a loose linkage and an anterior flange have markedly decreased the rates of aseptic humeral loosening [16, 42]. Ulnar component debonding and loosening can occur during hyperflexion stress with linked implants. Implant fracture and excessive polyethylene wear are more likely with heavy use of the limb and noncompliance with post-operative restrictions.

Unlinked designs have historically had problems with instability. Their design relies on the competency of the capsule, ligaments and muscle, and the support of the bony architecture [27, 28]. Capsuloligamentous insufficiency, bone loss, and component malposition can predispose the prosthesis to maltracking, subluxation, or dislocation. Advances in prosthetic design have led to ulno-humeral articulations with greater contact surface area and the addition of a radio-capitellar articulation. Balancing load distribution across both the ulna and radius should improve prosthetic survivorship. If the radial head is retained or replaced, precise tracking with the capitellum must be ensured, however. Maltracking of a radial head replacement may cause accelerated polyethylene wear or dislocation of a bipolar head. Finally, if precise tracking of the ulnohumeral joint cannot be achieved with an unlinked design, conversion to a linked prosthesis should be performed.

References

1. Dee R, Sweetnam DR (1970) Total replacement arthroplasty of the elbow joint for rheumatoid arthritis: two cases. Proc R Soc Med 63:653-655
2. Davis RF, Weiland AJ, Hungerford DS et al (1982) Nonconstrained total elbow arthroplasty. Clin Orthop 171:156-160
3. Kudo H, Iwano K (1990) Total elbow arthroplasty with a non-constrained surface-replacement prosthesis in patients who have rheumatoid arthritis. A long-term follow-up study. J Bone Joint Surg Am 72:355-362
4. O'Driscoll SW, King GJ (2001) Treatment of instability after total elbow arthroplasty. Orthop Clin North Am 32:679-695
5. Ring D, Koris M, Jupiter JB (2001) Instability after total elbow arthroplasty. Orthop Clin North Am 32:671-677
6. Schuind F, O'Driscoll S, Korinek S et al (1995) Loose-hinge total elbow arthroplasty. An experimental study of the effects of implant alignment on three-dimensional elbow kinematics. J Arthroplasty 10:670-678
7. O'Driscoll SW, An KN, Korinek S, Morrey BF (1992) Kinematics of semi-constrained total elbow arthroplasty. J Bone Joint Surg Br 74:297-299
8. Ramsey M, Neale PG, Morrey BF et al (2003) Kinematics and functional characteristics of the Pritchard ERS unlinked total elbow arthroplasty. J Shoulder Elbow Surg 12:385-390
9. Schneeberger AG, King GJ, Song SW et al (2000) Kinematics and laxity of the Souter-Strathclyde total elbow prosthesis. J Shoulder Elbow Surg 9:127-134
10. King GJ, Itoi E, Niebur GL et al (1994) Motion and laxity of the capitellocondylar total elbow prosthesis. J Bone Joint Surg Am 76:1000-1008
11. King GJ, Itoi E, Risung F et al (1993) Kinematic and stability of the Norway elbow. A cadaveric study. Acta Orthop Scand 64:657-663
12. Inagaki K, O'Driscoll SW, Neale PG et al (2002) Importance of a radial head component in Sorbie unlinked total elbow arthroplasty. Clin Orthop 400:123-131
13. Trail LA, Nuttall D, Stanley JK (2002) Comparison of survivorship between standard and long-stem souter-strathclyde total elbow arthroplasty. J Shoulder Elbow Surg 11:373-376
14. Trepman E, Vella IM, Ewald FC (1991) Radial head replacement in capitellocondylar total elbow arthroplasty 2- to 6-year follow-up evaluation in rheumatoid arthritis. J Arthroplasty 6:67-77

15. Trail IA, Nuttall D, Stanley JK (1999) Survivorship and radiological analysis of the standard Souter-Strathclyde total elbow arthroplasty. J Bone Joint Surg Br 81:80-84

16. Gill DR, Morrey BF (1998) The Coonrad-Morrey total elbow arthroplasty in patients who have rheumatoid arthritis. A ten to fifteen-year follow-up study. J Bone Joint Surg Am 80:1327-1335

17. Gschwend N, Simmen BR, Matejovsky Z (1996) Late complications in elbow arthroplasty. J Shoulder Elbow Surg 5:86-96

18. Kamineni S, Morrey BF (2004) Distal humeral fractures treated with noncustom total elbow replacement. J Bone Joint Surg Am 86:940-947

19. Garcia JA, Mykula R, Stanley D (2002) Complex fractures of the distal humerus in the elderly. The role of total elbow replacement as primary treatment. J Bone Joint Surg Br 84:812-816

20. Beredjiklian PK, Nalbantoglu U, Potter HG, Hotchkiss RN (1999) Prosthetic radial head components and proximal radial morphology: a mismatch. J Shoulder Elbow Surg 8:471-475

21. King GJ, Zarzour ZD, Patterson SD, Johnson JA (2001) An anthropometric study of the radial head: implications in the design of a prosthesis. J Arthroplasty 16:112-116

22. Morrey BF, Bryan RS (1982) Complications of total elbow arthroplasty. Clin Orthop 170:204-212

23. Bryan RS, Morrey BF (1982) Extensive posterior exposure of the elbow. A triceps-sparing approach. Clin Orthop 166:188-192

24. Weiland AJ, Weiss AP, Wills RP, Moore JR (1989) Capitellocondylar total elbow replacement. A long-term follow-up study. J Bone Joint Surg Am 71:217-222

25. Duck TR, Dunning CE, King GJ, Johnson JA (2003) Variability and repeatability of the flexion axis at the ulnohumeral joint. J Orthop Res 21:399-404

26. Hildebrand KA, Patterson SD, Regan WD et al (2000) Functional outcome of semiconstrained total elbow arthroplasty. J Bone Joint Surg Am 82:1379-1386

27. Ikavalko M, Lehto MU, Repo A et al (2002) The Souter-Strathclyde elbow arthroplasty. A clinical and radiological study of 525 consecutive cases. J Bone Joint Surg Br 84:77-82

28. Ewald FC, Simmons Jr ED, Sullivan JA et al (1993) Capitellocondylar total elbow replacement in rheumatoid arthritis. Long-term results. J Bone Joint Surg Am 75:498-507

29. van der Lugt JC, Geskus RB, Rozing PM (2004) Primary Souter-Strathclyde total elbow prosthesis in rheumatoid arthritis. J Bone Joint Surg Am 86:465-473

30. Figgie MP, Inglis AE, Mow CS, Figgie 3rd HE (1989) Salvage of non-union of supracondylar fracture of the humerus by total elbow arthroplasty. J Bone Joint Surg Am 71:1058-1065

31. Schneeberger AG, Adams R, Morrey BF (1997) Semiconstrained total elbow replacement for the treatment of posttraumatic osteoarthrosis. J Bone Joint Surg Am 79:1211-1222

32. Yamaguchi K, Adams RA, Morrey BF (1998) Infection after total elbow arthroplasty. J Bone Joint Surg Am 80:481-491

33. Kelly EW, Coghlan J, Bell S (2004) Five- to thirteen-year follow-up of the GSB III total elbow arthroplasty. J Shoulder Elbow Surg 13:434-440

34. Morrey BF, Adams RA (1995) Semiconstrained elbow replacement for distal humeral nonunion. J Bone Joint Surg Br 77:67-72

35. Pierce TD, Herndon JH (1998) The triceps preserving approach to total elbow arthroplasty. Clin Orthop 354:144-152

36. Spinner RJ, Morgenlander JC, Nunley JA (2000) Ulnar nerve function following total elbow arthroplasty: a prospective study comparing pre-operative and post-operative clinical and electrophysiologic evaluation in patients with rheumatoid arthritis. J Hand Surg Am 25:360-364

37. Ikavalko M, Belt EA, Kautiainen H, Lehto MU (2004) Souter arthroplasty for elbows with severe destruction. Clin Orthop 421:126-133

38. Tanaka N, Kudo H, Iwano K et al (2001) Kudo total elbow arthroplasty in patients with rheumatoid arthritis: a long-term follow-up study. J Bone Joint Surg Am 83:1506-1513

39. Willems K, De Smet L (2004) The Kudo total elbow arthroplasty in patients with rheumatoid arthritis. J Shoulder Elbow Surg 13:542-547

40. Moro JK, King GJ (2000) Total elbow arthroplasty in the treatment of posttraumatic conditions of the elbow. Clin Orthop 370:102-114

41. King GJ, Adams RA, Morrey BF (1997) Total elbow arthroplasty: revision with use of a non-custom semiconstrained prosthesis. J Bone Joint Surg Am 79:394-400

42. Ramsey ML, Adams RA, Morrey BF (1999) Instability of the elbow treated with semiconstrained total elbow arthroplasty. J Bone Joint Surg Am 81:38-47

CHAPTER 25

Total Elbow Arthroplasty for Post-traumatic Arthrosis

Introduction

Posttraumatic arthrosis of the elbow is often characterized by a chronic painful condition frequently associated with stiffness, joint deformity, contractures, bone loss, instability, numerous previous procedures resulting in a poor soft tissue envelope, and damaged and hypersensitive nerves [1]. Its treatment can therefore be difficult with an elevated number of complications.

Patients with posttraumatic arthrosis often are young and active. Before injury and development of posttraumatic arthrosis, these patients usually had a normal elbow. Some of them were sporty, or heavy workers. In contrast to patients with rheumatoid arthritis, the patients with posttraumatic arthrosis usually have normal joints except the involved elbow. The expectations of these patients often are high with the desire of returning to their previous level of activity. Therefore, posttraumatic arthrosis poses much more difficulties in the treatment than rheumatoid arthritis [2].

Only few options exist for the operative treatment of severe posttraumatic arthrosis. Arthrodesis reliably relieves pain [3] and restores a strong extremity. However, because of its great functional impairment [4], arthrodesis of the elbow rarely is considered a viable option [5, 6]. Interposition arthroplasty may be considered for a young patient, particularly one who has stiffness. Restoration of motion and relief of pain can be achieved with a reasonable but unpredictable rate of success [7-10]. However, interposition arthroplasty is not considered suitable for patients who perform strenuous physical labor [8]. Varying results have been reported for allograft replacement of the entire elbow joint [11, 12]. Concerns about the complication rate, continued degenerative changes, and fragmentation of the allograft may be the reasons why this procedure has not found wide acceptance.

For severe posttraumatic arthrosis, total elbow replacement has shown to be a suitable and reliable option of treatment. The indications, implants, results, and limitations are outlined below.

Implants and Literature Review

Hinged, Constrained Metal-On-Metal Implants

The results of highly constrained, linked metal-on-metal total elbow arthroplasties in the 1970^s were disappointing due to a high rate of early loosening [13, 14]. This was attributed to the rigid hinged implant mechanism transmitting high forces across the elbow joint directly to the prosthesis-bone interface.

Unlinked, Semiconstrained Resurfacing Implants

As these implants are not linked, part of the forces across the elbow joint are absorbed by the soft tissues, and not transmitted entirely to the prosthesis-bone interface. This may explain the lower loosening rates of these new resurfacing designs compared to the early linked, fully constrained devices [5, 15-25]. Yet, these unlinked implants were almost exclusively used for the treatment of rheumatoid arthritis. In addition, they require intact condyles and collateral ligaments for stability. Postoperative dislocations or instabilities were reported as predictable complications of these devices [5, 16-19, 21, 25]. This significantly limits their indications. Hence, preoperative deformity, asymmetric soft tissue contractures, bone loss, or marked instability are considered (relative) contraindications for use of these unlinked devices.

Linked, Semiconstrained Devices

These linked implants allow for a laxity within their mechanism similarly as the resurfacing devices. This diminishes the forces on the prosthesis-bone interface. Improved loosing rates were reported using these devices (see below) compared to the linked constrained implants. The great advantage of these prostheses is restoration of postoperative stability. Introduction of the linked semiconstrained implants changed the treatment of posttraumatic arthrosis and allowed for more reliable and satisfactory outcomes.

Early reports of linked semiconstrained prostheses often included only few cases of posttraumatic arthrosis [26-31]. In addition, several of these reports showed rather unfavorable results [26, 29-31]. In 1997, the first comprehensive series of semiconstrained Coonrad-Morrey total elbow replacements (Zimmer Corp., Warsaw, Indiana) for the treatment of posttraumatic arthrosis showed that this difficult pathology can be treated with artificial joint replacement. However, there seems to be important limits in the use of this implant [1].

Indications

For posttraumatic arthrosis, total joint replacement using the semiconstrained Coonrad-Morrey prosthesis is in our hands the treatment of choice in selected cases. These cases include advanced destruction of the ulnohumeral joint with marked narrowing or loss of the joint space, and for those patients who are older than 60 years. For patients younger than 60 years, total elbow replacement should be performed only with reservation, if no other suitable alternatives of operative treatment are available or for those in whom other reconstructive procedures have failed. For young patients with a severe posttraumatic arthrosis, interposition arthroplasty may be considered the treatment of first choice, rather than total joint replacement. In cases of failed interposition arthroplasty, total joint replacement is the treatment of choice for most patients.

Further Considerations

Age, Occupation, and Physical Activity

As the total elbow prosthesis is a mechanical device, it is subjected to wear, particularly of the polyethylene bushings. In a series at the Mayo Clinic, those with posttraumatic arthrosis who were younger than 60 years of age had a higher rate of complications (35% *vs* 17%) and, accordingly, a lower proportion of satisfactory results (78% compared to 89%) [1]. The prosthesis does not tolerate the stress of heavy physical work; thus, after total elbow replacement, we always advice the patients to avoid single-event lifting of objects that weigh more than 5 kg as well as repetitive lifting of any object that weighs more than 1 kg. Participation in heavy physical work and anticipated noncompliance are considered relative contraindications for this procedure. We discourage playing of golf and other impact sports.

Instability

Acute or posttraumatic instability is not a contraindication to elbow replacement that involves the use of the semiconstrained Coonrad-Morrey implant [1, 32], in fact, the condition is well managed with this device. Owing to its hinge design, this implant yields immediate and durable stability. This is also shown by the fact that during approach for joint replacement both collateral ligaments are released and no attempts are made to repair these ligaments without any adverse effects observed. In contrast to unlinked implants [33], the Coonrad-Morrey device also provides valgus-varus and axial stability without the tendency of the components to disassemble.

Bone Loss

Significant bone stock deficiency was present in 16 of the 41 patients in the series at the Mayo Clinic with posttraumatic arthrosis [1], and in 8 out of 16 patients in the series at Balgrist (Table 1) [32]. Only the humeral diaphysis is required to obtain secure fixation of the Coonrad-Morrey prosthesis. Rotational and anteroposterior stability is maintained by the anterior flange and bone graft. Thus, this implant requires neither the condyles nor the distal humerus for mechanical support. Therefore, nonunited parts of the distal humerus can be resected before insertion of the Coonrad-Morrey prosthesis, and their reconstruction is not required [34]. This facilitates enormously total elbow replacement and constitutes a great advantage over those total elbow prostheses that need the condyles for stability [28, 33]. If the bone loss extends into the supracondylar area and into the shaft of the humerus, the humeral component of the Coonrad-Morrey prosthesis can be cemented more proximally into the shaft. This results, however, in shortening of the humerus. If shortening exceeds 2 cm, it can cause weakening of the muscles crossing the elbow joint [35].

Traumatic loss of the proximal ulna is a difficult problem and requires reconstruction with allograft or autograft from the iliac crest to restore the site of insertion of the extensor mechanisms.

Table 1. Preoperative data of patients treated with Coonrad-Morrey Total Elbow Replacement for posttraumatic arthrosis at Mayo Clinic and at Balgrist (Department of Orthopaedic Surgery, University of Zurich)

Patient's data	Mayo Clinic n = 41	Balgrist n = 16
The average age of the patients at elbow replacement (years)	57 y (32-82)	59 y (26-79)
Period of treatment (year)	1981-1993	1996-2001
Previous surgery (number)	2.3 (0-7)	2 (0-6)
Significant bone stock deficiency with loss of at least 1 condyle (number of patients)	16	8
Significant joint or bone deformity (number of patients)	14	4
Preoperatively subluxed or dislocated elbow joint (number of patients)	17	7
Moderate (5°-20°) to severe varus-valgus instability (number of patients)	25	4
Mild to moderate ulnar neuropathy (number of patients)	6	4
Radial nerve palsy due to a complete traumatic laceration (number of patients)	1	1
Follow-up (years)	5 (2-12)	4 (2-7.5)

Deformity

Deformity is a feature often encountered in posttraumatic arthrosis expressed as angular abnormalities of more than 30° or translational problems. Long-standing deformity results in asymmetrical soft tissue contractures. Unlinked resurfacing total elbow prostheses usually cannot correct this type of deformity, and instability is common. Although hinged semiconstrained prostheses have the major advantage of being able to correct deformity, this correction may be at the expense of persistent or increased asymmetrical loads imparted by the distorted soft tissues, causing an increased wear of the prosthesis. Overall, in our experience, a marked preoperative deformity was associated with a significantly higher rate of complication (p = 0.02) [1]. Further, this deformity has recently been shown to be directly related to bushing wear of the articulation [36].

In cases of severe deformity, shortening of the distal humerus may be considered. The high asymmetrical loads of the soft tissues can be diminished by shortening the distal humerus accepting the disadvantage of weakening the muscles across the elbow joint as described above.

Technique

Coonrad-Morrey Total Elbow Prosthesis

This is a noncustom prosthesis with cement fixation of both stems. The humeral and the ulnar components have three interchangeable sizes each. The humeral stems are available in 10-, 15-, and 20-cm lengths with a standard short, and a long anterior flange useful for defects of the distal humerus. Fifteen-centimeter stems are usually used in patients with posttraumatic arthrosis. The prosthesis is made of a titanium alloy. The articulation consists of three high-density polyethylene bushings rotating around a cobalt-chrome pin. It allows a play of 7°-10° of varus and valgus and of 7° of rotation (Fig. 1) [37].

The operative technique for implantation of the semiconstrained Coonrad-Morrey prosthesis has been previously described [38]. However, some features deserve to be emphasized. A posterior midline incision is used, including posterior scars from previous procedures. Alternatively, prior medial and lateral incisions can be used for exposure. The ulnar nerve is always transposed anteri-

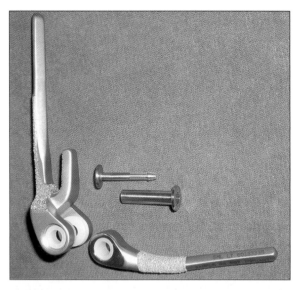

Fig. 1. Semiconstrained linked Coonrad-Morrey total elbow prosthesis consists of a hinge articulation which allows a play of 7°-10° of valgus-varus and of rotation. Sintered beads on the distal humeral component allow bone ingrowth and improve cement fixation. An anterior flange at the distal humeral component which, when incorporated with bone grafts, resists posterior displacement and torsion of the humeral stem. A layer of plasma spray coating improves cement fixation on the proximal ulnar component. Various lengths are available for the humeral stem: 10 cm (as shown on the picture, usually used for rheumatoid arthritis); 15 cm (recommended for posttraumatic arthrosis), 20 cm (for revision cases)

orly in a subcutaneous pocket. The recommended operative technique includes a triceps-sparing approach, which is accomplished by release and lateral reflection of the triceps from the olecranon in continuity with the ulnar periosteum and the fascia of the forearm along with the anconeus as described by Bryan and Morrey [39]. An intramedullary injecting system is used for optimal insertion of the cement containing some sort of antibiotics. An important element is the placement of a bone graft between the anterior flange and the distal part of the humerus to resist, after ingrowth, posterior displacement and rotational stresses on the humeral component. Usually, resection of the tip of the coronoid process is necessary to avoid impingement with the anterior flange, which would cause considerable distraction forces on the ulnar component [32]. Too deep insertion of the ulnar component is another potential cause of anterior impingement (Fig. 2). Significant bone stock deficiencies with lack of one or both epicondyles do not change or complicate the implantation of the humeral component. Nonunited condyles can be resected. If the entire distal humerus is deficient, the triceps doesn't need to be detached from the olecranon for the approach, as it has been described for total elbow arthroplasty in patients who have a nonunion of the distal humerus [34].

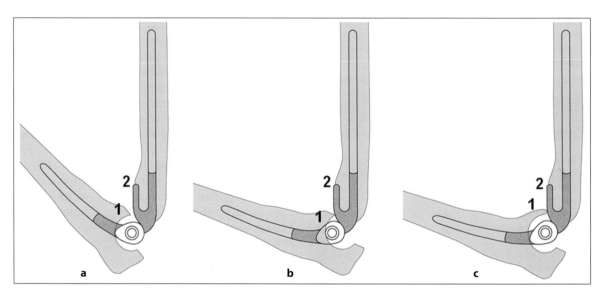

Fig. 2. (**a**) Correct depth of insertion of the ulnar component. The tip of the coronoid process (*1*) is resected. There is clearance between the coronoid process and the anterior flange of the humeral component (*2*). Flexion is unrestricted (reprinted with permission). (**b**) Too-deep insertion of the ulnar component resulting in anterior impingement between the coronoid process (*1*) and the anterior flange of the humeral component. Flexion is restricted (reprinted with permission). (**c**) Correct depth of insertion of the ulnar component but the coronoid osteophyte (*1*) has not been resected resulting in anterior impingement and restricted flexion (reprinted with permission)

Results

Experience at the Mayo Clinic

The Mayo experience was presented in 1997 and consists of 41 consecutive patients with post-traumatic arthrosis or dysfunction treated from 1981 to 1993 by semiconstrained Coonrad-Morrey elbow replacement (Figs. 3, 4) [1]. The patient data are shown on Table 1.

At the latest follow-up, using the Mayo elbow performance score, 16 patients out of 41 had an excellent result, 18 good, 5 fair, and 2 a poor outcome. Overall, 83% of all patients had a satisfactory objective outcome. Ninety-five percent of the patients with a functioning implant subjectively were considered to have a satisfactory outcome at the latest follow-up, excluding the 2 patients with an infection and 1 patient with a broken ulnar component. Preoperatively, 90% of the patients had moderate to severe pain. After surgery, 29 (76%) of 38 patients with a functioning implant had no or only mild pain (p < 0.0005). At follow-up, the mean arc of flexion-extension was 27°-131°, and the mean arc of pronation-supination was 66°-66°. Implantation of the semiconstrained elbow prosthesis resulted in nearly normal function: on an average, 4.8 out of the 5 activities of daily living could be performed by the patients.

There was not one case of aseptic loosening within the 12 years of follow-up. Almost no periarticular ossifications were observed. Only 4 patients showed ossifications of less than 1 cm in size with no clinical significance.

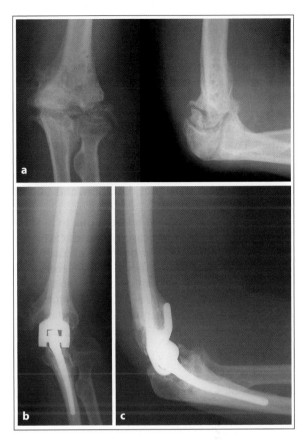

Fig. 3. (**a**) Preoperative radiographs of a 59-year-old patient with painful posttraumatic arthrosis after open reduction and internal fixation of a distal humerus fracture and two additional surgeries. (**b**) Anteroposterior and (**c**) lateral radiographs 11 years after Coonrad-Morrey total elbow replacement. Stable implant without signs of loosening. Functional range of flexion from 20° to 130°, and significant improvement of symptoms compared to preoperatively

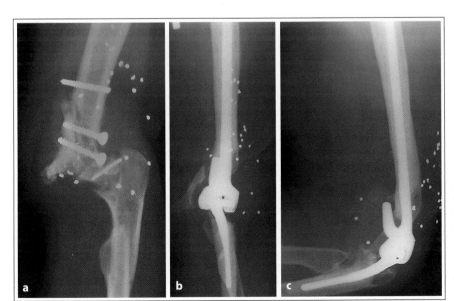

Fig. 4. (**a**) Preoperative anteroposterior radiograph of a patient after gun shot wound and important defect of distal humerus. (**b**) Anteroposterior and lateral (**c**) radiographs 14 years after insertion of a Coonrad-Morrey total elbow prosthesis. Stable elbow and implant without signs of loosening

Experience at Balgrist

The experience with the Coonrad-Morrey prosthesis used at Balgrist, Department of Orthopaedic Surgery of the University of Zurich included a similar series of 16 patients treated between 1996 and 2001 for posttraumatic arthrosis (Table 1) [32]. One patient had no radiological follow-up. Two patients had a history of previous infection of the elbow, 2 had previous latissimus dorsi pedicled graft coverage for soft tissue defects at the elbow, and 1 had a chronic triceps rupture.

At latest follow-up, or at revision due to loosening (1 case) or infection (1 case), 5 had an excellent, 7 good, 2 fair, and 2 a poor outcome according to the Mayo Elbow Performance Score. Overall, 75% were considered to have an objective satisfactory result. If at latest follow-up also the 2 patients after revision of their failed implants were included, 88% of the patients had a satisfactory objective outcome.

At follow-up, the mean arc of flexion was from 27° to 131°. Loosening with more than 2 mm of lucency around the entire interface was found in 2 humeral and 2 ulnar components of a total of 3 patients, resulting in a loosening rate of 19%.

A possible cause of ulnar loosening was attributed to impingement between the anterior flange of the humeral component and a long coronoid process in one patient (Fig. 2c).

Another case of early loosening occurred in a patient with a prior history of Staphylococcus aureus infection. Although the infection was considered eradicated at insertion of the prosthesis, persistent low-grade infection was still considered a possible cause for the loosening.

Inadequate cementation was observed in 2 humeral components; one of them was found loose at follow-up. In both cases with inadequate cementing, an anterograde cementing technique was used with direct injection of the cement using a syringe contrary to the recommendations of the manufacturer, which advises the use of an injecting system with retrograde insertion of the cement. Retrograde insertion of cement improves the degree of cement filling and the holding strength of the implants [40]. Since 1998, an advanced cementing technique has been used at Balgrist resulting consistently in adequate cementation, and no cases of loosening have been observed since then.

Complications

The number of complications (Table 2) was high. At the Mayo Clinic, 11 patients (27%) had major complications. Nine of them (22%) required an additional operation. Fracture of the ulnar component occurred in 5 patients (12%) (Fig. 5). Modification of the surface of the ulnar component from sintered beads to a pre-coat in 1995 and then to a plasma spray coating in 2000 increased the mechanical properties of the implant, and fatigue fractures of the proximal ulna have not been observed since then by the authors.

Table 2. Major complications with Coonrad-Morrey Total Elbow Replacement for posttraumatic arthrosis

Orthopaedic complication	Mayo Clinic n = 41	Balgrist n = 16	Comments	Treatment
Infection	2	1	*Pseudomonas aeruginosa* infection already present before joint replacement	Resection (2); staged exchange revision (1)
Fracture ulnar component	5	0	Traumatic injury (2); return to strenuous labor against advice of surgeon (2)	Replacement of ulnar component (4)
Worn bushings	2	0	Return to strenuous labor against advice of surgeon (2); preoperative deformity (2)	Exchange of bushings (2)
Mild persistent ulnar or median neuropathy	1	2		Decompression 1 week postoperatively (1)
Loosening	0	3	Poor cementing (1); anterior coronoid impingement (1); prior infection (1); eventually persistence of infection	Exchange revision (2)
Triceps rupture	1	1		Repair of triceps (2)
Hematoma	1	0		Evacuation (1)
Prolonged wound drainage	0	2	Hemodialysis (1)	Wound revision (2)
Other	3	1		Revisions (3)

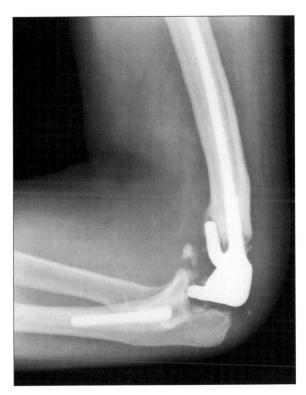

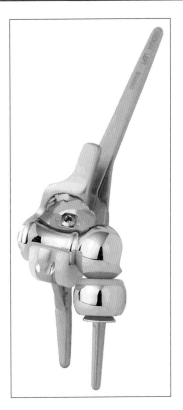

Fig. 5. Fracture of the ulnar component 2 years after implantation of the prosthesis in a 54-year-old construction worker. The ulnar component was exchanged resulting thereafter in an excellent result

Fig. 6. Latitude total elbow replacement with semiconstrained design can be used as linked or unlinked implant with optional insertion of a bipolar radial head prosthesis

Two patients presented with a particulate synovitis associated with worn bushings. They underwent a synovectomy and exchange of the bushings. All reoperations for a mechanical purpose resulted in a satisfactory outcome. There was not one case of loosening in the series of the Mayo Clinic.

Special concern has been expressed for bushing wear in younger and more active patients. To analyze polyethylene wear, all Coonrad-Morrey elbow prostheses performed at the Mayo Clinic from 1981 through 2000 for various indications (34% for trauma-related conditions) were retrospectively reviewed [36]. Out of 919 patients, only 12 (1.3%) had undergone an isolated exchange of the articular bushings as a result of polyethylene wear. Seven out of these 12 cases had posttraumatic arthrosis. Nine had extensive deformity. The bushings were revised at an average of 8 years after implantation. Polyethylene wear did not seem to be a major problem at the Mayo Clinic.

Newer implants such as the Latitude (Tornier-Zirst, Montbonnot, France) (Fig. 6) or the Discovery (Biomet, Warsaw, Indiana) have other polyethylene-metal designs aiming to increase longevity of the polyethylene and to allow higher loads on the prosthesis. Follow-up on these new designs will show whether the different contact surfaces of these new designs will succeed, or if eventually larger amounts of wear debris will result.

At Balgrist, there were 8 patients (50%) with totally 10 complications requiring 7 revisions. One patient with a prior *Pseudomonas aeruginosa* infection had recurrence of the infection after an infection-free period of 5 years. He required staged revision, resulting in an excellent result. Two wounds were successfully revised for aseptic, prolonged wound drainage of more than 7 days. As the soft tissue envelope is thin around the elbow, wound problems probably increase the risk of infection. The Authors therefore believe that aggressive wound management is important. The 2 patients with wound revisions had an uneventful recovery without development of an infection. Early loosening occurred in 3 patients as mentioned above.

Overall, although the complication rate was high, most of the complications did not influence the positive final outcome.

Summary

Severe post-traumatic arthrosis can be reliably and durably treated with a noncustomized, semiconstrained device. The patient's satisfaction is high. Function can reliably be restored. This represents a great improvement compared to the prior constrained implants with high loosening rates considering this very difficult group of patients. Correct cementation and surgical technique seems to be important. The rather high complication rate reflects the limitations of this procedure. Especially the mechanical complications indicate that, in younger patients, total elbow replacement may only be performed with reservation, and only for those who do not perform strenuous physical activities.

References

1. Schneeberger AG, Adams R, Morrey BF (1997) Semiconstrained total elbow replacement for the treatment of post-traumatic osteoarthrosis. J Bone Joint Surg Am 79:1211-1222
2. Gill DRJ, Morrey BF (1998) The Coonrad-Morrey total elbow arthroplasty in patients who have rheumatoid arthritis. A ten to fifteen-year follow-up study. J Bone Joint Surg Am 80:1327-1335
3. McAuliffe JA, Burkhalter WE, Ouellette EA, Carneiro RS (1992) Compression plate arthrodesis of the elbow. J Bone Joint Surg Br 74:300-304
4. O'Neill OR, Morrey BF, Tanaka S, An K-N (1992) Compensatory motion in the upper extremity after elbow arthrodesis. Clin Orthop 281:89-96
5. Ewald FC, Jacobs MA (1984) Total elbow arthroplasty. Clin Orthop 182:137-142
6. Morrey BF, Adams RA, Bryan RS (1991) Total replacement for post-traumatic arthritis of the elbow. J Bone Joint Surg Br 73:607-612
7. Froimson AI, Silva JE, Richey D (1976) Cutis arthroplasty of the elbow joint. J Bone Joint Surg Am 58:863-865
8. Knight RA, Zandt LV (1952) Arthroplasty of the elbow. J Bone Joint Surg Am 34:610-618
9. Morrey BF (1990) Post-traumatic contracture of the elbow. Operative treatment including distraction arthroplasty. J Bone Joint Surg Am 72:601-618
10. Tsuge K, Murakami T, Yasunaga Y, Kanaujia RR (1987) Arthroplasty of the elbow. J Bone Joint Surg Br 69:116-120
11. Allieu Y, Marck G, Chammas M, Desbonnet P, Raynaud J-P (2004) Allogreffes d'articulation totale du coude dans les pertes de substance ostéo-articulaires post-traumatiques étendues. Résultats à 12 ans de recul. Rev Chir Orthop 90:319-328
12. Urbaniak JR, Black KE Jr (1985) Cadaveric elbow allografts. A six year experience. Clin Orthop 197:131-140
13. Garrett JC, Ewald FC, Thomas WH, Sledge CB (1977) Loosening associated with GSB hinge total elbow replacement in patients with rheumatoid arthritis. Clin Orthop 127:170-174
14. Morrey BF, Bryan RS, Dobyns JH, Linscheid RL (1981) Total elbow arthroplasty. A five-year experience at the Mayo Clinic. J Bone Joint Surg Am 63:1050-1063
15. Allieu Y, Meyer ZU Reckendorf G, Daude O (1998) Long-term results of unconstrained Roper-Tuke elbow arthroplasty in patients with rheumatoid arthritis. J Shoulder Elbow Surg 7:560-564
16. Davis RF, Weiland AJ, Hungerford DS et al (1982) Nonconstrained total elbow arthroplasty. Clin Orthop 171:156-160
17. Kudo H, Iwano K, Nishino J (1999) Total elbow arthroplasty with use of a nonconstrained humeral component inserted without cement in patients who have rheumatoid arthritis. J Bone Joint Surg Am 81:1268-1280
18. Lowe LW, Miller AJ, Allum RL, Higginson DW (1984) The development of an unconstrained elbow arthroplasty. J Bone Joint Surg Br 66:243-247
19. Ruth JT, Wilde AH (1992) Capitellocondylar total elbow replacement. J Bone Joint Surg Am 74:95-100
20. Rydholm U, Tjörnstrand B, Petterson H, Lidgren L (1984) Surface replacement of the elbow in rheumatoid arthritis. J Bone Joint Surg Br 66:737-741
21. Soni RK, Cavendish ME (1984) A review of the Liverpool elbow prosthesis from 1974 to 1982. J Bone Joint Surg Br 66:248-253
22. Sourmelis SG, Burke FD, Varian JPW (1986) A review of total elbow arthroplasty and an early assessment of the Liverpool elbow prosthesis. J Bone Joint Surg Br 11:407-413
23. Trail IA, Nuttall D, Stanley JK (1999) Survivorship and radiological analysis of the standard Souter-Strathclyde total elbow arthroplasty. J Bone Joint Surg Br 81:80-84
24. Trancik T, Wilde AH, Borden LS (1987) Capitellocondylar total elbow arthroplasty. Two- to eight-year experience. Clin Orthop 223:175-180
25. Yanni ON, Fearn CBDA, Gallannaugh SC, Joshi R (2000) The Roper-Tuke total elbow arthroplasty. A 4- to 10-years results on an unconstrained prosthesis. J Bone Joint Surg Br 82:705-710
26. Brumfield RH Jr, Kuschner SH, Gellman H et al (1990) Total elbow arthroplasty. J Arthroplasty 5:359-363
27. Figgie HE III, Inglis AE, Ranawat CS, Rosenberg GM (1987) Results of total elbow arthroplasty as a salvage procedure for failed elbow reconstructive operations. Clin Orthop 219:185-193
28. Gschwend N, Loehr J, Ivosevic-Radovanovic D et al (1988) Semi-constrained elbow prosthesis with special reference to the GSB III prosthesis. Clin Orthop 232:104-111
29. Inglis AE, Pellicci PM (1980) Total elbow replacement. J Bone Joint Surg Am 62:1252-1258
30. Kasten MD, Skinner HB (1993) Total elbow arthroplasty. Clin Orthop 290:177-188
31. Kraay MJ, Figgie MP, Inglis AE et al (1994) Primary semiconstrained total elbow arthroplasty. J Bone Joint Surg Br 76:636-640
32. Schneeberger AG, Meyer DC, Yian EH (2007) Coonrad-Morrey total elbow replacement for primary and revision surgery: A 2 to 7.5 year follow-up study. J Shoulder Elbow Surg 16[Suppl 1]:S47-S59
33. Gschwend N, Scheier H, Bähler A, Simmen B (1996) GSB III elbow. In: Rüther W (ed) The elbow, endoprosthetic replacement and non-endoprosthetic procedures. Berlin Heidelberg, Springer, pp 83-98

34. Morrey BF, Adams RA (1995) Semi-constrained elbow replacement for distal humeral nonunion. J Bone Joint Surg Br 77:67-72

35. Hughes RE, Schneeberger AG, An K-N et al (1997) Reduction of triceps muscle force after shortening of the distal humerus. A computational model. J Shoulder Elbow Surg 6:444-448

36. Lee BP, Adams RA, Morrey BF (2005) Polyethylene wear after total elbow arthroplasty. J Bone Joint Surg Am 87:1080-1087

37. O'Driscoll SW, An K-N, Korinek S, Morrey BF (1992) Kinematics of semi-constrained total elbow arthroplasty. J Bone Joint Surg Br 74:297-299

38. Morrey BF, Adams RA (1993) Semi-constrained elbow replacement arthroplasty. Rational, technique, and results. In: Morrey BF (ed) The elbow and its disorders, 2nd ed. WB Saunders Company, pp 648-664

39. Bryan RS, Morrey BF (1982) Extensive posterior exposure of the elbow. A triceps-sparing approach. Clin Orthop 166:188-192

40. Faber KJ, Cordy ME, Milne AD et al (1997) Advanced cementing technique improves fixation in elbow arthroplasty. Clin Orthop 334:150-156

CHAPTER 26

Revision of Failed Elbow Arthroplasty

B.F. MORREY

1. A failed prosthesis will present either with or without a periprosthetic fracture.
2. If the integrity of the bone is not compromised by fracture, osteolysis or osteoporosis is commonly present.
3. Stiffness, scarring, and contracture of the soft tissue are common findings that can include the triceps, ulnar nerve, static deformity, and skin.

Loose implants may not be painful, so they should be followed carefully. Revision is offered, even if there is no pain, because extensive osteolysis can lead to fracture, making revision even more difficult.

Introduction

Over the last few years, our understanding of and techniques used to successfully revise failed arthroplasties have expanded considerably [1, 2]. A broad spectrum of clinical and pathological states is encountered with the failed total elbow arthroplasty. Several specific features of the presentation are considered as the management plan is formulated (Table 1).

Table 1. Surgical options for the failed total elbow arthroplasty are considered as functional restoring or as salvage procedures

Non-Implant Salvage
Fusion
Resection

Functional Restoration
Prosthetic Articulation
Allograft Replacement
Implant Insertion

Assessment

History. The most important historical information is compromised of the duration of implantation and the function early after implantation. An early failure from loosening may be due to sepsis. Hence, assessment for and excluding the possibility of sepsis is a most important consideration prior to any revision procedure, but especially in those with "early" unexplained or unanticipated failure.

Laboratory. The sedimentation rate and C-reactive protein studies are regularly employed along with aspiration of the joint if there is any question of sepsis.

Radiographic. The radiograph is, of course, most helpful for defining the exact cause of failure. In light of the radiographic appearance of the failure, the appropriate pre-operative plan is formulated. based primarily on the quality of the bone. In our practice, we do not offer surgery for radiolucent lines that are not painful. We do follow such patients and we do offer surgery if there is progressive resorption, bone loss, or impending fracture.

Implant Revision

The various options for reinsertion are predicated on the status and quality of bone and presence or absence of fracture. With increased longevity and increased use of elbow replacements by the orthopedic community, an increasing number of periprosthetic fractures are being seen. We have found it helpful to classify these according to site of involvement: Type I, metaphyseal; Type II, stem involvement; Type III, proximal or distal to the stem tip (Fig. 1). Management strategies are discussed below based on this classification [3].

Functional Restoration Revision Options

We offer a reinsertion revision in six circumstances depending on the above mentioned features of osseous competency. These options include:
- reinsertion into intact cement;
- reinsertion into the host bone;
- reimplantation into cancellous augmented host bone reinsertion;

- reimplantation into strut graft augmented host bone;
- use of a "composite" allograft;
- custom device reconstruction.

Technique of Reimplantation Revision

General Considerations

Pre-operative Planning and Implant Selection

The loose elbow implant may cause bone resorption. This may cause weak or absent triceps function due to resorption of the olecranon. The most important consideration is whether adequate fixation can be obtained with another stemmed implant given the amount and quality of the intact cement mantle. Hence, the most common special implant need is adequate stem length. The largest stemmed implant that comfortably fits in the bone stock is preferable. For humeral revisions, we use either the 15-long or 20 cm-length humeral stem of the Coonrad-Morrey design. Special long-stemmed ulnar components are also routinely available. The extended flange is especially helpful for deficient distal humeral bone stock. Custom devices are, thus, rarely needed with this system (Fig. 2).

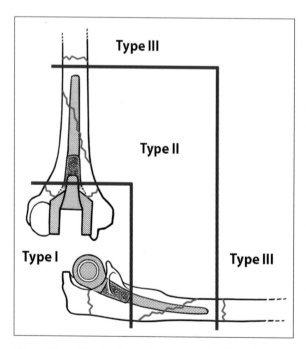

Fig. 1. Mayo Classification of periprosthetic elbow fractures. *Type I*, metaphyseal; *Type II*, involves stem; *Type III*, beyond stem. (Figure reproduced with permission, Mayo Foundation)

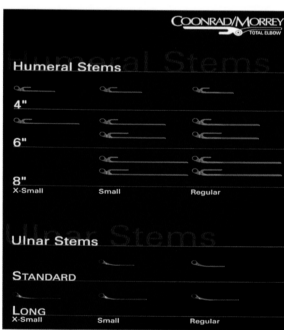

Fig. 2. Standard humeral and ulnar implants have considerable dimensional variety. The availability of the extended flange virtually eliminates the need for custom devices

Surgical Procedure

General Considerations and Prior Surgery

The surgical exposure is modified according to the patient's presentation [4]. Previous skin incisions are used as much as possible. The ulnar nerve is identified and decompressed if symptomatic or simply protected if not symptomatic. The management of the triceps is according to one of three methods: (1) the triceps is reflected (Mayo); (2) the triceps is split, particularly in patients in whom there have been multiple procedures with poor triceps tissue; or (3) the triceps is left attached to the ulna; after the joint or pseudarthrosis is resected and the ulna is rotated and displaced, adequate exposure is often attained even while leaving the triceps attached (Fig. 3).

Specific Technical Considerations

Preservation of Cement Mantle

If the bone-cement interface is intact the cement may be left and a new device re-cemented in the existing PMMA mantle.

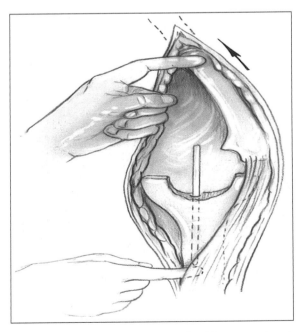

Fig. 3. In patients with loss of the distal humerus, the triceps can sometimes remain attached to the proximal ulna. The articulation is released and the ulna can simply be rolled out of the way, leaving the triceps attached medially or laterally

A high-speed bone burr with a 2 mm head and long extension shaft is helpful to remove cement between the implant and bone. Furthermore, if the bone-cement interface is secure, the cement cavity is expanded with the 4 mm "olive" burr to receive the revision implant stem. Cement injection systems are used to inject the cement down the canal. Typically, for revision surgery each component is cemented separately to minimize technical complications. Great care must be taken to avoid injury to the nerves. We graft cortical defects with autogenous or allograft bone to avoid extra-vasation of cement and lessen any stress riser effect in an attempt to prevent fracture.

Cement Removal and Reinsertion into Intact Bone

We use an esmarch technique to expose the humerus as proximally as necessary. Exposure or location and palpation of the radial nerve are necessary to avoid injury to this structure (Fig. 4). The humerus is then palpated in order to avoid violation of the cortex at the time of the cement removal.

The ulna is extensively exposed in a subcutaneous fashion for as great a distance as necessary to have adequate exposure and to avoid violation of the ulnar cortex. The medullary canal is first identified beyond the tip of the prior implant. If there is thinning at the tip of the implant, if a fracture has occurred, or if specific attention must be given to more distal insertion of the stem down the canal, the entire subcutaneous border of the ulna may be

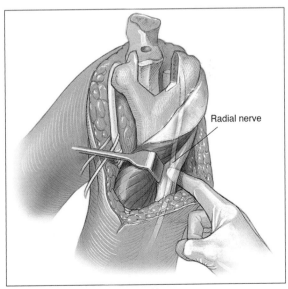

Radial nerve

Fig. 4. The humeral shaft is exposed sufficiently to palpate the radial nerve and lessen the likelihood of penetration

exposed to the extent necessary to avoid violation of the intact ulnar cortex.

Closure is carefully done with special care taken to assure triceps function and to avoid tension or pressure on the wound. After revision procedures, if an allograft has been used or if there has been extensive bone loss or a periprosthetic fracture has occurred. The elbow is placed in a splint in extension. After 4 to 6 weeks, the splint is removed and motion is begun. Because the range of motion after revision elbow replacement is virtually the same as that after primary joint replacement, early mobilization of the revision implant is not usually necessary.

Results

Reimplantation

There is little information with regard to the outcome of reimplantation of an artificial implant after a previously failed loose replacement [3]. Our initial experience with 42 patients followed an average of 5 years (range 2-11) [5] was reported in 1997. Approximately half of these patients had rheumatoid arthritis, and the other half post-traumatic arthritis as their underlying diagnosis (Fig. 5). At follow-up 38 of 42 were considered satisfactory outcomes [6].

Osseous Enhancement Options

If the process has caused resorption, osteolysis, or a periprosthetic fracture, an "augmentation" procedure is indicated in the form of impaction grafting or strut augmentation.

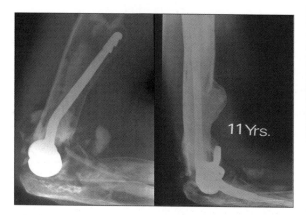

Fig. 5. Reinsertion into osseous envelope after cortical penetration of a loose humeral stem shows no evidence of loosening or lucency 11 years after 150-cm implant revision

Impaction Grafting

Indication. Expanded cortical bone of inadequate quality to provide a securely and reliable bone/cement interface. We attempt to attain at least 2 to 3 cm stem depth into intact bone.

Procedure. The extent of the expanded lytic bone is determined. The distance "D" of stem fixation that is attainable in the uninvolved bone is also determined. A rigid tube is placed in the expanded cortical portion of the bone. The elbow cement injector tube is cut at a distance "D" plus the length of cortical expansion. Cancellous bone or bone substitute is firmly packed around the outer tube (Fig. 6). Cement is injected into the intact canal

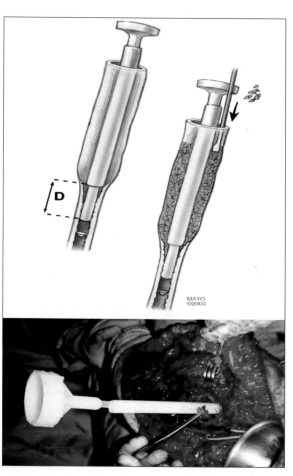

Fig. 6. For impaction grafting, a semi-rigid tube is inserted across the expanded osteolytic segment. The cement injector nozzle passes through the outer tube for a distance "D" into normal bone. Cancellous bone is firmly impacted around the tube. Cement is delivered into the intact bone for the distance "D". When the injector gun is withdrawn to the level of the outer tubes they are withdrawn together while continuing to inject cement into the void. The implant is then inserted

through an inner tube and withdrawn for the distance "D", after which the two tubes are withdrawn simultaneously while cement is injected in the region of the expanded cortex. The implant is then inserted. This technique may be used both for the humerus and ulna.

Results

The outcome of 12 patients who underwent revision total elbow arthroplasty with impaction grafting between 1993 and 1997. There were eight women and four men with a mean age of 60 years. All patients were followed for at least 2 years (range 25-113 months) with an average length of follow-up of 72 months. Seven of the patients had an initial diagnosis of rheumatoid arthritis, and five had post-traumatic arthritis. For three of the patients, impaction grafting was undertaken with the initial revision. The nine remaining patients had all undergone at least one prior revision without impaction grafting. Isolated impaction grafting on the ulnar side alone was undertaken in four elbows and on the humeral side alone in six patients. Two patients underwent impaction grafting of both the humerus and ulna. Six allograft struts were placed to span structural defects in five patients.

At the latest follow-up, eight of the elbows were intact after the index impaction grafting procedure (Fig. 7). Two elbows were revised for loosening and a third for fracture of an ulnar component. A fourth patient underwent a resection arthroplasty for infection. The eight remaining patients demonstrated marked radiographic improvement in bone quality in the region of impaction graft without clinical symptoms of loos-

ening. After further revision in three, at last follow-up five were rated excellent, four good, and three fair.

We conclude impaction grafting is a reliable technique to treat osteolysis associated with revision total elbow arthroplasty, however, complications can occur and the need for additional surgery is high.

Strut Grafting

This technique is especially useful for Type II and III periprosthetic fractures and for distal humeral or proximal ulnar bone loss. The most effective application to the humerus is that of an anterior strut that transverses the osteolysis or fracture and captures the flange anteriorly. A posterior strut is employed to enhance stability and to prevent the wire cutting through the host bone (Fig. 8). The radial nerve is exposed for humeral applications, and at least two circumferential wire fixation points are required around the normal host bone proximal to the fracture, and two around the osteolysis or expanded peri-articular bone distal to the fracture. The design of the Coonrad-Morrey implant allows restoration of the axis of rotation with a deficient humerus from the level of the olecranon fossa. The use of the extended flange and an anterior strut graft allows management of distal humeral deficiencies of up to 8 cm. If greater than 2 cm bone loss occurs proximal to the olecranon fossa, the length is accommodated by the

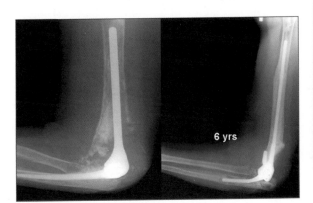

Fig. 7. Marked osteolysis effectively treated with impaction grafting at six years

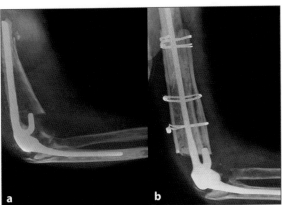

Fig. 8. a Patient with severe bone loss and fracture after failed Coonrad-Morrey implant. **b** At 2 years, the impaction graft with struts have been successful clinically and radiographically

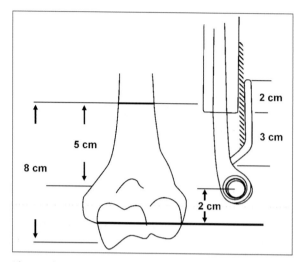

Fig. 9. The implant is routinely seated such that the distal 3 cm of humeral bone is not required for fixation of the implant. The extended flange allows an additional 3 cm bone loss and 2 cm of host bone is still covered by flange. If an additional 2 cm of bone is lost, the implant may be inserted further up the canal for about 2 cm. Hence, an 8 cm deficiency can be treated

extended flange (Fig. 9). The implant is simply inserted to the desired depth and the deficient bone is bridged by the flange and graft. If up to 5 cm bone loss is present proximal to the fossa, 3 cm is accommodated by the flange and strut graft and 2 cm shortening is accepted. The proper depth of insertion is determined by flexing the articulated trials with the elbow at 90° flexion; displace the ulna distally until tension limits further displacement and observe the depth of insertion of the humeral component at this point (Fig. 10).

Results

Humeral Reconstruction

Between 1991 and 1999, 11 humeral periprosthetic fractures around a loose component were treated with cortical strut allograft augmentation and revision arthroplasty using Coonrad-Morrey semiconstrained implants [7]. The indication for the initial arthroplasty had been rheumatoid arthritis in six cases and related to trauma in five cases. Six periprosthetic fractures presented after a primary and five after a revision arthroplasty. The average number of surgeries before occurrence of the fracture was 2.4 (range 1-5). Two parallel struts were used for fracture fixation in most cases. Patients were followed for a mean of 2.7 years (range 9 months-7 years).

Clinical and radiographic fracture union was obtained in 10 cases (Fig. 11); the only nonunion underwent an additional fixation procedure at another institution 9 months post-operatively. One patient required revision surgery for humeral aseptic loosening 7 years after fracture union; there were no other implant failures. Complications included an additional nondisplaced humeral periprosthetic fracture after surgery that failed to heal with closed treatment, one olecranon fracture, one permanent ulnar nerve injury and one triceps insufficiency. At most recent follow-up, seven of the eight patients with an intact reconstruction had a functional arc of motion and no or slight pain; one had moderate pain and limited motion.

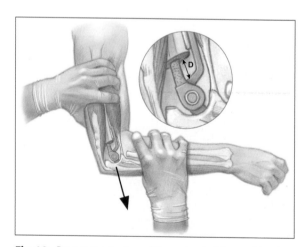

Fig. 10. Proper tensioning of the extended flanged implant occurs by observing flange position as the elbow is flexed 90° and distal pressure places flexors and extensors under tension. Reproduced with permission from the Mayo Foundation

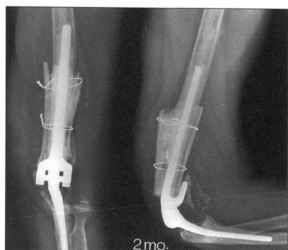

Fig. 11. Anterior and posterior struts effectively address deficient distal humeral bone

We have thus concluded that treatment of periprosthetic humeral fractures that present with a loose humeral component are effectively treated with revision elbow arthroplasty and strut allograft augmentation. The technique is associated with high rates of fracture union, implant survival and satisfactory clinical results. However, the complication rate is substantial.

Ulnar Reconstruction

Total elbow replacements with aseptic failure and proximal ulnar bone deficiency treated with allograft bone struts have also been reported [8]. The patients in this group had an average of 2.5 (range 1-4) prior surgical procedures. In addition to revision of the prosthetic components, the deficient bone stock was treated in one of four ways with allograft struts; 1) discrete cortical defects were contained; 2) periprosthetic fractures were splinted; 3) triceps attachment deficiency was reconstructed; and 4) expanded segments were augmented with struts and filled with impaction graft. The average follow-up was 4 years (range 2-11 years) in 21 patients (21 elbows).

The mean Elbow Performance Scores improved from 34 pre-operatively to 79 at the latest follow-up. Pain, stability and the activities of daily living scores improved most, with little change in motion (Fig. 12). Complications occurred in eight cases consisting of four soft-tissue and four osseous problems. Graft incorporation of up to 50% was present in three cases, 75% in five cases, and 100% in 13 cases.

We conclude most proximal ulnar bone stock deficiencies and fractures complicating revision total elbow surgery can be treated with allograft struts. Although a high complication rate may occur, discrete cortical lesions, periprosthetic fractures, and an expanded proximal ulna, which require augmentation with impaction grafting, are suitable for this technique. The technique has been unreliable, however, in restoring deficient olecranon bone stock.

Allograft Prosthetic Composite (APC) Reconstruction

In the past we have employed allograft prosthesis composites to treat deficiency both at the humerus and ulna. Overall the problem with interface union between the host and allograft bones has prompted us to limit the use of this surgical technique. However, this can be a successful option. In some instances of expanded bone, an allograft composite may be inserted into the thin shell of host bone. The major challenge is rigid fixation at the allograft/host bone interface.

Results. We recently documented our experience with this surgery [9]. Assessment of 16 cases revealed nine humeral and seven ulnar composites have been employed. We were surprised to learn that as a group these patients did rather well. Only two have been revised, leaving 88% still functioning a mean of 6 years after surgery (Fig. 13) [10].

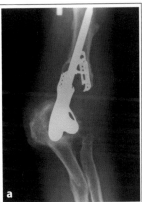
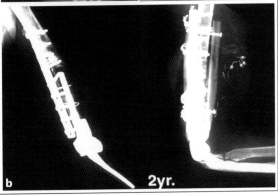

Fig. 13. (**a**) Massive bone loss of the distal humerus. (**b**) Composite allograft with plate fixation to control rotatory stability until the bone graft heals

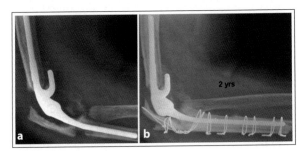

Fig. 12 a, b. Loose and fractured ulna with successful revision using strut augmentation

References

1. Blaine T, Adams R, Morrey BF (2001) Conversion of interposition arthroplasty to semiconstrained total elbow arthroplasty. AAOS, San Francisco, CA
2. Morrey BF, Bryan RS (1999) Revision total elbow arthroplasty. J Bone Joint Surg Am 69:523
3. O'Driscoll SW, Morrey BF (1999) Periprosthetic fractures about the elbow. Orthop Clinics North Am 30:319-325
4. Bryan RS, Morrey BF (1982) Extensive posterior exposure of the elbow: a triceps-sparing appraoch. Clin Orthop 166:188
5. Loebenberg MI, Adams R, O'Driscoll SW, Morrey BF (2005) Impaction grafting in revision total elbow arthroplasty. J Bone Joint Surg 87:99-106
6. King GJ, Adams RA, Morrey BF (1997) Total elbow arthroplasty: revision with use a non-custom semiconstrained prosthesis. J Bone Joint Surg Am 79:394-400
7. Sanchez Sotelo J, O'Driscoll SW, Morrey BF (2002) Periprosthetic humeral fracture after total elbow arthroplasty treatment with implant revision and strut allograft augmentation. J Bone Joint Surg Am 84:1642-1650
8. Kamineni S, Morrey BF (2004) Proximal ulnar reconstruction with strut allograft in revision total elbow arthroplasty. J Bone Joint Surg Am 86:1223-1229
9. Mansat P, Adams RA, Morrey BF (2004) Allograft-prosthesis composite for revision of catastrophic failure of total elbow arthroplasty. J Bone Joint Surg Am 86:724-735
10. Morrey BF, Adams RA (1995) Semiconstrained joint replacement arthroplasty for distal humeral nonunion. J Bone Joint Surg Br 77:67-72

CHAPTER 27

Elbow Nerve Tunnel Syndromes

A. CELLI, C. ROVESTA, M.C. MARONGIU

Introduction

The repetitive and stressing movements by athletes [1-5], wheelchair users [6], and manual workers [7-9] can cause overwork syndromes of articular and periarticular musculo-tendinous structures [10]. Terms like "lateral" and "medial epicondylalgia" characterize painful syndromes in the elbow, due to microtraumatic stress in the medial region (internal compartment) and in the lateral region (external compartment).

The etiology and pathogenesis of pain and functional limitation generally refer to three possible causes, often combined:

1. inflammatory and degenerative musculo-tendinous pathologies of the muscles that insert on the epicondyles;
2. osteo-articular pathologies: radial head and capitulum in the lateral side or medially the trochlea and olecranon;
3. nerve tunnel syndromes affecting the radial nerve on the lateral side of the elbow and the ulnar nerve on the medial side.

It is important to have a clinical approach which should be able to consider the joint and muscular-tendinous disease in close association with its neurological aspects.

Specific tests and pre-operative examinations should lead to the identification of the three local syndromes, either alone or combined, as well as their differentiation from proximal pathologies like vertebro-cervical syndrome and neurovascular disease in the cervico-axillary passage.

The Compartment Concept

Diagnosis of epicondylalgia may be helped by introducing the compartment concept in order to distinguish nerve tunnel pathology from osteo-articular and musculo-tendinous syndromes.

We define a "compartment" as the external, internal, anterior, or posterior anatomical sector where the osteoarticular, capsule-ligamentous, musculo-tendinous, and neurological structures can be simultaneously affected by microtraumatic overwork pathologies (Fig. 1).

This concept is useful not only for the classification of microtraumatic pathology in single sectors, but also because the compartment structures are often contemporaneously involved in the physiopathological process, as well as in the clinical presentation.

As a matter of fact, most nerve tunnel syndromes occur as a result of nearby osteo-articular or musculo-tendinous changes. Besides, clinical manifestations usually appear all together, and only through a careful semiological exams, can physicians estimate the pathological role of every anatomical element of a compartment. Consequently, treatment must consider not only the neurological loss, but also the surrounding compressing structures.

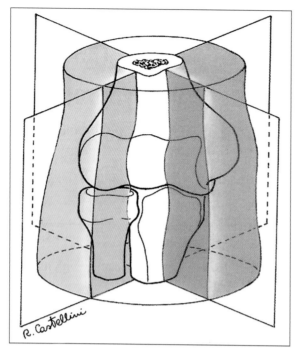

Fig. 1. The elbow compartments

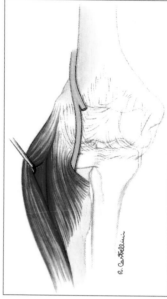

Fig. 2. The main structures of the lateral compartment

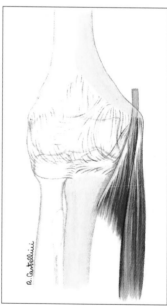

Fig. 3. The main structures of medial compartment

1. In the external compartment we find:
    – the radial-humeral joint;
    – the joint capsule, the radial collateral, and annular ligaments;
    – the lateral epicondylar muscles (extensor carpi radialis Iongus and brevis, supinator, and extensor digitorum communis);
    – the radial nerve and its two terminal branches (motor and sensory one) (Fig. 2).
2. In the internal compartment:
    – the ulno-humeral joint;
    – the joint capsule and ulnar collateral ligament;
    – the epitrochlear muscles (flexor carpi radialis and ulnaris, pronator teres. and flexor digitorum superficialis);
    – the ulnar nerve (Fig. 3).
3. In the anterior compartment:
    – the anterior ulno-humeral joint;
    – the pronator teres, flexor digitorum superficialis, and flexor carpi radialis muscles;
    – the median nerve.
4. In the posterior compartment:
    – the posterior ulno-humeral joint;
    – the triceps muscle.

Among the functional activities of the upper limb there are some common movements that overload the compartment structures.

Shoulder external rotation, elbow extension, forearm supination, or wrist extension can heavily stress the external compartment.

The overloading of the internal compartment occurs, however, in activities involving shoulder internal rotation, elbow flexion, forearm pronation, or wrist flexion.

Strain on the anterior compartment is determined by activities requiring repeated shoulder internal rotation, elbow flexion, forearm pronation, wrist extension, and finger flexion.

The posterior compartment is overworked in functional activities which demand repeated elbow extension in association with shoulder internal rotation and forearm supination.

Functional overloading in one compartment often affects nearby compartments whose structures are functionally linked.

It is easy to clinically observe how inflammatory and degenerative pathologies often develop in two compartments at once, with a combination of either the external and posterior or the internal and anterior compartments.

Our aim is to isolate and describe the diagnostic value of the clinical features and imaging study findings that can identify nerve tunnel syndrome in a painful elbow. In particular, this study will be focused on compression syndromes of the radial nerve (in the external compartment) and the ulnar nerve (in the internal compartment).

External Compartment Pathology: Radial Nerve Tunnel Syndrome

Radial tunnel syndrome has been identified at the beginning of the past century [11, 12] and described by many Italian [13-17] and foreign [18-23] authors, although it is an uncommon pathology (5%-8% of cases of lateral epicondylalgia) [24]. Nevertheless, finding an involvement of the Posterior Interosseous Nerve (PIN) in chronic lateral epicondylalgia is more frequent in our experience than what results from the above figures.

Chronic lateral epicondylalgia can be different combinations of the following three lesions:

1. insertional pathology of the lateral epicondylar muscles;
2. humero-radial joint disease;
3. compression of the radial nerve in the radial tunnel.

The Radial Tunnel

The "radial tunnel" [22] in the elbow is a possible site for nerve tunnel compression syndromes. The radial tunnel is defined as the space that begins proximally near the external bicipital groove and ends distally at the emergence of the motor branch of the radial nerve from the supinator muscle [25]. The radial tunnel can be divided into three levels: upper, middle, and lower.

In the upper portion (tunnel entrance) the nerve is located medially at the brachialis muscle and lies on the bottom of the lateral bicipital groove [26]. Afterwards the nerve splits into its sensory and motor branches; the latter, called Posterior Interosseous Nerve, heads posteriorly towards the ca-

pitulum and the joint capsule. In this area the nerve runs in a wide space and is unsheathed by loose connective tissue, which binds it to the nearby muscles, the joint capsule, and the radial collateral ligament (anterior bundle).

If microtrauma occurs, this loose connective tissue can be transformed into adherent and relatively inelastic fibrous tissue. The nerve then sticks to the joint capsule and may be compressed by the adherent bridles during elbow movement [14, 22, 27-31].

In the middle portion, the Posterior Interosseous Nerve is engaged below the extensor carpi brevis [32], whose arched free edge (spanning from the lateral epicondyle to the deep antibrachialis bundle and the aponeurosis of the flexor digitorum muscles) can be thicker and fibrotic (Figs. 4).

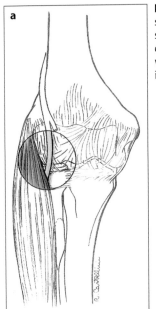

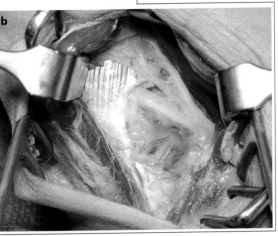

Fig. 4 a, b. The drawing shows the upper joint capsula and the arcade of the extensor carpi radialis sites where the PIN compression is possible

Authors have described many variations in the form and thickness of this fibrous septum which passes over the motor branch of the radial nerve. Forearm pronation tightens the aponeurosis just like the opposing wrist extension. Under such conditions, a thicker, inelastic fibrous arcade can compress the nerve [19, 20, 22, 23, 27-30, 33-35].

Neurolysis is mandatory in surgical treatment of lateral epicondylar pathologies with radial nerve compression. The success of surgical detachment of the extensor carpi radials brevis from the lateral epicondyle depends on the good release of the fibrous insertional arcade of this muscle, which is able to reduce the compression of the posterior interosseous nerve.

In the lower portion, the motor branch overtakes the arcade of the extensor carpi radialis brevis and then penetrates between the bundles of the superficial and deep heads of the supinator brevis muscle [19, 20, 22, 29, 36, 37]. The upper edge of the superficial head of the muscle is fibrous in about 30% of adults, while in the newborn this arcade is always muscular [37]. The fibrous arcade of the supinator brevis muscle has been called Frohse's Arcade [38], after the anatomist who described it in 1908 (Fig. 5).

In adults this arcade can be extensively fibrotic, because of a repeated pronation and supination of the forearm which produces a supinator brevis muscle overload. Pronation tightens the arcade and causes nerve compression, while supination releases it [30].

The superficial head of the supinator and its often fibrotic proximal bundles insert on the anterior surface of the lateral epicondyle, under the tendon of the extensor carpi radialis brevis and the radial collateral ligament (anterior bundle), or on the lateral surface of the annular ligament. Given this anatomical shape, it is easy to understand the role of the supinator brevis muscle, especially its superficial head, in the pathogenesis of lateral epicondylalgia. Actually, an insertional pathology in this area can affect the whole external compartment of the elbow, with clinical manifestations ascribable to syndromes of the lateral epicondyle, the motor branch of the radial nerve, and the capsule-ligamentous structures of the radio-humeral joint.

The final possible point of compression of the motor branch of the radial nerve is in its passage between the bellies of the superficial and deep heads of the supinator brevis muscle [23, 27-29, 35]. Such an instance is rare, and may happen when the deep head is congenitally underdeveloped ("exposed" area of the radial neck in 25% of cases according to Spinner) [35] or completely absent, as in one of our cases.

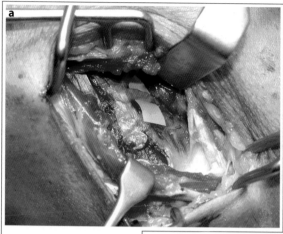

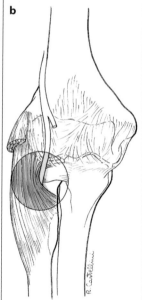

Fig. 5 a, b. In the lower site, the PIN compression is possible in the arcade of the supinator

In conclusion, it should be emphasized that nerve damage in the radial tunnel can occur in several places, but it raises mainly: in the fibrous arcade of the extensor carpi brevis; and (b) in the fibrous arcade of the supinator brevis muscle.

Clinical Diagnosis

The clinical diagnosis of posterior interosseous nerve compression in the radial tunnel is based on the presence of motor deficit in dependent muscles, featuring radiating pain from the elbow to the forearm and the hand, without objectively evident sensory loss [39].

Two clinical outcomes are possible. The first one is less common: pain can often hide a mild motor deficit; paresis is difficult to observe as well, this usually being a sign of more proximal nerve compression. Diagnosis becomes more difficult to reach in PIN tunnel syndromes in association with lateral epicondylitis symptoms [40, 41].

Based on a cadaveric study, Loh proposed (2004) a new clinical test, the Rule-of-Nine test, as a reliable method of diagnosing radial tunnel syndrome to improve the diagnostic accuracy in radial tunnel syndrome [42]. However, generally in this case the diagnosis is based on the character of the spontaneous or evoked pain, on the presence of motor deficit, the limitation of active and passive elbow movement, and the pre-operative examinations (X-ray, MRI, etc.).

The pain is localized in the lateral epicondylar region and it often radiates downwards from the postero-lateral surface of the forearm to the wrist. Many authors consider this feature very important for the diagnosis of nerve compression. Daytime pain does not subside with rest and it sharpens at night [22, 28, 29, 37, 43-45]. Otherwise, we consider as secondary aspects both the particular kind of localization and the rhythm of the spontaneous pain for the diagnosis of nerve compression, because the posterior interosseous nerve is a muscular nerve whose sensory component is proprioceptive.

Pain in such cases is dull, poorly localized, and it affects the lateral epicondyle and its muscles following the distribution of the proprioceptive receptors; that is why it can be similar to musculo-tendinous and osteoarticular diseases.

Pain evoked by pressure on the supinator canal at the radial head is considered a specific sign, differentiated from lateral epicondylar pain, evoked by pressure on the lateral epicondyle.

The pain produced by opposing supination with elbow extension is considered specific since the nerve is tensed up by the elbow extension, and therefore compressed by the forced contraction of the supinator muscle. Reawakening of pain by passive pronation with extended elbow has got the same meaning: shifting of the radius associated to the tension of a fully supinator extension can cause nerve compression.

Many authors suppose these three pain-evoking tests to be typical in nerve tunnel syndrome [20, 27, 29, 45, 46]. In our experience they are reliable but not specific signs of posterior interosseous nerve compression in patients with lateral epicondylalgia. In fact, we believe that the nerve tunnel syndrome is often associated with pathology of the musculotendinous structures of the external compartment, so that all tests engaging this compartment evoke pain, as they always affect the nearby muscular and osteoarticular structures as well as the nerve.

Roles' sign is considered specific for nerve tunnel syndrome by many authors [20, 22, 29, 47]: it consists in opposed extension of the third finger which causes pain. In truth we agree with Allieu [43], Comtet [27], and Howard [48], who consider it aspecific, given its presence in many routine lateral epicondylar syndromes. Unfortunately it does not indicate motor branch compression below the extensor carpi radialis brevis arcade, as Roles suggested, but it simply expresses the presence of an insertional pathology of this muscle and the extensor digitorum communis. The involvement of the extensor digitorum muscle in the lateral epicondylar insertion is shown by the pain sprung from the opposed extension of the third (Maudsley's test) and fourth fingers [49], while the extension of the second and fifth fingers is painless, because of the separation of their extensor muscles. The character of the spontaneous and evoked pain cannot be sufficient to reach a diagnosis of PIN tunnel syndrome. The clinical manifestations become typical when pain is accompanied by functional limitation and paresis of the muscles innervated below the point of compression (individual or common extensors, thumb extensors, etc.). Paralysis is progressive and does not feature a sensory deficit in the radial nerve dermatome.

Patients usually complain of a weakening of the metacarpo-phalangeal extension as well as a thumb extension and abduction.

Wrist extension is preserved in order to protect the integrity of the nerve branches directed to the extensor muscles of the radius, but it is achieved with radial deviation due to extensor carpi ulnaris insufficiency [12].

The EMG confirms the presence and site of neuromuscular damage [50, 51], and it is therefore important for the differential diagnosis. Also MR imaging is a useful method for evaluating nerve disease. It can portray the normal anatomy and identify unsuspected space-occupying masses [52]. Nevertheless, in spontaneous paralysis of the PIN and serious paretic damage, it is always advisable to consider other causes of neurological lesions, caused by multiple neuropathies of metabolic, toxic, or infective origin. In their primary phases these forms may affect only a single nerve and localize themselves where microtraumatic damage can be done (nerve tunnel syndromes); afterwards neurological harm will subsequently manifest itself in various and often symmetrical sites.

At last, we have to pay attention to particular local anatomical conditions: a tendinofibrous Frohse's arcade, an "exposed" area of the radial neck (25% of cases according to Spinner), local deformations such as lymphomas [47, 53] or ganglia [54], arthroplasty [55], fractures [56], and fibrotic triceps [57].

Discussions

At the Clinica Ortopedica dell'Università di Modena the clinical and therapeutic interest in PIN tunnel syndromes dates back more than 30 years [13,16].

From our experience with lateral epicondylar pathology, we find it useful to analyze the current pathogenetic and therapeutic problems in diagnosis of PIN tunnel syndromes.

Lateral epicondylalgia must be considered a syndrome without a definite cause and whose pathogenesis remains obscure [34].

It can follow an isolated trauma or repeated microtrauma inflicted during athletic or occupational activity. Functional overloading causes pathological changes in all structures that make up the external compartment. Three types of lesions, either alone or combined, can cause lateral epicondylalgia:
1. insertional pathology;
2. radio-humeral joint disease;
3. PIN compression syndromes.

Insertional pathology is the most frequent cause of lateral epicondylalgia. Around the sick osteotendinous junction many anatomical structures are involved and often affected, giving the primary pathology peculiar clinical and pathological aspects [58]. These kind of events can explain lateral epicondylalgia pathogenesis. If the beginning pathology affects the osteotendinous structures, it may subsequently involve both the radio-humeral joint and the PIN.

At that point the clinical presentation becomes confused, and a superficial clinical evaluation is unlikely to reveal all the various pathological aspects. This is a frequent situation in lateral epicondylalgia, where the insertional pathology can be the sufficient condition for the development of nerve tunnel syndromes. This is true firstly because of the relationship between the tendinous arcade that forms the proximal insertion of the extensor carpi radialis brevis and the PIN, and secondly because of the role of the supinator brevis muscle in the external compartment.

The extensor carpi radialis brevis muscle inserts on the lateral epicondyle and has a thick fibrous lamina that inserts on the joint capsule and the annular ligament. The PIN is connected to this insertional arcade. Our observations of both living patients and cadavers show how this thick fibrous lamina tenses up in fully forearm supination, and then relaxes in pronation. The nerve is compressed in supination, and the resulting damage may be increased by the presence of fibrotic changes causing hardening and retraction of the tendinous lamina. The extensor carpi radialis brevis is not assisted by the extensor

carpi radialis longus during contraction in a flexed elbow with supinated forearm and extended wrist. The supinator brevis muscle bears the entire responsibility of forearm supination, and is thus overworked in manual work requiring repeated forearm supination against resistance. The nearby muscles do not help supination while the elbow is extended, if it is flexed yet; supination is powered by the contraction of the biceps and the supinator muscles. Pronation, however, is carried out by the pronator teres and helped by wrist flexors, particularly the flexor carpi ulnaris muscle, through the entire range of elbow flexion and extension. The supinator brevis muscle is therefore overworked in the functional positions of the upper limb.

Consequently we believe that insertional syndromes are frequent, and they could be the main pathogenetic factor in all types of lateral epicondylalgia whose symptoms are determined by nerve tunnel syndromes The superficial head of the supinator brevis muscle inserts on the lateral epicondyle, the capsule, and the radial collateral ligament, and has a direct relationship with the PIN (Fig. 6). As result, osteotendinous pathology of the supinator brevis can eventually provoke neurological musculotendinous, and joint disease. In these cases, lateral epicondylalgia is often resistant to standard medical and physical therapy and

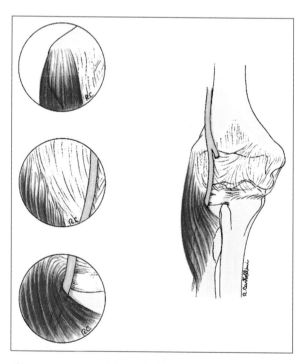

Fig. 6. The superficial head of the supinator muscle is inserted on the lateral epicondyle, the capsula and the lateral collateral ligaments are in direct contact with the PIN

must therefore be subjected to surgery, which should aim to treat the osteotendinous, osteoarticular, and neurological pathologies all at once.

Surgical intervention consists of isolating and freeing the portion of the radial nerve inside the radial tunnel. Exploration can be done through either a parallel or a zigzag incision [29]. Either a posterior or an antero-lateral approach can be used to expose the radial nerve and the Frohse's arcade [30]. The posterior approach aims at reaching the nerve by passing through the extensor carpi radialis brevis anteriorly, behind the extensor digitorum communis [29]; the nerve can also be reached by passing through the extensor carpi radialis longus and brevis. Such an incision can be lengthened proximally in case of possible lateral epicondylar muscle detachment [22, 30, 34, 38]. The antero-lateral approach requires a rectilinear, zigzag, or S-shaped incision made distally at the bend of the elbow and medially at the brachioradialis. The advantage of this approach consists of isolating the nerve proximally, and therefore hastening mobilization. This approach, however, implies the isolation of numerous intramuscular neurovascular bundles along the course of the nerve and it leaves a prominent scar. The incision in the arcade of the extensor radialis brevis muscle is transverse, while the section of Frohse's Arcade is longitudinal and parallel to the nerve. In this operation we have used the following procedure for over 20 years:

1. anesthesia (local or general) without curarization;
2. limb ischemia with a tourniquet;
3. 5 cm lateral incision starting at the lateral epicondyle and heading distally toward the radial styloid process (Fig. 7);
4. isolation of the lateral cutaneous nerve of the forearm in the subcutaneous tissue above the antibrachial fascia (Fig. 8);

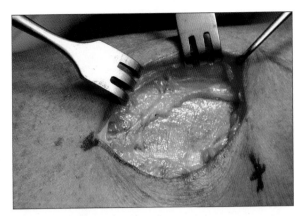

Fig. 8. The lateral cutaneous nerve is isolated in the subcutaneous tissue

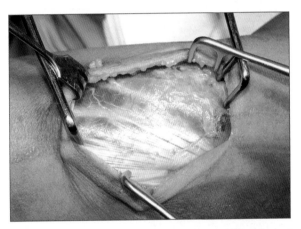

Fig. 9. The space between the extensor carpi brevis and longus is identified

5. recognition of the passage between the extensor carpi radialis longus and brevis muscles (Fig. 9);
6. singling out of the two terminal branches (sensory and motor one) of the radial nerve, then isolation of the nervous branch that innervates the extensor carpi radialis brevis;
7. recognition of the fibrous tendinous arcade of the extensor carpi radialis brevis and its section or detachment from the lateral epicondyle (Fig. 10);
8. singling out of the Frohse's arcade, of the PIN, and the anterior recurrent vein and artery of the elbow (Fig. 11);
9. section of the fibrous arcade of the supinator brevis and possible detachment of the supinator from the lateral epicondyle. This allows the exploration of the humero-radial joint (Fig. 12);
10. neurolysis of the PIN thanks to optics;

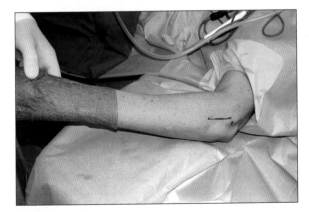

Fig. 7. Lateral skin incision

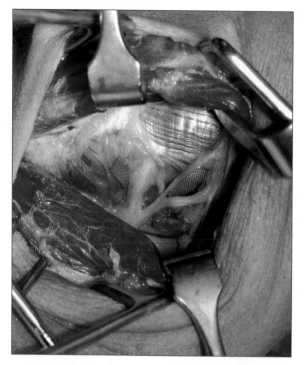

Fig. 10. The branches of the radial nerve are identified

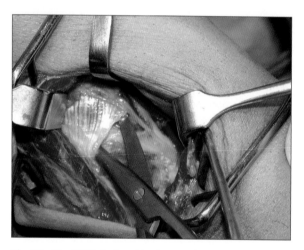

Fig. 11. The PIN is isolated in the arcade

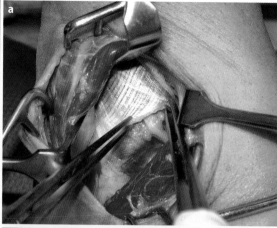

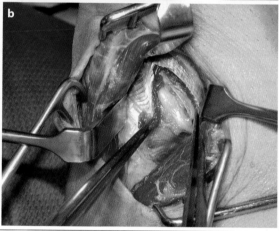

Fig. 12 a, b. The section of the arcade is performed and the neurolysis of the nerve can be done

Internal Compartment Pathology: Ulnar Nerve Tunnel Syndrome

Many studies dedicated to ulnar nerve tunnel syndrome over the last 50 years [59-61] have given us a thorough knowledge of its physio-pathogenetic and clinical aspects. Starting from the first observations of Panas (1878) and Andrae (1889), both foreign [62-71] and Italian [16, 28, 72, 73] physicians have described the different pathological and clinical aspects as well as the surgical treatment [62, 65, 66, 74-89]. Nevertheless, there are still some unresolved clinical and surgical problems. The differential diagnosis can be difficult: C8-T1 spinal compression, primary lower trunk compression and the secondary medial trunk at the interscalenic and costo-clavicular passage form a remarkable range of similar pathologies [90-99].

Surgical neurolysis is unanimously considered the fittest treatment, but the choice of method is still controversial.

The Cubital Tunnel

The ulnar nerve passes from the posterior portion of the arm to the medial portion of the forearm inside the cubital tunnel, an osteofibrous canal where true kinetic anatomy is achieved [64, 100-102], allowing the nerve to change its position according to the different movements of the elbow [103].

The osteofibrous tunnel carrying the ulnar nerve is split into two anatomical parts with different functional characteristics (Fig. 13).

The proximal portion is a true triangular osteofibrous canal bordered by:
- the posterior surface of the epitrochlea, on the front;
- the medial surface of olecranon, on the back;
- a thick fibrous bundle called the epitrochlear-olecranon ligament.

This ligament, which is transversely tensed from the epitrochlea to the olecranon, is a rudimentary epitrochleo-ulnar muscle that is present in many mammals, where it is categorized as a regressive anomaly (Gruber's muscle). In the proximal tract of the cubital tunnel, the nerve is surrounded by loose cellular tissue and accompanied by the posterior recurrent ulnar artery. A small serous bursa allows the nerve to slide over the posterior surface of the epitrochlea, thus avoiding traction or compression during elbow movement.

In the distal portion of the tunnel [104] the nerve emerges from the elbow region and it runs down the forearm. This portion of the tunnel is an osteofibrous opening whose floor is formed by the olecranon and the ulnar collateral ligament; the roof is the fibrous arcade that joins the two heads of the flexor carpi ulnaris, both inserted on the epitrochlea and olecranon (Fig. 14). Anglo-Saxon physicians call this

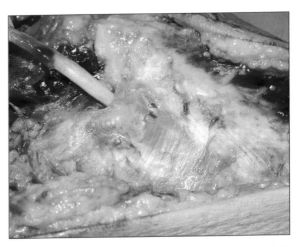

Fig. 14. The ulnar nerve in the arcade of the flexor carpi ulnaris

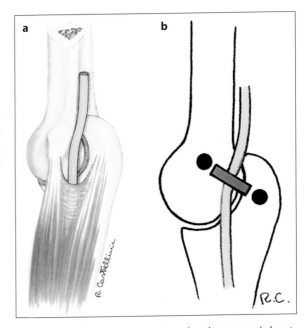

Fig. 15 a, b. During the extension the ulnar nerve is located centrally in the groove under the arcade of Osborne

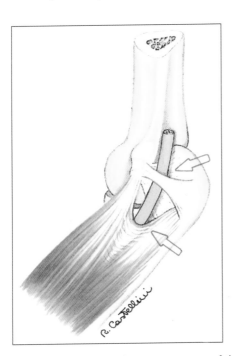

Fig. 13. The drawing shows the two segments of the cubital tunnel (the epitrochlear-olecranon ligament and the arcade of the flexor carpi ulnaris) where the ulnar nerve compression is possible

fibrous arcade, which becomes the epitrochlear-olecranon ligament, Osborne's arcade, after the author who discovered its pathogenicity and coined the term "cubital tunnel syndrome". Osborne [65, 66] describes the structure of this fibrous membrane, pointing out the potential harmfulness of the transversal fibers that close the opening of the canal, since the position of the ulnar nerve varies during elbow flexion and extension. Mansat [64] described the dynamic anatomy of the ulnar nerve in elbow flexion (Fig. 15). During these movements the nerve tightens and lengthens about 5 mm for every 45° of flexion; it also shifts toward the antero-medial portion of the groove and tends to dislocate anteriorly (Fig. 16). This shift is possible in the proximal part near the epitrochlear-olecranon groove, but it becomes critical in the distal part near the cubital tunnel. In fact, the two heads of the flexor carpi ulnaris that insert on the epitrochlea and the olecranon move apart, putting stress on the fibrous arcade that joins them [64-66, 71]. The epitrochlear head then compresses and hooks the ulnar nerve. This harmful mechanism is powered by the decrease in height (about 2.5 mm) and volume of the cubital tunnel, which provokes three- to six-fold increase in the intraneural head of the flexor carpi ulnaris pressure. These observations indicate that true primary ulnar

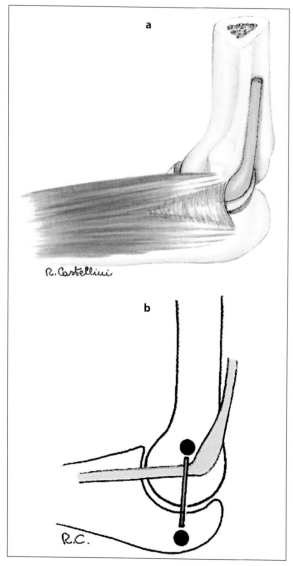

Fig. 16 a, b. During the flexion the nerve tends to dislocate anteriorly, coming in contact with the epitroclear head of the flexor carpi ulnaris

nerve tunnel syndrome occurs near the arcade of the flexor carpi ulnaris. In this area, as a matter of fact, even under normal conditions the nerve is subjected to compression, strain, and intraneural hemodynamic changes during elbow flexion. The whole can lead to neuropathy with peri- and intraneural fibrosis. Elbow flexion can also be used as a clinical test (cubital maneuver). In nerve compression pathologies occurring in the arcade of the flexor carpi ulnaris, the simple bending of the elbow is able to bring on paresis in the hand regions innervated by ulnar nerve. This maneuver can be made easier by the complete abduction of the shoulder and hyperextension of the wrist, as to pull the nerve taut. Compression pathology of the ulnar nerve in the internal compartment of the elbow can occur in two sites: (1) the epitrochlear-olecranon groove, and (2) the fibrous arcade of the flexor carpi ulnaris.

The epitrochlear-olecranon groove is predisposed to this pathology because of congenital and/or acquired factors. First, in this area the nerve is free and unsheathed by loose, well-vascularized cellular tissue [105]. Secondarily, in many cases the looseness of the epitrochlear-olecranon bundle allows the nerve to dislocate in front of the epitrochlea [67]. The commonest congenital factors capable of changing this space are constitutional cubital valgus deformity, epitrochlear-olecranon ligament hypertrophy, epitrochlear and anconeus muscle persistence, and congenital overlooseness of the ligament.

Acquired factors that can provoke the onset of ulnar neuropathy are traumatic and degenerative lesions that cause valgus deformity in the elbow as well as the formation of bone spurs in the groove. Both articular sensorial diseases (especially in rheumatoid arthritis) and local disease with reactive bursitis can occupy the epitrochlear-olecranon space and cause nerve compression. Yet the most likely causing compression structure in overwork syndromes of the internal compartment is surely [43, 65, 66] the arcade of the flexor carpi ulnaris. The specific etiology is caused by repeated occupational or athletic movements that produce hypertrophy of the flexor carpi ulnaris and the thickening of the proximal insertional arcade, resulting in chronic compression of the ulnar nerve. Even though the arthritic changes in the humero-cubital joint do not cause compression in the groove, they may encourage primary neuropathy in the flexor carpi ulnaris since they limit the movement of the nerve during elbow flexion and extension. This leads Allieu [43] to declare that the elderly patient's hand made thin by interosseous muscle hypotrophy is partially a result of compression pathology of the ulnar nerve, which over time is exacerbated by arthritis and repeated microtrauma.

Clinical Diagnosis

Clinically, the syndrome presents sensory and motor deficit of the ulnar nerve [106, 107]. McGowan [86] distinguishes three successive phases. The first is characterized by subjective sensory deficit with episodic paresis, often in the little finger. Slight hypoesthesia may be present. In the second phase the paresis becomes painful, the hypoesthesia is more severe, and an initial muscular deficit appears with mild hypotrophy of the hypothenar and interosseous muscles.

Amyotrophy of the first interosseous space is often the first sign [43].

The patient shows a weakened grip, especially between the thumb and forefinger (first-degree Froment sign). In the third phase the sensory and motor deficits are more significant. The clinical manifestation becomes typical and it collects all signs of ulnar nerve paresis in the hand [108]. Marked hyposthenia is accompanied by muscular deficits and either hypotrophy or atrophy. Nevertheless, the "ulnar hand" is inconstant, often mild compared to traumatic nervous lesions. Local signs may be revealed, such as the search for the ulnar pain focal point through palpation or percussion at the cubital tunnel; the positivity of the cubital maneuver (awakening of pain during passive elbow flexion) is similar to the Phalen test used for carpal tunnel syndrome [109]. The complementary examinations are based chiefly on EMG [57, 110-114]: it shows not only the neurogenic harm to the intrinsic hand muscles (innervated by ulnar nerve), but also the decrease in conduction time, which can help localize the compression site. It should be pointed out that, in case of primary pathology, the decrease in conduction time may become evident after stress tests of the flexor carpi ulnaris. Both routine and tangential X-rays can show possible epitrochlear-olecranon groove changes. MRI may provide useful information on the movement of the nerve and its relationship with the nearby tissues in different degrees of elbow flexion [114, 115]. Ultrasound can sometimes be helpful [116-118].

The differential diagnosis should be made with other possible sites of nerve compression in the upper limb. The spinal character of C8-T1 compression and irritative pathologies in cervicobrachialgia as well as the typical peripheral motor character of ulnar nerve compression in Guyon's canal allow easy differentiation of these pathologies from nerve compression in the elbow. The differential diagnosis with the outlet syndrome is more difficult. The following clinical observations make this diagnosis easier:

1. Compression syndrome of the ulnar nerve in the elbow is more common in males [100] and in those who suffer repeated microtrauma in athletic [119, 120] or occupational activity [121-123]. Outlet syndrome is more common in females who exhibit hyperkyphosis during shoulder adduction. Painful subacromial pathology may also be present.

2. In the ulnar nerve compression, hand paresis can be evoked by passive elbow flexion [124]. In the outlet syndrome, however, it can be brought on by upper limb abduction and dynamic tests that modify the costo-ciavicular and interscalenic spaces (Adson, Wright, etc.).

3. In elbow syndromes the paresis primarily affects the hand, while in the outlet syndrome the distribution of the medial cutaneous nerve of the forearm is also affected (Fig. 17).

4. Tinel's sign [112, 125] is present at the proximal insertion of the flexor carpi ulnaris in elbow syndromes, in the supra- or subclavicular region in the outlet syndrome.

5. Sensory and motor deficits are typical of the ulnar nerve in elbow compression syndromes: intrinsic hand muscles show deficits, while the

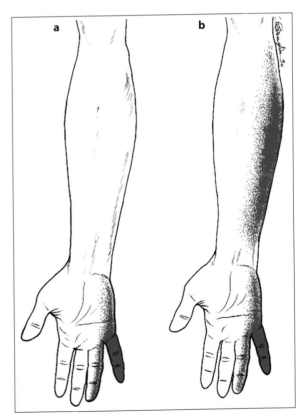

Fig. 17. The drawing shows the distribution of the paresis in the (**a**) tunnel syndromes of the ulnar nerve and in the (**b**) out-let syndrome

flexor carpi ulnaris and the flexor profundus of the little finger are rarely affected. In costo-clavicular syndromes, however, there is a sensory-motor deficit in the entire C8-T1 distribution.

6. In the diagnosis of compression neuropathy of the elbow, EMG is the most indicative exam, while in costo-clavicular compression syndrome the EMG can be confirmed with hemodynamic exams (Doppler, arteriogram).

Treatment

The primary stages of nerve tunnel syndrome (Mc-Gowan's phase 1) can be treated conservatively. Reducing manual work, the use of a brace, and local and general medical treatment can slow down the evolution of the disease. Surgical treatment is indicated in the subsequent stages, however, due to the clinical and instrumental evidence of nervous harm (phases 2 and 3).

Treatment should have two main goals:
1. nerve decompression;
2. improvement of peri- and intraneural circulatory conditions.

Many different techniques have been proposed to achieve these aims in the past 70 years, since Platt [67] described the nerve anteposition technique. All authors, however, tend to emphasize the significance of the following three stages of surgery: the section of the epitrochlear-olecranon ligament, the section of the arcade of the flexor carpi ulnaris, and finally the lateral neurolysis with epinerviotomy. The proposed techniques can be divided into three groups:
1. techniques including only the above three stages [126-129];
2. techniques adding anteposition of the nerve [104, 130, 131];
3. techniques adding medial epicondylectomy [77, 82, 83, 132-135].

Foster [79], Lugnegard [136], and Adelaar [137] compared the studies in which these methods were used, concluding that the results are very lightly influenced by the choice of technique. Recently, a new arthroscopic approach has been proposed with positive results [138-140].

In the light of our experience, we do not believe that a standard surgical technique can be identified [141, 142]. We do not consider anteposition to be primary in all cases [61]. The essential elements are the section of both the arcade of the flexor carpi ulnaris and the epitrochlear-olecranal ligament in order to check the condition of both the nerve and the perinervous tissue in the space behind the epitrochlea. Therefore, if there are no congenital or acquired malformations of the epitrochlear-olecranon groove and the compression is identified at the arcade of the flexor carpi ulnaris, the following procedure should be followed:

– section of the arcade of the flexor carpi ulnaris, which should be wide and lengthened distally (Fig. 18). Care must be taken not to injure it at the collateral nervous branch, headed for the muscle that detaches from the posterior wall of the nerve and is therefore protected by the head of the muscle inserting on the olecranon;
– section of the epitrochlear-olecranon ligament;
– anterior longitudinal epinerviotomy with the aid of optic magnification, taking care not to cut off the arterial and venous epineurial circulation. It is often necessary to perform the epinerviotomy near the arcade of the flexor carpi ulnaris, where the nerve compression can be observed, rather than in the epitrochlear-olecranon groove.

Anteposition is necessary in cases of cubitus valgus, bone spurs inside the groove, inability of the groove to hold the nerve which tends to dislocate during elbow flexion, or further surgery to treat chronic neuropathy [143-146]. Moreover, anteposition must be accurately performed; the main stages are as follows:

– isolation of the nerve by opening the groove and widely sectioning the proximal (Struthers' Arcade [147, 148]) and distal (arcade of the FCU) fibrous structures;
– detachment of the nerve from the bottom of the groove while attempting to save the loose perinervous tissue that contains venous and arterial vessels;

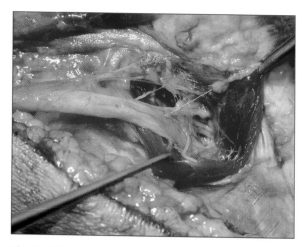

Fig. 18. The arcade of the flexor carpi ulnaris is opened and the ulnar nerve neurolysis can be done until to the first motor branch

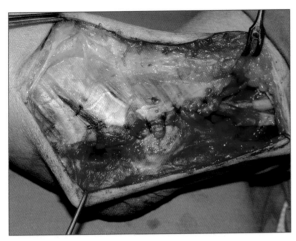

Fig. 19. The submuscular anteposition of the ulnar nerve can be performed

the PIN in addition to lateral epicondylar insertional disease, or the former plus radio-humeral joint disease. Supinator muscle (at its insertion point), PIN (in Frohse's Arcade), and the radio-humeral joint (on the radial collateral and annular ligaments) are all anatomically connected to lateral epicondylalgia; therefore, microtraumatic phlogistic pathology may explain the different tendinous, neurological, and articular manifestations of many types of lateral epicondylalgia. Surgical treatment should be reserved to forms with clinical signs of peripheral nerve damage, resistant to standard therapy. A lateral approach provides an anatomical route to the supinator muscle that runs between the extensor carpi longus and brevis muscles. In this way insertional, compression, and osteoarticular syndromes can all be treated simultaneously.

- insertion of the nerve in well-vascularized tissue protected by the bone surface. In order to achieve this we prefer to perform anteposition in the flexor carpi ulnaris belly (Fig. 19) rather than in the subcutaneous tissue.

The detachment of the epitrochlear head of this muscle is done at the tendinous insertion, even if some authors [77, 83] prefer to chip off a piece of bone from the epitrochlea. At the end of the operation, elbow flexion and extension should cause no compression of the muscle-covered nerve.

Conclusions

Among the painful pathologies of the elbow, tunnel syndromes with nerve compression must be generally considered a product of regional musculotendinous inflammation.

Ulnar nerve pathology in the elbow is common, although diagnosis is often difficult. In its primary phases, the arcade of the flexor carpi ulnaris is the true site of compression. Tinel's sign in the area indicates nerve damage and the EMG confirms the diagnosis. The success of surgical treatment depends on both its timeliness and the correct choice of technique, which is based on the presence of congenital or acquired malformations of the epitrochlear-olecranal groove. Whatever method is chosen, it should aim to free the nerve in the osteofibrous groove of the flexor carpi ulnaris.

Isolated pathology of the motor branch of the radial nerve in the elbow is very rare. Lateral epicondylalgia may be manifested by pathologic and clinical signs of either radial tunnel syndrome of

References

1. Cabrera JM, McCue FC 3rd (1986) Nonosseous athletic injuries of the elbow, forearm, and hand. Clin Sports Med 5:681-700
2. Izzi J, Dennison D, Noerdlinger M et al (2001) Nerve injuries of the elbow, wrist, and hand in athletes. Clin Sports Med 20:203-217
3. Plancher KD, Peterson RK, Steichen JB (1996) Compressive neuropathies and tendinopathies in the athletic elbow and wrist. Clin Sports Med 15:331-371
4. Wang FC, Crielaard JM (2001) Entrapment neuropathies in sports medicine. Rev Med Liege 56:382-390
5. Akuthota V, Plastaras C, Lindberg K et al (2005) The effect of long-distance bicycling on ulnar and median nerves: An electrophysiologic evaluation of cyclist palsy. Am J Sports Med 33:1224-1230
6. Boninger ML, Robertson RN, Wolff M, Cooper RA (1996) Upper limb nerve entrapments in elite wheelchair racers. Am J Phys Med Rehabil 75:170-176
7. Lawrence T, Mobbs P, Fortems Y, Stanley JK (1995) Radial tunnel syndrome: A retrospective review of 30 decompressions of the radial nerve. J Hand Surg Br 20:454-459
8. Roquelaure Y, Raimbeau G, Dano C et al (2000) Occupational risk factors for radial tunnel syndrome in industrial workers. Scand J Work Environ Health 26:507-513
9. Roquelaure Y, Raimbeau G, Saint-Cast Y et al (2003) Occupational risk factors for radial tunnel syndrome in factory workers. Chir Main 22:293-298
10. Allieu Y, Amara B (2002) Nerve entrapment syndrome of the elbow and forearm. Ann Chir Plast Esthet 47(1):36-46
11. Heyse-Moore GH (1983) Resistant tennis elbow. J Hand Surg Br 9:64-66
12. Sunderland S (1968) Nerves and nerve injuries. Livingstone, London
13. Bedeschi P Celli L (1979) Lesioni dei nervi periferici da sport. GIOT 5:323-329
14. Frignani R, Marchetti N (1967) Sulla sindrome dissociata del nervo radiale nella doccia di torsione del gomito. Riv Chir Mano 6:38-41

15. Laus S, Galli G (1976) Paralisi dissociate del nervo radiale da compressione nel muscolo breve supinatore. Riv Chir Mano 4:166-170

16. Luppino T, Celli L, Vaccari A (1971) Ulteriore contributo alla conoscenza delle sindromi compressive del nervo radiale alla doccia di torsione del gomito. Boil Soc Med Chir di Modena 71

17. Marchetti N et al (1978) Sindromi nervose canalicolari degli arti ad eziologia non traumatica Liviana Ed, Padova

18. Capener N (1966) The vulnerability of the posterior interosseous nerve of the forearm. J Bone Joint Surg Br 48:770

19. Kopell HP, Thompson WAL (1963) Peripheral entrapment neuropathies. Williams and Wilkins Company, Baltimore

20. Lister GD, Belsole RB, Kleinert HE (1979) The radial tunnel syndrome. J Hand Surg 4:52-59

21. Nirschl RP, Petfrone FA (1979) Tennis elbow: The surgical treatment of lateral epicondylitis. Bone Jont Surg Am 61:832-839

22. Roles NC, Maudsley RH (1972) Radial tunnel syndrome. Resistant tennis elbow as a nerve entrapment. J Bone Joint Surg Br 54:499-508

23. Sponseller PD, Engber WD (1983) Double entrapment radial tunnel syndrome. J Hand Surg 8:420-423

24. Werner C (1979) Lateral elbow pain and posterior interosseous nerve entrapment. Acta Orthop Scand 174:1

25. Riffaud L, Morandi X, Godey B et al (1999) Anatomic bases for the compression and neurolysis of the deep branch of the radial nerve. In: The radial tunnel. Surg Radiol Anat 21:229-233

26. Kalb K, Gruber P, Landsleitner B (1999) Compression syndrome of the radial nerve in the area of the supinator groove. Experiences with 110 patients. Handchir Mikrochir Plast Chir 31:303-310

27. Comtet JJ, Chambaud D, Genety J (1976) La compression de la branche postérieur du nerf radiai. Nouv Presse Med 5:1111-1114

28. Comtet JJ, Lalain Moyen B, Genety J et al (1985) Les epicondylalgies avec compression de la branche postérieure du nerf radial. Rev Chir Orthop 71:89-93

29. Eversmann WW (1988) Entrapment and compression neuropathies. In: Green DP (ed) Operative hand surgery. Churchill Livingstone

30. Palazzi S, Palazzi C, Raimondi P, Aramburo F (1983) Syndromes compressifs du nerf radiai In: Syndrome canalaire du membre supérieur. Monographie du GEM Expansion Scientifique Francaise, Paris, pp 41-54

31. Sharrad WJW (1966) Posterior interosseous neuritis. J Bone Joint Surg Br 48:777-780

32. Erak S, Day R, Wang A (2004) The role of supinator in the pathogenesis of chronic lateral elbow pain: A biomechanical study. J Hand Surg Br 29:461-464

33. Narakas A (1974) Epicondylite et nerf radial. Med Hyg 22:2067

34. Narakas A (1979) Le traitement chirurgical de l'epicondylalgie. In: Coude et médecine de rééducation. Masson, pp 129-139

35. Spinner M (1972) The radial nerve In: Injuries to the major branches of peripheral nerves of forearm.WB Saunders, Philadelphia

36. Mosser JJ, Deflassieux M, Aupecle P, Piganiol G (1978) Compression de la branche postérieure du nerf radiai par un tumeur benigne de la region du coude. J Chir 115:515-522

37. Spinner M (1968) The arcade of Frohse and its relationship to posterior interosseous nerve paralysis. J Bone Joint Surg Br 50:809-812

38. Frohse F, Frankel M (1908) Die Muskeln des menschlichen Armes. Iena Fischer

39. Sarhadi NS, Korday SN, Bainbridge LC (1999) Radial tunnel syndrome: Diagnosis and management. J Hand Surg Br 24:139-140

40. Bak K, Torholm C (1996) Supinator syndrome: Entrapment of the posterior interosseous nerve. Ugeskr Laeger 158:2275

41. Vollinger M, Partecke BD (1998) The supinator syndrome. Handchir Mikrochir Plast Chir 30:103-108

42. Loh YC, Lam WL, Stanley JK, Soames RW (2004) A new clinical test for radial tunnel syndrome – The Rule-of-Nine test: A cadaveric study. J Orthop Surg (Hong Kong) 12:83-86

43. Allieu Y (1976) Compressions nerveuses non traumatiques du membre supérieur Cahiers d'enseignement de la SOFCOT Conferences d'enseignemen sous la direction di J Duparc Expansion Scientifique Francaise Paris

44. Mansat M (1986) Syndromes canalaires et des defilés Enc Med Chir Paris, 15005, A10-A11

45. Serre H, Simon L, Claustre I (1966) L'origine canaliculaire de certains syndromes du membre supérieur. Rev Rhum 33:231-246

46. Ritts GD, Wood MB, Linscheid RL (1987) Radial tunnel syndrome A ten-year surgical experience. Clin Orthop Rei Res 219:201-205

47. Moss SH, Switzer HE (1983) Radial tunnel syndrome: A spectrum of clinical presentations. J Hand Surg 8:414-420

48. Howard FM (1980) Controversies in nerve entrapment syndromes in the forearm and wrist In: Controversies in hand surgery, pp 110-115

49. Fairbank SR, Corelett RJ (2002) The role of the extensor digitorum communis muscle in lateral epicondylitis. J Hand Surg Br 27:405-409

50. Albrecht S, Cordis R, Kleihues H, Noack W (1997) Pathoanatomic findings in radiohumeral epicondylopathy. A combined anatomic and electromyographic study. Arch Orthop Trauma Surg 116:157-163

51. Milcan A, Ozge A, Sahin G et al (2004) The role of electrophysiologic tests in the early diagnosis of posterior interosseous neuropathy in patients thought to have lateral epicondylitis. Acta Orthop Traumatol Turc 38:326-329

52. Rosenberg ZS, Bencardino J, Beltran J (1997) MR features of nerve disorders at the elbow. Magn Reson Imaging Clin N Am 5:545-565

53. Malcapi C, Grassi G (1975) I lipomi profondi degli arti e la sindrome di compressione del nervo radiale da lipoma dell'avambraccio. Mi Ortop 26:551-570

54. Ferrini L (1974) Paralisi dissociata parziale del nervo radiale al gomito da ganglio artrogeno. Chir Org Mov 63:153-157

55. Zook J, Ward WG Sr (2001) Intraosseous radial nerve entrapment complicating total elbow revision. J Arthroplasty 16:919-922

56. Rommens PM, Blum J, Runkel M (1998) Retrograde nailing of humeral shaft fractures. Clin Orthop Relat Res 350:26-39

57. Midroni G, Moulton R (2001) Radial entrapment neuropathy due to chronic injection-induced triceps fibrosis. Muscle Nerve 24:134-137

58. Perugia L, Postacchini F, Ippolito E (1981) Tendinopatia inserzionale degli estensori della mano (epicondilite-"ten-

nis elbow") Tendinopatia inserzionale dei flessori della mano e pronatori dell'avambraccio (epitrocleite-epicondilite mediale) In: I tendini, biologia/patologia/clinica Masson Italia Ed, Milano

59. Bartels RH, Menovsky T, Van Overbeeke JJ, Verhagen WI (1998) Surgical management of ulnar nerve compression at the elbow: An analysis of the literature. J Neurosurg 89:722-727

60. Bartels RH (2001) History of the surgical treatment of ulnar nerve compression at the elbow. Neurosurgery 49:391-399, discussion 399-400

61. Nathan PA, Istvan JA, Meadows KD (2005) Intermediate and long-term outcomes following simple decompression of the ulnar nerve at the elbow. Chir Main 24:29-34

62. Durandeau A, Chavoix JB, Geneste R (1986) A propos de 91 compressions du nerfcubital au niveau du coude. Rev Chir Orthop 2:240-242

63. Feindel W, Stratford J (1958) Cubital tunnel compression in tardy uinar palsy. Can Med Ass 78:351

64. Mansat M, Guiraud B, Cjanet M, Testut MF (1978) Le tunnel cubital et les paralysies cubitales idiopathiques au niveau du coude. Pathologie des nerfs périphériques P Fabre

65. Osborne O (1970) Compression neuritis of the ulnar nerve at the elbow. The Hand 2:10-13

66. Osborne O (1957) The surgical treatment of tardy ulnar neuritis. J Bone Joint Surg Br 39:1-82

67. Platt H (1926) The pathogenesis and treatment of traumatic neuritis of the ulnar nerve in postcondylar groove. Br J Surg 13:409-413

68. Roullet J (1983) Syndrome compressif du nerf cubital au coude. Monografia GEM, pp 74-95

69. Sunderland S (1968) Nerves and nerve injuries. Livingstone, London

70. Vanderpool DW, Chalmers J, Lamb DW, Whiston TB (1968) Peripheral compression lesions of the ulnar nerve. J Bone Joint Surg Br 50:792-803

71. Wadsworth TO (1977) The external compression syndrome of the ulnar nerve at the cubital tunnel. Clin Orthop 124:189-204

72. Altissimi M, Pecorelli F, Pimpinelli G (1986) La compressione del nervo ulnare al gomito. GIOT 12:413-418

73. Calandriello B, Colì O, Pedemonte P (1960) Patologia del nervo ulnare alla doccia epitrocleare. Arc Puttl, pp 120-125

74. Adelaar RS, Foster WC, Mc Dowel C (1984) The treatment of the cubital tunnel syndrome. J Hand Surg Am 9:90-95

75. Benoit BG, Preston DN, Atack DM, Da Silva MD (1987) Neurolysis combined with the application of a silastic envelope for ulnar nerve entrapment at the elbow. Neurosurg 20:594-598

76. Chaise F, Bouchet T, Sedel L, Witvoet J (1983) Résultats de la liberation chirurgicale du nerf cubitale dans les syndromes du défilé retro-epitrochléen. J Chir 120:251-255

77. Craven PR, Green DP (1980) Cubital tunnel syndrome. Treatment by medial epicondylectomy. J Bone Joint Surg Am 62:986-989

78. Dimond ML, Lister GD (1985) Cubital tunnel syndrome treated by long-arm splintage. J Hand Surg Am 10:430

79. Foster RJ, Edshage MD (1981) Factors related to the outcome of surgically managed compressive ulnar neuropathy at the elbow level. Hand Surg 6:181-192

80. Froimson AI, Zahrawi MD (1980) Treatment of compression neuropathy of the ulnar nerve at the elbow by epicondylectomy and neurolysis. J Hand Surg 5:391-395

81. Kamhin M, Ganel A, Rosenberg B, Engel J (1980) Anterior transposition of the ulnar nerve. Acta Orthop Scand 51:475-478

82. Jones RE, Gauntt C (1979) Medial epicondylectomy for ulnar nerve compression syndrome at the elbow. Clin Orthop 139:174-178

83. King T, Morgan FP (1959) Late results of removing the medial humeral epicondyle for traumatic ulnar neuritis. J Bone Joint Surg Br 41:51-55

84. Learmonth JK (1942) A technique for transplanting the ulnar nerve. Surg Gynec Obstet 75:792-793

85. Macnicol MF (1979) The results of operation for ulnar neuritis. J Bone Joint Surg Br 61:159-164

86. McGowan AJ (1950) The results of transposition of the ulnar nerve for traumatic neuritis. J Bone Joint Surg Br 32:293-301

87. Ogata K, Manske PR, Lesker PA (1985) The effects of surgical dissection on regional bloodflow to the ulnar nerve in the cubital tunnel. Clin Orthop 193:195-198

88. Payan I (1970) Anterior transposition of the ulnar nerve: An electrophysiological study. J Neurol Neurosurg 33:157-165

89. San Martin S, Bueno C, Montes C et al (2000) The most significative parameters for the diagnosis of focal neuropathy of the cubital nerve in the elbow. Rev Neurol 31:720-723

90. Acosta JA, Hoffman SN, Raynor EM et al (2003) Ulnar neuropathy in the forearm: A possible complication of diabetes mellitus. Muscle Nerve 28:40-45

91. Aszmann OC, Kress KM, Dellon AL (2000) Results of decompression of peripheral nerves in diabetics: A prospective, blinded study. Plast Reconstr Surg 106:816-822

92. Fikry T, Saidi H, Madhar M et al (2004) Cubital tunnel syndrome and heterotopic ossification. Eight case reports. Chir Main 23:109-113

93. Hager D, Schoffl H (2001) Traumatically-induced dislocation of the ulnar nerve. Unfallchirurg 104:1186-1188

94. Landau ME, Barner KC, Campbell WW (2005) Effect of body mass index on ulnar nerve conduction velocity, ulnar neuropathy at the elbow, and carpal tunnel syndrome. Muscle Nerve 32:360-363

95. Ming Chan K, Thompson S, Amirjani N et al (2003) Compression of the ulnar nerve at the elbow by an intraneural ganglion. J Clin Neurosci 10:245-248

96. Mouthon L, Halimi C, Muller GP et al (2000) Systemic scleroderma associated with bilateral ulnar nerve entrapment at the elbow. Rheumatology (Oxford) 39:682-683

97. Richardson JK, Jamieson SC (2004) Cigarette smoking and ulnar mononeuropathy at the elbow. Am J Phys Med Rehabil 83:730-734

98. Wang HC, Tsai MD (1996) Compressive ulnar neuropathy in the proximal forearm caused by a gouty tophus. Muscle Nerve 19:525-527

99. Zemel NP (2000) Ulnar neuropathy with and without elbow instability. Hand Clin 16:487-495

100. Contreras MG, Warner MA, Charbonneau WJ, Cahill DR (0000) Anatomy of the ulnar nerve at the elbow: Potential relationship of acute ulnar neuropathy to gender differences. Clin Anat 11:372-378

101. Gonzalez MH, Lotfi P, Bendre A et al (2001) The ulnar nerve at the elbow and its local branching: An anatomic study. J Hand Surg Br 26:142-144

102. Oswald TA (1998) Anatomic considerations in evaluation of the proximal ulnar nerve. Phys Med Rehabil Clin N Am 9:777-794

103. Green JR Jr, Rayan GM (1999) The cubital tunnel: Anatomic, histologic, and biomechanical study. J Shoulder Elbow Surg 8:466-470

104. Degeorges R, Masquelet AC (2002) The cubital tunnel: Anatomical study of its distal part. Surg Radiol Anat 24:169-176

105. Testut L (1923) Anatomia umana. Utet

106. Huang JH, Samadani U, Zager EL (2004) Ulnar nerve entrapment neuropathy at the elbow: Simple decompression. Neurosurgery 55:1150-1153

107. Kalb RL (1998) Evaluation and treatment of elbow pain. Hosp Pract (Off Ed) 1533:176, 181-182, 185

108. Padua L, Aprile I, Mazza O et al (2001) Neurophysiological classification of ulnar entrapment across the elbow. Neurol Sci 22:11-16

109. Greenwald D, Moffitt M, Cooper B (1999) Effective surgical treatment of cubital tunnel syndrome based on provocative clinical testing without electrodiagnostics. Plast Reconstr Surg 104:215-218

110. Izzi J, Dennison D, Noerdlinger M et al (2001) Nerve injuries of the elbow, wrist, and hand in athletes. Clin Sports Med 20:203-217

111. Herrmann DN, Preston DC, McIntosh KA, Logigian EL (2001) Localization of ulnar neuropathy with conduction block across the elbow. Muscle Nerve 24:698-700

112. Kingery WS, Park KS, Wu PB, Date ES (1995) Electromyographic motor Tinel's sign in ulnar mononeuropathies at the elbow. Am J Phys Med Rehabil 74:419-426

113. Merlevede K, Theys P, van Hees J (2000) Diagnosis of ulnar neuropathy: A new approach. Muscle Nerve 23:478-481

114. Mobbs RJ, Rogan C, Blum P (2003) Entrapment neuropathy of the ulnar nerve by a constriction band: The role of MRI. J Clin Neurosci 10:374-375

115. Kijowski R, Tuite M, Sanford M (2005) Magnetic resonance imaging of the elbow Part II: Abnormalities of the ligaments, tendons, and nerves. Skeletal Radiol 34:1-18

116. Martinoli C, Bianchi S, Zamorani MP, Zunzunegui JL, Derchi LE (2001) Ultrasound of the elbow. Eur J Ultrasound 14:21-27

117. Backhaus M, Schmidt WA, Mellerowicz H et al (2002) Technical aspects and value of arthrosonography in rheumatologic diagnosis 4: Ultrasound of the elbow. Z Rheumatol 61:415-425

118. Park GY, Kim JM, Lee SM (2004) The ultrasonographic and electrodiagnostic findings of ulnar neuropathy at the elbow. Arch Phys Med Rehabil 85:1000-1005

119. Aoki M, Takasaki H, Muraki T et al (2005) Strain on the ulnar nerve at the elbow and wrist during throwing motion. J Bone Joint Surg Am 87:2508-2514

120. Chen FS, Rokito AS, Jobe FW (2001) Medial elbow problems in the overhead-throwing athlete. J Am Acad Orthop Surg 9:99-113

121. Amirjani N, Thompson S, Satkunam L et al (2003) The impact of ulnar nerve compression at the elbow on the hand function of heavy manual workers. Neurorehabil Neural Repair 17:118-123

122. Bonfiglioli R, Lodi V, Tabanelli S, Violante FS (1996) Entrapment of the ulnar nerve at the elbow caused by repetitive movements: Description of a clinical case. Med Lav 87:147-151

123. Descatha A, Leclerc A, Chastang JF, Roquelaure Y (2004) Study Group on Repetitive Work Incidence of ulnar nerve entrapment at the elbow in repetitive work. Scand J Work Environ Health 30:234-240

124. Rosati M, Martignoni R, Spagnolli G et al (1998) Clinical validity of the elbow flexion test for the diagnosis of ulnar nerve compression at the cubital tunnel. Acta Orthop Belg 64:366-370

125. Montagna P, Liguori R (2000) The motor tinel sign: A useful sign in entrapment neuropathy? Muscle Nerve 23:976-978

126. Bartels RH, Termeer EH, van der Wilt GJ et al (2005) Simple decompression or anterior subcutaneous transposition for ulnar neuropathy at the elbow: A cost-minimization analysis-Part 2. Neurosurgery 56:531-536, discussion 531-536

127. Bartels RH, Verhagen WI, van der Wilt GJ et al (2005) Prospective randomized controlled study comparing simple decompression versus anterior subcutaneous transposition for idiopathic neuropathy of the ulnar nerve at the elbow: Part 1. Neurosurgery 56:522-530, discussion 522-530

128. Idler RS (1996) General principles of patient evaluation and nonoperative management of cubital syndrome. Hand Clin 12:397-403

129. Luch AL (1998) Release of ulnar nerve compression at the elbow through a transverse incision. J Shoulder Elbow Surg 7:38-42

130. Loy S, Bhatia A, Asfazadourian H, Oberlin C (1997) Ulnar nerve fascicle transfer onto to the biceps muscle nerve in C5-C6 or C5-C6-C7 avulsions of the brachial plexus. Eighteen cases. Ann Chir Main Memb Super 16:275-284

131. Paternostro-Sluga T, Ciovika R, Turkof E et al (2001) Short segment stimulation of the anterior transposed ulnar nerve at the elbow. Arch Phys Med Rehabil 82:1171-1175

132. Dinh PT, Gupta R (2005) Subtotal medial epicondylectomy as a surgical option for treatment of cubital tunnel syndrome. Tech Hand Up Extrem Surg 9:52-59

133. Efstathopoulos DG, Themistocleous GS, Papagelopoulos PJ et al (2006) Outcome of partial medial epicondylectomy for cubital tunnel syndrome. Clin Orthop Relat Res 444:134-139

134. Tsujino A, Itoh Y, Hayashi K (1996) Excursion of the ulnar nerve at the elbow following epicondylectomy or transposition. J Hand Surg Br 21:255-256

135. Xarchas KC (2003) Partial medial epicondylectomy for cubital tunnel syndrome: Outcome and complications. J Shoulder Elbow Surg 12:205

136. Lugnegard H, Juhlin L, Nilsson BJ (1982) Ulnar neuropathy at the elbow treated with decompression. Scand J Plast Reconstr Surg 16:195-200

137. Adelaar RS, Foster WC, Mc Dowel C (1984) The treatment of the cubital tunnel syndrome. J Hand Surg Am 9:90-95

138. Nakao Y, Takayama S, Toyama Y (2001) Cubital tunnel release with lift-type endoscopic surgery. Hand Surg 6:199-203

139. Porcellini G, Paladini P, Campi F, Merolla G (2005) Arthroscopic neurolysis of the ulnar nerve at the elbow. Chir Organi Mov 90:191-200

140. Tsai TM, Chen IC, Majd ME, Lim BH (1999) Cubital tunnel release with endoscopic assistance: Results of a new technique. J Hand Surg Am 24:21-29

141. Kim DH, Han K, Tiel RL et al (2003) Surgical outcomes of 654 ulnar nerve lesions. J Neurosurg 98:993-1004

142. Rochet S, Obert L, Lepage D et al (2004) Should we divide Osborn's ligament during epicondylectomy and in situ decompression of the ulnar nerve? Chir Main 23:131-136

143. Bartels RH, Grotenhuis JA (2004) Anterior submuscular transposition of the ulnar nerve for post-operative focal neuropathy at the elbow. J Bone Joint Surg Br 86:998-1001

144. Caputo AE, Watson HK (2000) Subcutaneous anterior transposition of the ulnar nerve for failed decompression of cubital tunnel syndrome. J Hand Surg Am 25:544-551

145. Kleinman WB (1999) Cubital tunnel syndrome: Anterior transposition as a logical approach to complete nerve decompression. J Hand Surg Am 24:886-897

146. Matei CI, Logigian EL, Shefner JM (2004) Evaluation of patients with recurrent symptoms after ulnar nerve transposition. Muscle Nerve 30:493-496

147. De Jesus R, Dellon AL (2003) Historic origin of the "Arcade of Struthers." J Hand Surg Am 28:528-531

148. Siqueira MG, Martins RS (2005) The controversial arcade of Struthers Surg Neurol 64 1:17-20

Suggested Readings

Akuthota V, Plastaras C, Lindberg K et al (2005) The effect of long-distance bicycling on ulnar and median nerves: An electrophysiologic evaluation of cyclist palsy. Am J Sports Med 33:1224-1230

Catalano F, Di Lazzaro A, De Santis E (1980) La neuropatia del nervo ulnare alla doccia epitrocleare. Arch Putti 30:143-153

Dellon AL, Coert JH (2004) Results of the musculofascial lengthening technique for submuscular transposition of the ulnar nerve at the elbow. J Bone Joint Surg Am Am 86:169-179

Durandeau A, Chavoix JB, Geneste R (1986) A propos de 91 compressions du nerf cubital au niveau du coude. Rev Chir Orthop 2:240-242

Durandeau A, Geneste R (1988) Un syndrome canalaire rare: La paralysie du nerf interosseux postérieur A propos de 10 cas. Rev Chir Orthop 74:156-157

Fragiadakis Fg, Lamb DW (1970) An unusual cause of ulnar nerve compression. The Hand 2:14-15

Gervasio O, Gambardella G (2004) Anterior submuscular transposition of the ulnar nerve in severe cubital tunnel syndrome. Personal experience. J Neurosurg Sci 48:113-116

Harrelson JM (1975) Hypertrophy of the FUC as a cause of ulnar nerve compression in the distal part of the forearm. J Bone Joint Surg Am 57:553-555

Heyse-Moore GH (1983) Resistant tennis elbow. J Hand Surg Br 9:64-66

Jillapalli D, Bradshaw DY, Shefner JM (2003) Motor unit number estimation in the evaluation of focal conduction block. Muscle Nerve 27:676-681

Jones RE, Gauntt C (1979) Medial epicondylectomy for ulnar nerve compression syndrome at the elbow. Clin Orthop 139:174-178

Kaplan PE (1984) Posterior interosseous neuropathies: Natural history. Arch Phys Med Rehab 65:399-400

Kenesi Cl, Ficat C (1973) Traitement chirurgical de l'epicondylalgie. Rev Rhum 40:347-351

King T, Morgan FP (1959) Late results of removing the medial humeral epicondyle for traumatic ulnar neuritis. J Bone Joint Surg Br 41:51-55

Kitzinger HB, Aszmann OC, Moser VL, Frey M (2005) Significance of electroneurographic parameters in the diagnosis of chronic neuropathy of the ulnar nerve at the elbow. Handchir Mikrochir Plast Chir 37:276-281

Lawrence T, Mobbs P, Fortems Y, Stanley JK (1995) Radial tunnel syndrome. A retrospective review of 30 decompressions of the radial nerve. J Hand Surg Br 20:454-459

Luppino T, Celli L, Vaccari A (1971) Considerazioni anatomo-cliniche sulle sindromi compressive canalicolari del nervo ulnare al gomito e al polso. Boll Soc Med Chir di Modena 71:1-11

Mondelli M, Giannini F, Morana P, Rossi S (2004) Ulnar neuropathy at the elbow: Predictive value of clinical and electrophysiological measurements for surgical outcome. Electromyogr Clin Neurophysiol 44:349-356

Mulholland RC (1966) Non-traumatic progressive paralysis of the posterior interosseous nerve. J Bone Joint Surg Br 48:781-785

Nawrot P, Romanowski L, Nowakowski A (2004) History of the surgical treatment of cubital tunnel syndrome. Chir Narzadow Ruchu Ortop Pol 69:135-137

Nouhan R, Kleinert JM (1997) Ulnar nerve decompression by transposing the nerve and Z-lengthening the flexor-pronator mass: Clinical outcome. J Hand Surg Am 22:127-131

Plancher KD, Peterson RK, Steichen JB (1996) Compressive neuropathies and tendinopathies in the athletic elbow and wrist. Clin Sports Med 15:331-371

Scaraglio C, Pisu G, Bignotti B (1988) La sindrome da compressione del nervo radiale all'arcata di Frohse. Mi Ortop Traum 39:55-58

Seradge H (1997) Cubital tunnel release and medial epicondylectomy: Effect of timing of mobilization. J Hand Surg Am 22:863-866

Van Rossum I, Buruma OJS, Kampi-Iuisen, Onvlee GJ (1978) Tennis elbow-A radial tunnel syndrome? J Bone Joint Surg Br 60:197-198

Wang FC, Crielaard JM (2001) Entrapment neuropathies in sports medicine. Rev Med Liege 56:382-390

Werner CO (1979) Lateral elbow pain and posterior interosseous nerve entrapment. Acta Orthop Scand 174:1-62

Younge DH, Moise P (1994) The radial tunnel syndrome. Int Orthop 18:268-270

CHAPTER 28
Traumatic Isolated Lesions of Musculocutaneous Nerve

C. Rovesta, M.C. Marongiu, G. Bonanno, A. Celli, L. Celli

Introduction

Isolated proximal lesion of musculocutaneous nerve causes a palsy of main flexors of the elbow (biceps and brachialis anterior muscles) but brachioradialis (innervated by radial nerve), epitroclear, and epicondilar muscles are able to maintain a flexion against gravity. For this reason sometimes diagnosis is neither easy nor early [1].

Anatomy

The muscolocutaneous nerve rises from the lateral cord of the brachial plexus and is made of nerve fibers originating from C5 and C6. It pierces the coracobrachialis muscle (perforating the nerve of Casserio) after innervating and then travels distally in the interval between the biceps and the brachialis anterior muscle. It gives off motor branches to the biceps in the midarm and to the brachialis more distally. Finally, it passes through the deep fascia of the elbow and where it becomes the lateral cutaneous nerve of the forearm (Fig. 1) [2].

Anatomical anomalies of this nerve aren't rare: fibers originate from C7 in 20% of cases; in 14% it surrounds the belly of the coracobrachialis without perforating it, and in 3%-6% of the population it originates directly from the median nerve [3, 4].

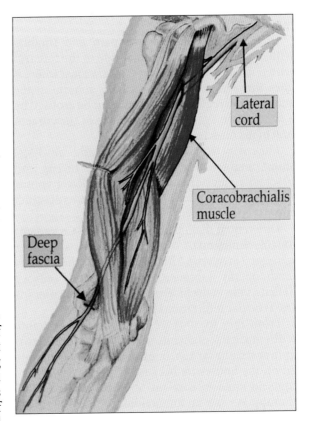

Fig. 1. Musculocutaneous nerve origins from lateral cord and passes trough coracobrachialis muscle and then runs between the biceps and brachialis anterior muscles and the terminal sensitive ramus becomes subcutaneous passing through the deep brachial fascia

Types of Lesions

In our experience and in literature, an isolated lesion of the musculocutaneous nerve can be realized by a repeated microtrauma, an indirect trauma, or a direct trauma of the nerve. These possibilities can present different problems for early and differential diagnosis and treatment [5].

Repeated Microtrauma (Nerve Tunnel Syndrome)

Hypertrophy or strong repetitive contraction of coracobrachialis muscle, acts as a "tongs mechanism," stretching the nerve which passes through it. Overuse and hypertrophy of biceps and anterior brachialis muscles can contribute to the onset of a compression syndrome [6]. The risk of compression is even higher with shoulder in abduction and retroposition because of a tense coracobrachialis muscle [7].

The clinical picture shows pain and tingling with hypoesthesia in the radial side of the forearm with positive Tinel sign over the nerve just where it goes through the coracobrachialis muscle in the subcoracoid region (Fig. 2). Pain can be aroused by a contraction against the resistance of the coracobrachialis muscle.

Muscular trophism is normal and an EMG shows slight neural damage in the biceps and brachialis anterior muscles with a slower motor and sensory conduction in Erb's point-axilla tract compared to the contralateral limb [8].

Differential diagnosis is made with C6 radiculopathy (movement of spine arouses pain, other muscles involved), long head of the biceps tendinopathy (absence of motor and sensory deficit), pain in the biceps sulcus (subsides after intra-articular infiltration) [9].

From 1983 to 2003 we observed four patients with musculocutaneous tunnel syndrome (two gymnasts, one farmer, one housewife). We operated on the housewife because of persisting symptoms in spite of rest and medical and physical therapy. We saw an anomalous course of axillary artery which pierced the coracobrachialis muscle with the musculocutaneous nerve, which appeared compressed.

A combination of neurolysis and arteriolysis led to a complete remission of pain.

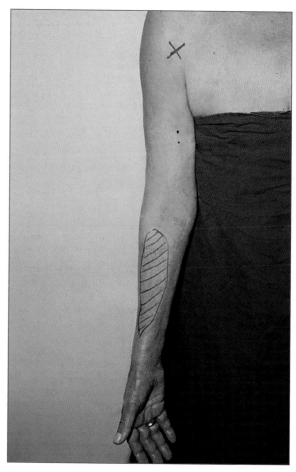

Fig. 2. In nerve tunnel syndrome at coracobrachialis level, patient presents tingling and hypoesthesia in the radial side of forearm and Tinel sign in the subcoracoid region

Indirect Trauma

The musculocutaneous nerve has its main point of attachment at its entrance into the coracobrachialis muscle, plus two others at its origin from the lateral cord and its entrance into the brachial fascia. Movements that pull these points away from each other cause traction of the nerve (for example, abduction and retroposition of the shoulder or extrarotation and retroposition of the shoulder).

The rapid and violent retroposition of the shoulder with the arm abducted and extrarotated, results in a stretching of the nerve and a tension of the coracobrachialis muscle with a possible lesion of the musculocutaneous nerve [10]. The clinical picture shows a subjective pain on the antero-lateral surface of the arm and lateral portion of the forearm with hypoesthesia, tingling, and diminished strength in flexion of the elbow.

A severe hypotrophy of the flexor muscle in anterior part of the arm is seen, but the flexion against gravity of the elbow is maintained (active brachioradialis and epitrochlear muscles) Tinel sign is positive in the subcoracoid region and EMG reveals neurologic deficiency in the biceps and brachialis anterior muscle [11].

Differential diagnosis is made with lesion of the plexus and traction of C5–C6 roots (in this situation the abduction, extrarotation, and elbow flexion is lost). If there is a rupture of the biceps tendon (proximal or distal) the muscle is retracted and there is no sensitive deficit. EMG is negative [12].

We observed ten patients (mean age 28.5 years) all with trauma in retroposition of the shoulder. Two cases had a spontaneous recovery and eight were operated. All lesions were from the origin of the nerve to its exit from the coracobrachialis muscle, with a big neuroma in continuity in four cases. We performed two neurolysis and six grafts with sural nerve.

The outcome (follow-up 8.3 years, minimum 1.8 maximum 13 years) was excellent or good in six patients (biceps M4–M5) and fair in two patients (biceps M2-M3)

Direct Trauma

Protected by the humerus and flexor muscles, the nerve can be traumatized by humeral fractures, gun shot (Fig. 3), deep glass wound, iatrogenic lesions during surgery for internal fixation of humeral fracture, and more commonly operations for anterior instability (inadvertent section of the nerve, stretching of the nerve during the transfer of the tip of the coracoid) [13, 14].

When the nerve perforates the coracobrachialis muscle proximally (distance from the coracoid apex to the entrance of the nerve minor of 5 cm), and if the coracoid apex is shifted on the glenoid, the nerve is tractioned [15].

In the clinical picture, the size of sensory and motor deficiency derives from seriousness of the lesion and we can observe results from rapidly regressing simple tingling in the lateral forearm, to anesthesia and complete atrophy of the biceps and brachialis anterior muscles (Fig. 4).

We observed 14 patients: one gun shot, two deep wound, four fractures of humerus, seven iatrogenic lesions in surgery of the shoulder (six of which operated for anterior instability). There was a spontaneous recovery in eight patients and surgical treatment in six patients (4 neurolysis and 2 grafts).

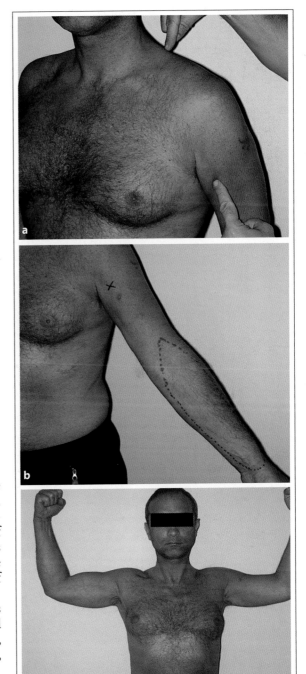

Fig. 3. B.A., male age 47 years. Gun shot with lesion of musculocutaneous nerve. (**a**) Entrance hole of the bullet in the arm and exit in scapular region. (**b**) Tinel sign proximal to the entrance hole and hypoesthesia in radial side of the forearm. (**c**) Hypotrophy of flexor of the elbow

The outcome (follow-up of 7.3 years, minimum 3 years, maximum 11.7 years) was fair in two patients (biceps M2-M3) and good or excellent in four patients (biceps M4-M5).

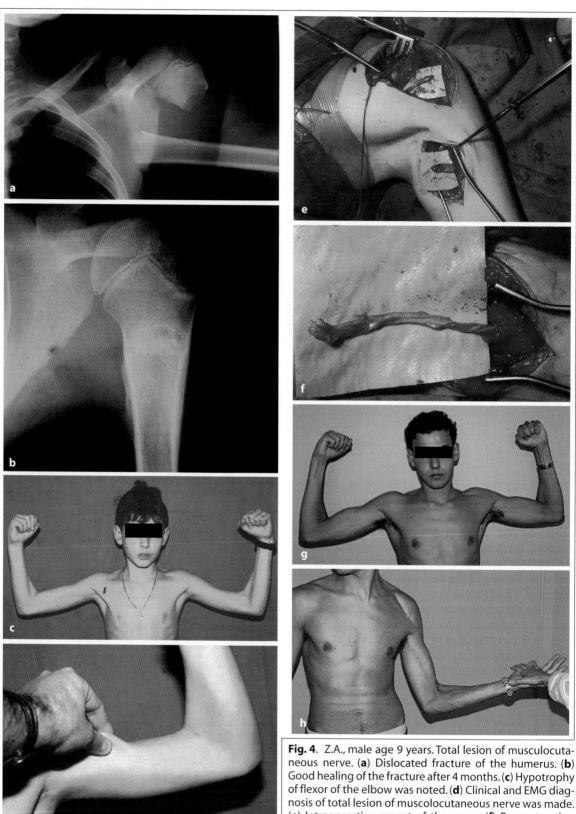

Fig. 4. Z.A., male age 9 years. Total lesion of musculocutaneous nerve. (**a**) Dislocated fracture of the humerus. (**b**) Good healing of the fracture after 4 months. (**c**) Hypotrophy of flexor of the elbow was noted. (**d**) Clinical and EMG diagnosis of total lesion of muscolocutaneous nerve was made. (**e**) Intraoperative aspect of the nerve. (**f**) Reconstruction with 2 grafts of sural nerve 8 cm long. (**g**) Control of the patients after 10 years with a complete muscular recovery, (**h**) and also normal strength

Conclusions

Traumatic isolated lesions of the musculocutaneous nerve are often carried out in passage through the coracobrachialis muscle, particularly with a compression and stretching mechanism. Repeated microtrauma (canalicular syndrome) is rare and it is often solved with rest and correcting sportive or working movements.

Indirect trauma after violent retroposition of the abducted and extrarotated shoulder often is initially confused with radicular lesion (C5–C6) or muscolotendineous lesion.

Direct trauma is not rare during surgery of the shoulder: we have to avoid direct lesion by suture or equipment of synthesis. In the correction of instability, before transferring the coracoid apex, we have to isolate and protect the musculocutaneous nerve, considering variations in anatomy and level of piercing. If the distance from the coracoid is <5 cm, we must consider the possibility of stretching the muscolocutaneous nerve. The outcomes of surgical reconstruction are good or excellent in more than 70% of patients.

References

1. Celli L, Rovesta C, Balli A, Marongiu MC (1992) Isolated traumatic lesions of the musculocutaneous nerve in the elbow. Springer-Verlag Heidelberg Berlin New York, pp 139-145
2. Osborne AW, Bonney G (2000) The musculocutaneus nerve. J Bone Joint Surg Br 82:1140-1142
3. Sunderland S (1978) Nerves and nerve injuries. Churchill Livingstone, Edinburgh
4. Gelbermann RH (1991) Operative nerve repair and reconstruction. Lippincott, pp 1165-1166
5. Yilmaz C, Gskandari MM, Colak M (2005) Traumatic musculocutaneus neuropathy: a case report. Arch Orthop Trauma Surg 125:414-416
6. Braddom RL, Wolfe C (1978) Musculocutaneous nerve injury after heavy exercise. Arch Phys Med Rehabil 5:383
7. Pecina M, Bojanic J (1993) Muscolocutaneous nerve entrapment in the upper arm. Int Orthop 17:232-234
8. Trojaborg W (1976) Motor and sensory conduction in the musculocutaneous nerve. J Neurol Neurosurg Psychiatr 39:890-899
9. Lugli MG, Rovesta C, Celli L (1986) Sindromi canalicolari del nervo muscolocutaneo. Atti XII congresso nazionale SIRC. Monduzzi Editore, Bologna 1:169-174
10. Jerosch J, Castro WHM, Colemont J (1989) A lesion of the musculocutaneus nerve. A rare complication of anterior shoulder dislocation. Acta Orthop Belg 55:230-232
11. Auzou P, Le Ber I, Ozsancakc C, Mannequin D (2000) Isolated truncular paralysis of the musculocutaneous nerve of the upper limb. Rev Chir Orthop Reparatrice Apparat Mot 86:188-192
12. Pitkow RB (1978) Partial neuropraxia of the biceps brachii motor nerve simulating tendon rupture. J Bone Joint Surg Am 60:1148
13. Weidmann E, Huggler AH (1978) Die lesion des nervus musculo-cutaneus bei der operativen behandlung der habituellen schulterluxation. Orthopade 7:192-193
14. Bach BR, O'Brien SJ, Warren RF, Leighton M (1988) An unusual neurological complication of the Bristow procedure. J Bone Joint Surg Am 70:458-460
15. Bartosh RH, Dugdale TW, Nielsen R (1992) Isolated musculocutaneous nerve injury complicating closed fracture of the clavicle: a case report. Am J Sport Med 20:356-359

CHAPTER 29

The Traumatic Nerve-Vascular Lesions

R. Adani, G. Leo, L. Tarallo

Introduction

The elbow represents an important point of passage between vascular (brachial artery) and nervous (median, radial, and ulnar nerve) structures, susceptible to direct trauma when there is intra-articular trauma to an elbow.

Vascular Injury

Dislocation of the elbow is a common orthopaedic injury, third in occurrence after glenohumeral and patellar femoral dislocations. Arterial injury associated with elbow dislocation is rare; arterial damage is generally associated with compound injuries [1]. Many reports have described such problems as occurring in the presence of open or closed reduction, anterior or posterior dislocations, and other associated upper extremity fractures [2-5]. The usual vessel injured is the brachial artery. It is important to use clinical parameters for evaluation of vascular compromise, but objective studies are also important for diagnostic classification. Loss of pulse does not preclude attempted closed reduction, but if arterial flow is not re-established after reduction, confirmed by the absence of the wrist pulse and with the hand poorly perfused, the patient should be prepared for surgical exploration. Controversy still remains regarding the optimal management of an absent radial pulse in an otherwise well-perfused hand [6]. Moreover, the presence of pulses alone does not ensure adequate circulation to the hand or perfusion of the forearm musculature. The role of angiography in the treatment of these patients is not clear. Shaw et al. [7] noted the risk of arteriography to be the following: prolongation of ischemic time between fracture and reduction, arterial damage at the catheter insertion site, and allergy to contrast material. Sabharwal et al. [6] suggested arteriography for better defining the location and extent of the vascular injury and the presence of a collateral circulation. The assessment of brachial artery patency by noninvasive imaging in now possible with the use of MRA [8]. This technique has been shown to be more sensitive than angiography in evaluating peripheral circulation, eventually associated with color-flow duplex ultrasound. By combining these techniques, both anatomically and hemodynamically significant information are obtained. The brachial artery can be found kinked; often there is associated spasm that may respond to local treatment. Nevertheless, the majority of the cases require repair of the damaged lumen with resection and end-to-end anastomosis, removal of thrombus with thrombectomy or intra-arterial thrombolysis with urokinase infusion, or brachial artery reconstruction using an interposition vein graft, generally employing the saphenous vein (Fig. 1).

All attempts should be done to restore arterial flow rather than ligating the brachial artery. Occasionally no graft is needed; however, if a full elbow mobility after vessel reconstruction is attempted, the brachial artery must have adequate length to permit full extension of the elbow. If perfusion of

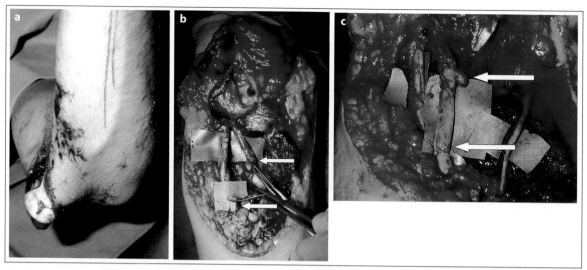

Fig. 1. Open elbow dislocation (**a**) with brachial artery laceration (*arrows* point to the transected brachial artery) (**b**).The repair of the artery was performed using an interposition vein graft (*arrows* points to the reconstructed brachial artery) (**c**)

the forearm and hand has been poor because of prolonged ischemic time, forearm fasciotomy should be done during the vascular repair to decrease compartment pressure and to prevent Volkmann's contracture (Fig. 2) [9].

In conclusion, many factors influence the final result of fractures and/or elbow dislocations with ischemia; clinical findings must be carefully evaluated and correlated with information obtained by laboratory instruments (Fig. 3).

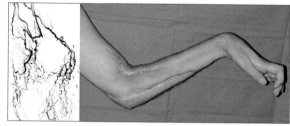

Fig. 2. Long-term result of inadequate perfusion around the elbow (confirmed by angiography)

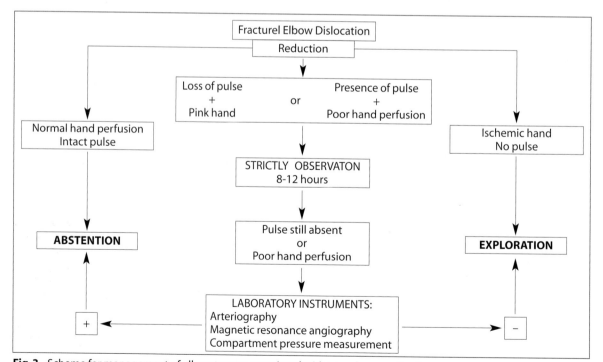

Fig. 3. Scheme for management of elbow trauma associated with vascular complication

Nerve Injury

The median, ulnar, radial, and anterior interosseous nerves are all susceptible to injury at the time of elbow dislocation.

Median nerve injury after dislocation of the elbow is unusual; however, various cases have been reported in the literature in the recent years [10-24].

Fourrier et al. [14] and Hallet [15] described 3 types of median nerve entrapment that may accompany elbow dislocation.

In type 1 (Fig. 4 a, b) the nerve dislocates behind the medial epicondyle and is entrapped in the humero-ulnar joint. There must have been a medi-

al epicondyle fracture at the time of elbow dislocation or a rupture of the medial collateral ligament and so at injury or during reduction the nerve slips into the joint. The ligament subsequently repairs by fibrosis and the nerve is permanently trapped.

In type 2 (Fig. 4 c, d) after fracture of the medial epicondyle (in children the epiphysis of the epicondyle is torn off by the common flexor origin), the nerve slips into the fracture site and becomes entrapped by the medial epicondyle; finally it becomes surrounded in fracture callus as healing occurs.

A type 3 (Fig. 4 e, f) happens in the absence of a medial epicondylar fracture when the nerve is looped within the humero-ulnar joint.

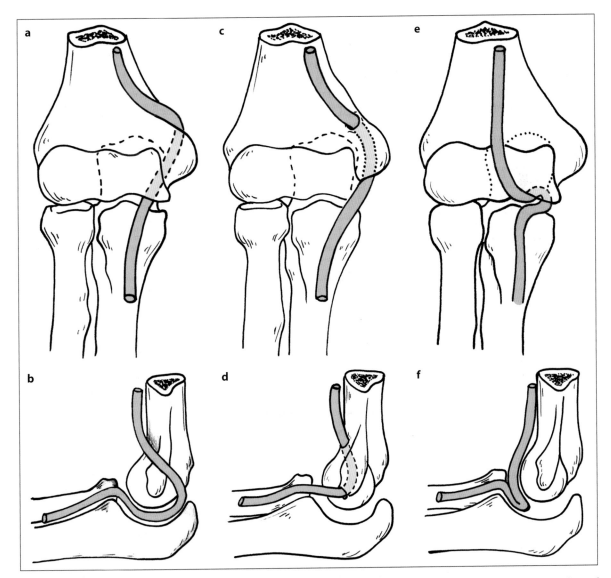

Fig. 4. (**a, b**) The nerve is displaced posterior to the medial epicondyle and becomes adherent to the posterior surface of the humerus alongside the ulnar nerve. (**c, d**) The nerve is embedded in medial epicondyle fracture callus and passes through a bony tunnel. (**e, f**) The nerve is looped into the front of the elbow

Pritchard et al. [12] proposed that the nerve may loop into the humero-ulnar joint through a tear of the medial capsule or the anterior joint capsule and the brachialis muscle, and after reduction may remain entrapped by the flare of the medial epicondyle.

In 1994, Al-Qattan et al. [23] reported a case of posterior elbow dislocation with the median nerve both encased within the healing medial epicondylar fracture and entrapped intra-articularly, which they suggested to be classified as type 4.

The origin of the flexor-pronator muscle group from the medial epicondyle prevents posterior displacement of the median nerve during dislocation of the elbow. Since the medial epicondyle is more likely to be avulsed before physeal closure, it is quite common that most of the cases reported of median nerve entrapment after dislocation have been in children (Fig. 5) [20].

The best cure for median nerve entrapment is prevention. When reducing the dislocation it is necessary to displace the upper end of the forearm medially before laterally rotating it, bringing it forward and then flexing it to allow the nerve to return to its proper anterior position [16, 21, 23].

Recognition of median nerve entrapment after reduction of elbow dislocations is often delayed; in most cases the neurovascular damage was not discovered before reduction. Median nerve deficit is usually recognized after reduction of the dislocation [12, 15, 17, 18, 21, 24] and the injury of the median nerve, with the exception of a few cases [19, 20] was managed expectantly for several weeks to months, because this was assumed to be a traction injury [19, 24].

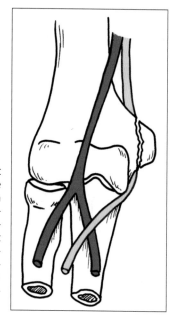

Fig. 5. It is evident that an essential part of the mechanism of median nerve entrapment following elbow joint dislocation is detachment of the proximal insertion of the flexor muscles (which in children includes the medial epicondyle)

Pain, although frequently severe at the time of dislocation, is usually mild once the elbow dislocation has been reduced [17]. Hallet [15] reported that median nerve entrapment does not cause pain; others have noted severe pain in the arms of patients after nerve entrapment [11, 12]. Since pain is not a characteristic sign of entrapment the diagnosis depends on finding sensory loss in the areas of the hand innervated by the median nerve, and weakness in the long flexors of the thumb and index finger. The most difficult diagnosis is probably the isolated anterior interosseous nerve palsy, because no sensory loss is noted.

The Tinel's sign may be positive at the elbow; other associated signs include difficulty in reducing the elbow and limitation of motion immediately after reduction [18, 19]. Delays in diagnosis have been attributed to several factors: entrapment of the median nerve is a rare condition that usually occurs in young patients who are sometimes more difficult to interview and examine, the displacement of the medial epicondyle may be difficult to define, and finally when a neurological deficit is present, it has often been attributed to a neurapraxic lesion [25]. For these reasons the key to early diagnosis is a high degree of suspicion combined with thorough and repeated neurological examinations [19], before and after closed reduction [25].

Radiographically, the diagnosis of median nerve entrapment should be considered in a patient who has a fracture of the medial epicondyle or a widened medial joint space after reduction.

Every median nerve injury in association with an elbow dislocation must be viewed as very probably representing entrapment of the nerve if more than mild hyperesthesia is present, and especially if pain is present [17]. In this case, exploration and decompression of the nerve is indicated [12, 15, 17].

Matev [26] described a radiographic sign consisting of a focal cortical depression on the ulnar side of the distal humeral metaphysis with interruption of the periosteal reaction. This sign is present only after 3 months from the initial injury and is caused by healing around the nerve which passes through a bony tunnel formed by a fracture of the epicondyle in type 1 and 2; Matev's sign was later reported also by other authors [17, 24, 25].

In addition to clinical and radiographic signs, and electromyographic studies (EMG may be helpful in demonstrating signs of denervation 6 weeks after injury), the magnetic resonance imaging may be useful in the early and late diagnosis of the median nerve entrapment [27].

MRI evaluates the course of the median nerve and can prevent the late diagnosis of intra-articular median nerve entrapment. Muscle atrophy revealed by MRI should be a clue to nerve entrapment when seen in the setting of reduced elbow dislocation [27].

When entrapment is diagnosed the nerve should be explored surgically and freed from bone or joint [15]; if the nerve is intact and there is evidence, after nerve stimulation of motor conduction, neurolysis is indicated [10, 11, 12, 17, 18].

If the median nerve is replaced by scar with absence of motor conduction, resection of the damaged nerve and reastomosis are indicated [26].

Longstanding compression usually results in severe structural damage to a nerve, necessitating reconstruction with excision and microsurgical repair with grafts [23, 24] (Figs. 6, 7).

Ulnar nerve injuries are more common than median nerve injuries in association with elbow dislocation [15, 28]. The valgus displacement that occurs during dislocation can also put the ulnar nerve under tension. Usually after performing closed reduc-

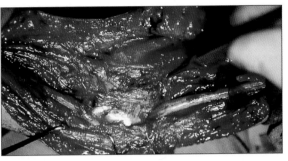

Fig. 7. Type 2 of Hallet classification. The median nerve was incarcerated is an associated fracture of the medial humeral epicondyle

tion of the elbow the ulnar neuropathy resolves immediately. In case of an associated medial epicondylar fracture, ulnar anterior transposition should be performed at the time of reduction [29].

Intra-articular entrapment of the radial nerve in association with dislocation of the elbow is very rare [30-32]. The radial head is displaced posteriorly and the radial nerve is displaced laterally and posteriorly around the lateral epicondyle; the radial nerve can enter the radio capitellar joint through the disrupted posterior capsule [32].

Fracture of the medial epicondyle or epitrochlea is more frequent than fracture of the lateral epicondyle. This fragment can be, in the child and adolescent, avulsed from the humerus during a posterior dislocation of the elbow [33]. The epicondylar fragment is lodged between the medial articular surface of the trochlea and ulna, inhibiting reduction and the ulnar nerve can became trapped within this fragment (Fig. 8). In cases in

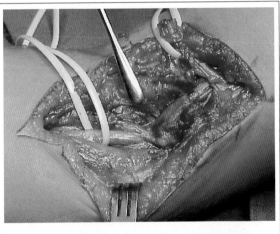

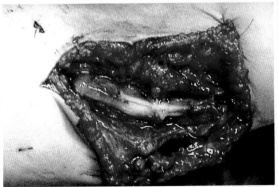

Fig. 6. Type 1 of Hallet classification. The median nerve was isolated in the distal arm and in the forearm and traced towards the joint (the median nerve is being held with lops). The nerve was transacted proximal to its entrapment and distal to its point of emergence from the elbow joint resulting in a 4 cm nerve gap. The nerve was reconstructed using sural nerve grafts. (Figures reproduced with permission from R. Luchetti, M.D.)

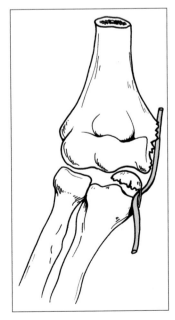

Fig. 8. Intra-articular displacement of epitrochlea and entrapment within joint after reduction of dislocation of elbow. The fragment displaced and rotated can compress the ulnar nerve

which the medial epicondyle has been displaced into the joint, the risk of ulnar nerve involvement is quite high. For this reason the function of the ulnar nerve must be carefully assessed.

If the dysfunction is complete, the ulnar nerve is probably compressed by the fragment and the ulnar nerve must be explored surgically [34].

The fragment should be removed from the joint and reattached to the distal medial humerus (Fig. 9); ulnar nerve transposition has been performed at the time of reduction.

Neural injuries associated with displaced supracondylar humeral fractures in children are fairly common. The incidence of nerve injuries has been estimated to be approximately 7% of cases [34]. The median, ulnar, and radial nerves course adjacent to the elbow joint and each one can be involved. The most commonly injured nerve is the radial (41%), followed by median nerve (36%); the ulnar nerve is involved in 23% of cases [34].

The insult to the nerve can occur at the time of injury by direct trauma from bony fragments, traction, or entrapment between fracture fragments; nerve in-

juries can also occur secondary to treatment by manipulation, traction, or percutaneous pinning [35,36].

Injury to the brachial artery has been reported in as many as 10% of displaced supracondylar fractures [37].

In type 3 fractures, using the Gartland classification system [38], there is no continuity between fracture fragments. Usually, during supracondylar fractures the brachialis muscle protects the anterior or neurovascular structures from injury but in case of severe displacement either medial or lateral, the spike can penetrate the brachialis muscle; this results in a much higher incidence of neurovascular complications with type 3 extension fractures [39].

With postero-lateral displacement of the distal fragment the spike penetrates medially and the median nerve and the brachial artery may be entrapped [34, 35, 40, 41]. If the distal spike penetrates the brachialis muscle laterally, with the distal fragment displaced postero-medially, the radial nerve may be entrapped [34, 42, 43]. It seems that posteromedially displaced fractures are slightly more likely to be associated with neural compromise [40].

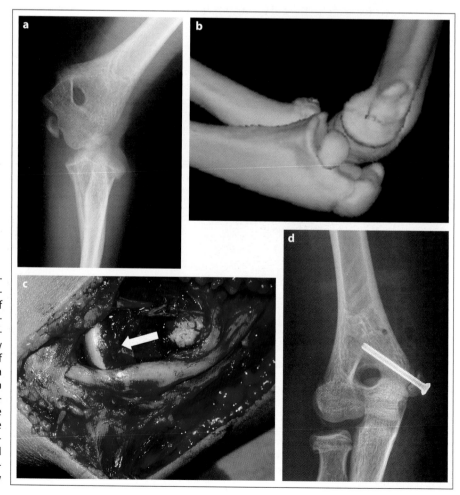

Fig. 9. (**a**) Antero-posterior view showing a posterolateral dislocation of the elbow with the presence of the medial epicondyle within the elbow joint. (**b**) Entrapment of the fragment between humerus and olecranon confirmed by CT examination. (**c**) Severe ulnar nerve compression due to the dislocated epicondyle fragment. (**d**) Reduction and internal fixation of the medial epicondyle with screw

Flexion-type supracondylar fractures are rare; a major complication of this type of fracture is injury to the ulnar nerve by the sharp spike of the proximal fragment when the distal fragment is displaced antero-medially [34].

When the fractures are closed, reducible, and not associated with vascular damage, closed treatment of the fracture and initial observation of the neural injury is the treatment of choice [34, 35, 40, 42, 44].

Most injuries are neurapraxic and will resolve spontaneously by 6 months with an average of 2-3 months [34, 35, 40, 41, 44, 45].

Brown and Zinar [46] suggest a waiting period of 6 months before doing electromyography to determine if exploration is warranted.

The indications for open exploration include vascular damage, open injury, irreducible fracture, and neural injury (Fig. 10). In this case the fracture is reduced and the involved nerve identified; if the nerve is found to be in anatomical continuity neurolysis is performed with major neural recovery [45]. Also, if open reduction is performed for fracture alignment, exploration of the involved nerve is appropriate [40].

Occasionally, however, there have been few cases of complete transection of the nerve, usually the radial one [40, 42, 43, 45]. If the nerve has been transacted, repair or nerve grafting is needed.

Neurological deficit involving the radial, ulnar, and median nerve associated with supracondylar fractures must be recognized. In the case of median nerve involvement isolated to the anterior interosseous branch, the clinical findings are subtle [35, 40, 41].

Neurological deficit may be overlooked if the motor function is not specifically tested. Children will commonly complain of numbness, but will rarely notice a minimal motor loss, especially when

it is painful to move [35]. Flexor pollicis longus and flexor digitorum profundus to the index finger should be carefully tested.

Given specific fracture displacement patterns, one is more aware of the potential for specific nerve dysfunction and a diligent search can be made to document this loss before surgery [39].

The posterior interosseous nerve is the nerve most commonly injured following Monteggia fracture dislocations [47]. The posterior interosseous nerve is the deep branch of the radial nerve; it crosses the radio capitellar joint and enters the substance of the supinator muscle mass between the superficial and deep layers. Anterior dislocation of the radial head may result in a traction injury to the posterior interosseous nerve as it passes dorsolaterally around the proximal radius causing a paresis of the nerve [48, 49] (Fig. 11).

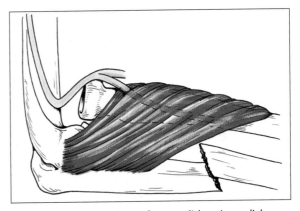

Fig. 11. Anterior Monteggia fracture dislocation radial nerve is depicted dividing into superficial and posterior interosseous nerves, the latter then coursing around the radial neck

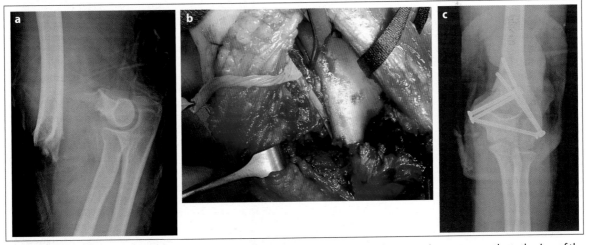

Fig. 10. (**a**) Severe postero-medial supracondylar fracture. (**b**) Exposure of the fractures demonstrates the tethering of the radial nerve over the sharp lateral spike of the proximal humerus. (**c**) Post-operative view: an open reduction was performed with screws

Posterior interosseous nerve palsy as a result of Monteggia fracture can be caused by a direct trauma [48, 50], compression of the nerve in the arcade of Frohse [51], entrapment between the radius and ulna [52], stretching by the laterally dislocated radial head [53], and tardy palsy due to scarring from an old, unreduced radial head [54]. The arcade of Frohse may be thinner and therefore more pliable in children [51] and this can explain the rapid resolution of posterior nerve injury in children, usually about 9 weeks after reduction [48, 50, 55].

In children, prolonged observation (minimum 6 months) seems indicated before exploration of the posterior interosseous nerve injury [55]. Spinner [51] recommends exploration of the nerve within 2 months if no clinical or electromyography recovery is noted; this may be more appropriate in adult patients than in children.

The operative approach includes neurolysis of the posterior interosseous nerve eventually combined with excision of the radial head in cases of tardy radial nerve injury associated with radial head dislocation [54, 56].

The association of median or ulnar nerve injuries with Monteggia fracture is low [47, 48, 50, 57].

Patients with injuries to the elbow should have careful neurological exams. The neurological complications presented are not common but also not rare and must be recognized and promptly treated.

References

1. Manouel M, Minkowitz B, Shimotsu G et al (1993) Brachial artery laceration with closed posterior elbow dislocation in an eight year old. Clin Orthop 296:109-112
2. Louis DR, Ricciardi JE, Spengler DA (1974) Arterial injury: A classification of posterior elbow dislocation. J Bone Joint Surg Am 56:1631-1636
3. Grimer RJ, Brooks S (1985) Brachial artery damage accompanying closed posterior dislocation of the elbow. J Bone Joint Surg Br 67:378-381
4. Endean ED, Veldenz HC, Schwarcz TH, Hyde GL (1992) Recognition of arterial injury in elbow dislocation. J Vasc Surg 16:402-406
5. Squires NA, Tomaino MM (2003) Brachial artery rupture without median nerve dysfunction after closed elbow dislocation. Am J Orthop 32:298-300
6. Sabharwal S, Tredwell SJ, Beauchamp RD et al (1997) Management of pulseless prink hand in pediatric supracondylar fractures of humerus. J Pediatr Orthop 17:303-310
7. Shaw BA, Kasser JR, Emans JB, Rand FF (1990) Management of vascular injuries in displaced supracondylar fractures without arteriography. J Orthop Trauma 1:25-29
8. Swan JS, Carroll TJ, Kennell TW et al (2002) Time-resolved three-dimensional contrast-enhanced MR angiography of the peripheral vessels. Radiology 225:43-52
9. Mubarak SJ, Wallace CD (2000) Complications of the supracondylar fractures of the elbow. In: Morrey BF (ed) The elbow and its disorders. WB Saunders, Philadelphia, pp 201-218
10. Mannerfelt L (1968) Median nerve entrapment after dislocation of the elbow. J Bone Joint Surg Br 50:152-155
11. Steiger RN, Larrick RB, Meyer TL (1969) Median nerve entrapment following elbow dislocation in children. J Bone Joint Surg Am 51:381-385
12. Pritchard DJ, Linscheid RL, Svien HJ (1973) Intra-articular median nerve entrapment with dislocation of the elbow. Clin Orthop 90:100-103
13. Bonvallet JM (1977) Paralysis of the median nerve after impaction in a dislocation of the elbow. Ann Chir 31:345-349
14. Fourrier P, Levai JP, Collin JP (1977) Incarceration du nerf median au cours d'une luxation du coude. Rev Chir Orthop 63:13-16
15. Hallet J (1981) Entrapment of the median nerve after dislocation of the elbow. J Bone Joint Surg Br 63:408-412
16. Strange Clair St FG (1982) Entrapment of the median nerve after dislocation of the elbow. J Bone Joint Surg Br 64:224-225
17. Green NE (1983) Entrapment of the median nerve following elbow dislocation. J Pediatr Orthop 3:384-386
18. Pritchett JW (1984) Entrapment of the median nerve after dislocation of the elbow. J Pediatr Orthop 4:752-753
19. Danielsson LG (1986) Median nerve entrapment in elbow dislocation. Acta Orthop Scand 57:450-452
20. Floyd WE, Gebhardt MC, Emans JB (1987) Intra-articular entrapment of the median nerve after elbow dislocation in children. J Hand Surg Am 12:704-707
21. Boe S, Holst-Nielsen F (1987) Intra-articular entrapment of the median nerve after dislocation of the elbow. J Hand Surg Br 12:356-358
22. Tropet Y, Menez D, Brientini JM et al (1989) Entrapment of the median nerve after dislocation of the elbow. Acta Orthop Belg 55:217-221
23. Al-Qattan MM, Zuker RM, Weinberg MJ (1994) Type 4 median nerve entrapment after elbow dislocation. J Hand Surg Br 19:613-615
24. Rao SB, Crawford AH (1995) Median nerve entrapment after dislocation of the elbow in children. Clin Orthop 312:232-237
25. Noonan KJ, Blair WF (1995) Chronic median nerve entrapment after posterior fracture-dislocation of the elbow. J Bone Joint Surg Am 77:1572-1575
26. Matev I (1976) A radiological sign of entrapment of the median nerve in the elbow joint after posterior dislocation. J Bone Joint Surg Br 58:353-355
27. Akansel G, Dalbayrak S, Yilmaz M et al (2003) MRI demonstration of intra-articular median nerve entrapment after elbow dislocation. Skeletal Radiol 32:537-541
28. Galbraith KA, McCullough CJ (1979) Acute nerve injury as a complication of closed fractures or dislocations of the elbow. Injury 11:159-164
29. O'Driscoll SW (2000) Elbow dislocations. In: Morrey BF (ed) The elbow and its disorders. WB Saunders, Philadelphia, pp 409-420
30. Watson-Jones R (1930) Primary nerve lesions in injuries of the elbow and wrist. J Bone Joint Surg 12:121-140
31. Motta A, Callea C, Poli G (1978) Radial nerve paralysis caused by articular interposition in dislocation of the elbow. Chir Organi Mov 64:113-115

32. Su Liu G, Jupiter JB (2004) Posterolateral rotatory elbow subluxation with intra-articular entrapment of the radial nerve. J Bone Joint Surg Am 86:603-606

33. Hotchkiss R (1996) Fractures and dislocations of the elbow. In: Rockwood CA, Green DP (eds) Rockwood and Green's fractures in adult. Lippincott-Raven, Philadelphia, pp 929-1024

34. Wilkins KE, Beatty JH, Chambers HG et al (1996) Fractures and dislocations of the elbow. In: Rockwood CA, Wilkins KE, Beatty JH (ed) Fractures in children. Lippincott-Raven, Philadelphia, pp 653-904

35. Jones ET, Louis DS (1980) Median nerve injuries associated with supracondylar fractures of the humerus in children. Clin Orthop 150:181-186

36. Kekomaki M, Luoma R, Rikalainen H (1984) Operative reduction and fixation of a difficult supracondylar extension fracture of the humerus. J Pediatr Orthop 4:13-15

37. Ashbell TS, Kleinert HE, Kutz JE (1967) Vascular injuries about the elbow. Clin Orthop 50:107-127

38. Gartland JJ (1959) Management of supracondylar fractures of the humerus in children. Surg Gynecol Obstet 109:145-154

39. Lyons S, Quinn M, Stanitski CL (2000) Neurovascular injuries in type 3 humeral supracondylar fractures in children. Clin Orthop 376:62-67

40. McGraw JJ, Akbarnia BA, Hanel DP, Keppler L, Burdge RE (1986) Neurological complications resulting from supracondylar fractures of the humerus in children. J Pediatr Orthop 6:647-650

41. Spinner M, Schreiber S (1969) Anterior interosseous nerve paralysis as a complication of supracondylar fractures of the humerus in children. J Bone Joint Surg Am 51:1584-1590

42. Banskota A, Volz RG (1984) Traumatic laceration of the radial nerve following supracondylar fracture of the elbow. Clin Orthop 184:150-152

43. Martin DF, Tolo VT, Sellers DS (1989) Radial nerve laceration and retraction associated with a supracondylar fracture of the humerus. J Hand Surg Am 14:542-545

44. Pirone AM, Graham AK, Krajbich JI (1988) Management of displaced extension type supracondylar fractures of the humerus in children. J Bone Joint Surg Am 70:641-650

45. Culp WR, Osterman AL, Davidson RS et al (1990) Neural injuries associated with supracondylar fractures of the humerus in children. J Bone Joint Surg Am 72:1211-1215

46. Brown IC, Zinar DH (1995) Traumatic and iatrogenic neurological complications after supracondylar humerus fractures in children. J Pediatr Orthop 15:440-443

47. Jessing P (1975) Monteggia lesions and their complicating nerve damage. Acta Orthop Scand 46:601-609

48. Stein F, Gabrias SL, Deffer PA (1971) Nerve injuries complicating Monteggia lesions. J Bone Joint Surg Am 53:1432-1436

49. Merv Letts R (2000) Dislocations of the child's elbow. In: Morrey BF (ed) The elbow and its disorders. WB Saunders, Philadelphia, pp 261-286

50. Spinner M, Freundlich BD, Teicher J (1968) Posterior interosseous nerve palsy as a complication of Monteggia fractures in children. Clin Orthop 58:141-145

51. Spinner M (1968) The arcade of Frohse and its relationship to posterior interosseous nerve paralysis. J Bone Joint Surg Br 50:809-812

52. Morris A (1975) Irreducible Monteggia lesion with radial entrapment. J Bone Joint Surg Am 56:1744-1746

53. Spar I (1977) A neurologic complication following Monteggia fracture. Clin Orthop 122:207-209

54. Lichter R, Jacobsen T (1975) Tardy palsy of the posterior interosseous nerve with a Monteggia fracture. J Bone Joint Surg Am 57:124-125

55. Olney BW, Menelaus MB (1989) Monteggia and equivalent lesions in childhood. J Pediatr Orthop 9:219-223

56. Holst-Nielsen F, Jensen V (1984) Tardy posterior interosseous nerve palsy. J Hand Surg Am 7:572-575

57. Chen W-S (1992) Late neuropathy in chronic dislocation of the radial head. Acta Orthop Scand 63:343-344

CHAPTER 30

The Utility of Continuous Axial Brachial Plexus Catheters after Surgery

F. GAZZOTTI, L.V. INDRIZZI, G. MAGNI, E. BERTELLINI, A. TASSI

Theory: The Post-operative Elbow Contracture

Surgery of elbow lesions is a challenging and demanding procedure. In recent years, an aggressive approach to the treatment of even chronic lesions around the elbow joint in combination with more specific surgical techniques and advanced post-operative rehabilitation have increased the indications for surgical intervention and improved the final outcome [1-3].

The development of joint contracture remains a well-recognized complication of elbow surgery and can unfortunately be quite common. The precise causes of the propensity of this joint for ankylosis are poorly understood.

Elbow stiffness has been classified in a number of ways, but a consistent feature is capsular contracture, even when the contracture of the elbow joint develops as a result of a more complicated process involving contractures of joint capsule, ligamentous structures, musculotendinous structures, intra-articular adhesion, and ectopic ossification.

The contracted elbow is defined as an elbow with a reduction in extension greater than 30° and/or flexion less than 120°. Although supination and pronation are often reduced as well, this will not be considered here further, as contracture of the elbow is not related to forearm rotation. Stiffness of the elbow can cause substantial disability and actually impairs hand function, limiting the ability to put one's hand in the volume of a sphere in space, as the hand movement is highly dependent on elbow extension and flexion and forearm rotation. A 50% reduction of elbow motion can reduce the upper extremity function by almost 80%.

The stiffness following surgery or injury to a joint can be determined by intrinsic and extrinsic factors but develops as a progression of four stages: bleeding, edema, granulation tissue, and fibrosis. Continuous passive motion (CPM) properly applied during the first two stages of stiffness acts to pump blood and edema fluid away from the joint and peri-articular tissues. This allows maintenance of normal peri-articular soft tissue compliance. CPM is thus effective in preventing the development of stiffness if full motion is applied immediately following surgery and continued until swelling that limits the full motion of the joint no longer develops. This concept has been applied successfully to elbow rehabilitation: early and efficient rehabilitation is necessary for preventing the initial or delayed accumulation of peri-articular interstitial fluids, improving outcome after elbow surgery. Without CPM, any improvement achieved with surgery could be lost and stiffness can follow or worsen [4,5].

The rehabilitation of elbow injuries presents numerous challenges, among the most important of which is pain control. Regardless of the anesthesia technique used for elbow surgery, the post-operative analgesia remains one of the most relevant problems, because it is the most limiting factor of the rehabilitation therapy. Pain depends on several factors: the site and the extent of the surgery, the preoperative health condition of the patient (including use of, e.g., analgesic or antidepressant drugs), etc. Normally after elbow surgery the pain is moderate to severe for 36-48 hours at rest, but during movement pain increases enormously and becomes the major factor compromising early physical therapy.

Thus post-operative analgesia in orthopedic procedures on the elbow is mandatory not only as an ethical issue but also, perhaps most importantly, to permit continuous and aggressive physical therapy preventing the stiffness. In fact the aim of any analgesic technique should not only be to lessen pain but also to facilitate earlier mobilization and to reduce peri-operative complications.

Anesthesia *vs* Analgesia

In orthopedics, the choice between regional and general anesthesia in most cases depends on all or some of the following factors: patient preference, state of health of the patient, expertise of the anesthesiologist, duration and surgical position of the procedure, and surgeon's preference and practice pattern in the hospital.

In general, most extremity procedures can be performed using regional anesthesia alone or with light sedation. More complicated operations may be performed under general anesthesia alone or, alternatively, using combined techniques such as a regional anesthetic supplemented with light general anesthesia.

Orthopedic procedures for the arm can be performed with a variety of brachial plexus block techniques, using intravenous regional anesthesia or combinations of individual nerve blocks in the arm. The selection depends on the site and type of surgery, the anesthesiologist's experience and preference, and technical device availability in the hospital.

In particular, elbow surgery can be performed by either infraclavicular or supraclavicular or axillary block (although T1-T2 intercostobrachial nerve block in the axilla may be necessary as a supplement to axillary block if medial incisions are made in the upper arm) [6-9].

However, the anesthesia techniques discussed above are a different issue from post-operative pain control, although, not surprisingly, anesthesia techniques can influence the analgesic requirements and the likelihood of collateral effects, such as emesis, in the early post-operative period. In upper limb surgery, for example, single-injection brachial plexus blocks, even with long-acting local anesthetics, can provide almost 12 hours of analgesia,

which can be sufficient to eliminate the need for narcotics with good analgesia (only in ambulatory patients with low or moderate pain).

Although opioid analgesics will continue to play an important role in pain management, the use of both local anesthetic agents and NSAIDs is assuming an even greater role, mostly in orthopedic surgery, which lends itself to regional anesthesia-analgesia [10, 11].

The analgesia can in theory be made to last indefinitely (or in any case much more than the 12 hours achieved with a single injection of local anesthetics) by the introduction of continuous infusion of the same drug(s) through a catheter placed very close to the neural structures, in the same position where the single-shot regional block should be performed.

A number of different regional techniques have been tried for controlling pain after elbow surgery with the catheter positioning at different levels of the brachial plexus: interscalene, supraclavicular, infraclavicular, and axillary approaches. The application of a continuous infusion of local anesthetic through an infraclavicular catheter is actually the best technique available to achieve pain relief at rest and on movement after this type of surgery, and to continue the analgesia as needed.

If post-operative pain service is available in the hospital, the best way to optimize the pain therapy will be based on continuous infusion of local anesthetic associated with patient-controlled regional analgesia (PCRA) modalities. Local anesthetic boluses or continuous infusion can provide profound analgesia, with advantages over parenteral opioids that include earlier mobilization with an improved rate of rehabilitation, reduced catabolism, improved bowel function, higher arterial oxygen tension, and fewer pulmonary complications.

Thus to optimize the analgesia, clinicians should be able to effectively treat post-operative pain using a combination of a peripheral analgesia technique and NSAIDs (and, only if necessary, a low dose of narcotics) with a multimodal approach to pain characterized by fewer side effects and better results than those achieved with narcotic analgesia alone.

Practice

As noted above, catheters for pain control in elbow surgery have been placed by different practitioners at different levels along the brachial plexus perivascular sheath: interscalene, supraclavicular, infraclavicular, and axillary, with different and interesting results.

A review of the literature reveals that the number of anecdotal reports of complications is greater following supraclavicular techniques, although the axillary approach is used more often. The potential for serious complications (such as pneumothorax, local anesthetic toxicity, central neural toxicity, etc.) after brachial plexus anesthesia appears to be greater with the approaches above the clavicle.

With an interscalene block the brachial plexus is approached at the level of the roots and primary trunks. The inferior trunk (C8-T1), which is deeper, is often incompletely involved and so the ulnar and median nerves are rarely blocked, and to obtain good pain control for elbow surgery it is mandatory to use an axillary block. This block is also frequently prone to collateral effects such as Horner's syndrome, recurrent laryngeal nerve block, and, mostly, ipsilateral phrenic block. This is why this block is contraindicated in patients with advanced lung disease and significant impairment of pulmonary function. However of all possible complications the risk of central neural blockade and pneumothorax appear to be higher after the interscalene approach.

Of all the sites of access to the brachial plexus, the supraclavicular block is the one that allows the greatest diffusion as the brachial plexus cords are very close together at the site of injection, but it is also the one with the greatest risk of pneumothorax, because of the closeness of the parietal pleura to the neurological structures involved in the block. The risk of pneumothorax has deterred many anesthesiologists from using the supraclavicular approach and is most likely the reason that infraclavicular approaches are more popular. We do not use the supraclavicular approach, for these reasons.

At the level of the axilla, the different nerves of the brachial plexus are individualized and a continuous infusion does not always provide complete upper limb analgesia, because diffusion of the local anesthetic solution can be incomplete. The axillary approach is not devoid of complications. In common with other supraclavicular techniques, local anesthetic toxicity, nerve injury and failure are the most common complications. There are also some very specific complications unique to the axillary approach: vascular complications such as vasospasm, hematoma, and venous and arterial thrombus. The axillary artery may be accidentally or deliberately penetrated, and there are a few anecdotal reports of loss of circulation to the upper extremity after the transarterial approach. Vasospasm is thought to be the most likely cause of the problem. Hematoma formation has been associated with nerve injury.

In addition, there is a high risk (mostly during rehabilitation movement) of secondary displacement of the catheter introduced and essential for the continuous infusion of local anesthetics; this is the main reason why, although some authors still prefer this technique, we do not find it suitable for elbow post-operative analgesia [12-14].

With the infraclavicular placement of a catheter for continuous infusion, the brachial plexus is approached at the level of the cords just where they give origin to the nerves, and thus it is possible to obtain good analgesia for elbow surgery [15-18]. Furthermore with this approach the plexus is joined quite deeply (4-7 cm) and in a position where it is also very easy to firmly stabilize the catheter for a long time in a comfortable way [19, 20]. There is no risk of pneumothorax or central neural blockade. Normally the patients find this technique more comfortable and less painful than the axillary block, especially in trauma cases in which upper limb mobilization is not needed to perform the block; it has also been successfully applied for acute pain management in children [21]. The only disadvantage is the impossibility of achieving compression after a vascular puncture, but ruling out patients with coagulation abnormalities dramatically reduces the risk of hematoma formation.

The combined use of ultrasound and nerve stimulation for the localization of the brachial plexus during infraclavicular block was recently evaluated, with good results. The needle and subsequently the catheter were positioned posterior to the artery until distal muscle stimulation was obtained. Injection through the catheter resulted in local anesthetic spread posterior to the artery and successful block. Ultrasound guidance during infraclavicular brachial plexus block enables direct visualization of the needle/catheter tip location and confirmation of appropriate local anesthetic spread [22], lowering the risk of vascular puncture.

This is why, among the different approaches which have been described, the infraclavicular brachial plexus block for us is the simplest and the safest to perform and the most suitable for the reliable insertion of a catheter to be maintained in place for a long period.

Technical Aspects

Position

The patient lies supine with the head turned slightly to the opposite side of the arm to be blocked.

Whereas according to Raj's original technique the arm should be abducted 90° from the chest wall, with our approach the arm is adducted or even abducted but not over 45° from the chest wall and if possible flexed at the elbow.

Landmarks

Of all the different ways and landmarks described to perform this technique, the simplest, safest, and most reliable approach is based on coracoid process identification [23]. The coracoid process of the scapula must be identified after palpation and marked in the infraclavicular region. A point on the skin about 2 cm medial and about 2 cm caudal to the tip of the coracoid process identifies the brachial plexus below. The axillary artery pulse in the axilla is marked, ideally at the point where the pulse disappears under the pectoralis major muscle [24].

Technique

Using an aseptic technique, after skin cleaning, a skin wheal of local anesthetic is raised just inferior and medial to the coracoid process, 2 cm medially and below the coracoid process (Fig. 1); next a 120-mm cannulated needle (MULTIPLEX) (Fig. 2) connected to an electrical nerve stimulator (ENS) with 1.0 mA current and 2 Hz impulse frequency, and to the ground electrode on the chest, is introduced through the skin wheal vertically with a slightly lateral and caudal direction, with an angle of 0° to 15° toward the axilla, until the evocation of a muscular contraction (twitch) (Fig. 3). The average depth of the needle insertion required to reach the brachial plexus is 5.1 cm (2.25 to 7.75 cm in men and 2.1 to 6.5 cm in women) with the arm abducted not more than 45°. Greater abduction of the arm will make the performance of the technique easier because the brachial plexus depth is reduced and the cords are more spread, but this implies a normal joint functionality. This technique is particularly useful and advantageous when the abduction of the arm is limited or painful. As the needle connected to the ENS approaches the cords of the brachial plexus, twitch of the muscles supplied by those fibers will occur. Flexion or extension of the elbow, wrist, or fingers and external or internal rotation of the forearm confirms that the needle point is in close proximity to the nerve fibers of the brachial plexus. The needle should be advanced slowly until the maximum muscle movements are observed.

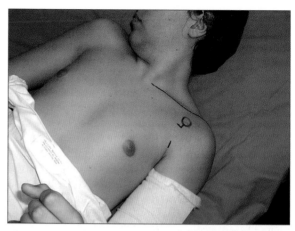

Fig. 1. The coracoid process of the scapula is identified and marked in the infraclavicular region: a point on the skin about 2 cm medial and caudal to the tip of the coracoid process identifies the brachial plexus below

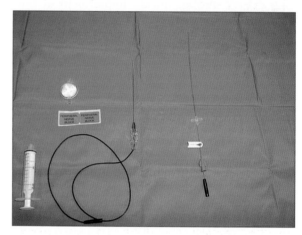

Fig. 2. Materials needed for the continuous block with stimulating catheter

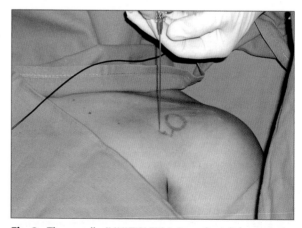

Fig. 3. The needle (MULTIPLEX) is introduced through the skin wheal vertically in a slightly lateral and caudal direction, with an angle of 0°-15° toward the axilla, until the evocation of a muscular contraction

The best twitch is the twitch of the muscles supplied by the cord innervating the sensitive zone involved by surgical treatment. The best twitch, in the case of elbow surgery, is represented by the contraction of the muscles supplied by the radial nerve (triceps muscle, etc.) [25, 26]; when the best twitch is found the current should be decreased until a muscle response is still elicited, in the corresponding innervation area, with a 0.2-0.3 mA current [27]; afterwards the split cannula must be cautiously disconnected from the needle and left inside while the needle is gently withdrawn and removed (Fig. 4).

The stimulating catheter connected to the ENS is then introduced through the cannula held firmly by one hand of the anesthesiologist (Fig. 5).

As the muscular twitch reappears even with a low current of 0.2-0.3 mA, the split cannula can be very carefully withdrawn; if the twitch it still remains, it is possible to fix the catheter and to remove the stimulating wire inside the catheter (Fig. 6). After repeated aspiration tests and connection of the filter, the catheter must be sterilely draped (Fig. 7). It is possible to start the local anesthetic injection pre- or post-operatively (see below). This type of approach is very well accepted by patients, even young ones (Fig. 8). In any case, prior to performing this technique, the patient, according to the procedures of monitored anesthesia care (MAC), may be lightly sedated with a small amount of a short-acting benzodiazepine such as midazo-

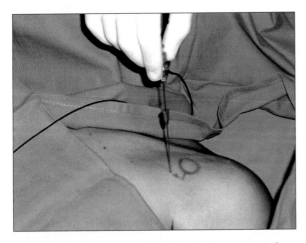

Fig. 4. When the best twitch is found, the current is lowered until a muscle response is still elicited with a 0.2-0.3 mA current; afterwards the split cannula must be cautiously disconnected from the needle and left inside while the needle is gently withdrawn and removed

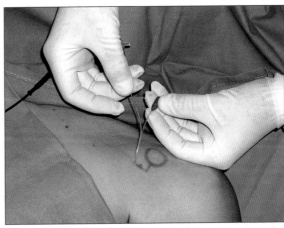

Fig. 6. As the muscular twitch reappears even with a low current of 0.2-0.3 mA, the split cannula can be very carefully withdrawn and if the twitch still remains, it is possible to fix the catheter and to remove the stimulating wire inside the catheter

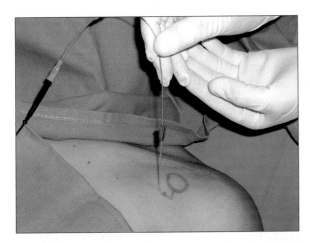

Fig. 5. The stimulating catheter connected to the ENS is then introduced through the cannula firmly held by one hand of the anesthesiologist

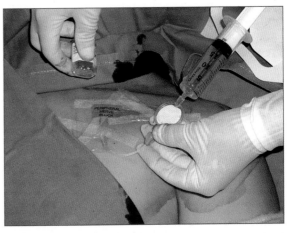

Fig. 7. After repeated aspiration tests and connection of the filter, the catheter must be sterilely draped. It is possible to start the local anesthetic injection pre- or post-operatively

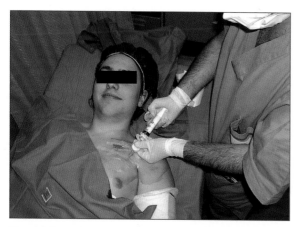

Fig. 8. This type of approach is very well accepted by patients, even young ones

lam, and/or fentanyl with the purpose of relieving anxiety and improving comfort.

If post-operative pain service is available, the best way to optimize the pain therapy will be based on a continuous infusion of local anesthetic associated with PCRA modalities using very simple electronic or disposable pumps.

Limitations

There are not many limitations to the use of catheter techniques for post-operative analgesia after elbow surgery. First, as noted earlier, their use is contingent on an effective pain service operating with the cooperation of the nurses and orthopedic surgeons, and obviously an anesthesiologist experienced in regional anesthesia techniques is necessary. Secondly, a patient's refusal and all the contraindications to regional anesthesia are also relevant in this case: an uncooperative patient, a previous adverse reaction to a local anesthetics, local or systemic infection, uncorrected metabolic derangement, and, most commonly, the clotting formation disorders, since vascular puncture and eventually hematoma formation are the most frequent complications of this approach. The control of hematomas can be more difficult compared with other techniques (axillary or interscalene) [12].

The final complicating factor relates to persistent upper extremity nerve injury.

Patients who are at risk of developing a compartment syndrome should not receive a continuous infusion of local anesthetic, because this may mask the early diagnostic signs (excessive pain, numbness, or muscle weakness).

A related problem concerns the use of regional analgesia in patients who are at risk of developing nerve injuries during and immediately after surgery, particularly after complicated elbow surgery. For obvious anatomical reasons, elbow surgery, mostly when it is complicated by chronic lesions and severe stiffness, frequently involves one or more of the three major nerves supplying the forearm and the hand (ulnar, radial, and median nerves); the most often involved is undoubtedly the ulnar nerve.

Moreover, continuous brachial plexus blocks may theoretically increase the incidence of neurologic complications because of catheter-induced mechanical trauma and local anesthetic toxicity, although in one report [14], the risk of neurologic complications associated with continuous block was described as similar to that of the single-dose techniques.

In these cases it is very important to place the catheter using electrical nerve stimulation before the surgery, but to start the local anesthetic infusion only after the end of the surgical procedure when, with the patient completely awake, it is possible to perform an accurate neurological examination of all the nerves supplying the arm and to identify any nerve injury related to the surgery. In this way it is possible to avoid confusion, to focus on early detection of potential neurological deterioration, and to assign the legal responsibility for the neurological damage.

Also for this reason in our hospital we prefer to use a stimulating catheter, which, despite the higher cost, should theoretically lower the incidence of anesthesia-related neurological injuries since it is possible with its use to know more reliably where the tip of the catheter is. However, there are as yet insufficient data [28] to determine whether stimulating catheters are safer, and more studies are necessary to establish which is the best approach to continuous regional anesthesia.

Finally, the presence of a catheter anywhere in the body exposes patients to the risk of accidental injection of a medication into the wrong site.

In summary, the most common complications reported after continuous brachial plexus sheath catheterization are local anesthetic toxicity, nerve injury, and (nerve) block failure.

Conclusions

Since 1946, when Ansbro first described continuous brachial plexus anesthesia, the majority of reports on continuous methods of brachial plexus anesthesia have described axillary catheterization. However, continuous techniques are continuously evolving, and in recent years reports of an infraclavicular approach have increased to the point where it is now widely accepted as the gold standard for elbow surgery post-operative analgesia.

The importance of the continuous axial brachial plexus block after surgery is based on its capacity to enable pain-free, very early continuous physical therapy so as to maximize the advantages gained with the surgery, giving a patient physical and psychological well being, with cooperation among the staff involved in the surgical procedure (nurses, physical therapists, anesthesiologists, and surgeons).

The continuous infraclavicular brachial plexus block, with stimulating catheters, is probably the best technique to reach a good and reliable post-operative analgesia after elbow surgery, even for long periods. However, the results are enhanced by its combination with conventional pain therapy. Thus to optimize the analgesia a multimodal approach is suitable – a combination of local anesthetic continuous infusion and boluses on demand, plus anti-inflammatory drugs (NSAIDs) and eventually narcotics can provide profound analgesia, with advantages over narcotic analgesia alone.

References

1. Morrey BF (2005) The post-traumatic stiff elbow. Clin Orthop Relat Res 431:26-35
2. Jupiter JB, O'Driscoll SW, Cohen MS (2003) The assessment and management of the stiff elbow. Instr Course Lect 52:93-111
3. Sojbjerg JO (1996) The stiff elbow. Acta Orthop Scand 67:626-631
4. O'Driscoll SW, Giori NJ (2000) Continuous passive motion (CPM): theory and principles of clinical application. J Rehabil Res Dev 37:179-188
5. Chinchalkar SJ, Szekeres M (2004) Rehabilitation of elbow trauma. Hand Clin 20:363-374
6. Koscielniak-Nielsen ZJ, Rotboll Nielsen P, Risby Mortensen C (2000) A comparison of coracoid and axillary approaches to the brachial plexus. Acta Anaesthesiol Scand 44:274-279
7. Parikh RK, Rymaszewski LR, Scott NB (1995) Prolonged postoperative analgesia for arthrolysis of the elbow joint. Br J Anaesth 74:469-471
8. Schroeder LE, Horlocker TT, Schroeder DR (1996) The efficacy of axillary block for surgical procedures about the elbow. Anesth Analg 83:747-751
9. Brown AR (2002) Anaesthesia for procedures of the hand and elbow. Best Pract Res Clin Anaesthesiol 16:227-246
10. Hadzic A, Arliss J, Kerimoglu B et al (2004) A comparison of infraclavicular nerve block versus general anesthesia for hand and wrist day-case surgeries. Anesthesiology 101:127-132
11. White PF (1995) Management of postoperative pain and emesis. Can J Anaesth 42:1053-1055
12. Kang SB, Rumball KM, Ettinger RS (2003) Continuous axillary brachial plexus analgesia in a patient with severe hemophilia. J Clin Anesth 15:38-40
13. Mezzatesta JP, Scott DA, Schweitzer SA et al (1997) Continuous axillary brachial plexus block for postoperative pain relief. Intermittent bolus versus continuous infusion. Reg Anesth 22:357-362
14. Bergman BD, Hebl JR, Kent J, Horlocker TT (2003) Neurologic complications of 405 consecutive continuous axillary catheters. Anesth Analg 96:247-252
15. Schreiber T, Ullrich K, Paplow B et al (2002) The use of the infraclavicular plexus catheter for the treatment of postoperative and chronic pain. Anaesthesist 51:16-22
16. Ilfeld BM, Morey TE, Enneking FK (2003) Continuous infraclavicular perineural infusion with clonidine plus ropivacaine compared with ropivacaine alone: a randomized double-blinded, controlled study. Anesth Analg 97:706-712
17. Ilfeld BM, Morey TE, Enneking FK (2004) Infraclavicular perineural local anesthetic infusion: a comparison of three dosing regimens for postoperative analgesia. Anesthesiology 100:395-402
18. Desroches J (2003) The infraclavicular brachial plexus block by the coracoid approach is clinically effective: an observational study of 150 patients. Can J Anaesth 50:253-257
19. van Oven H, Agnoletti V, Borghi B et al (2001) [Patient controlled regional analgesia (PCRA) in surgery of stiff elbow: elastomeric vs. electronic pump]. Minerva Anestesiol 67:117-120
20. Ilfeld BM, Morey TE, Enneking FK (2002) Continuous infraclavicular brachial plexus block for postoperative pain control at home: a randomized double-blinded, placebo-controlled study. Anesthesiology 96:1297-1304
21. Dadure C, Raux O, Capdevila X et al (2003) Continuous infraclavicular brachial plexus block for acute pain management in children. Anesth Analg 97:691-693
22. Porter JM, McCartney CJ, Chan VW (2005) Needle placement and injection posterior to the axillary artery may predict successful infraclavicular brachial plexus block: report of three cases. Can J Anaesth 52:69-73
23. Wilson JL, Brown DL, Wong GY et al (1998) Infraclavicular brachial plexus block: parasagittal anatomy important to the coracoid technique. Anesth Analg 87:870-873
24. Grossi P, Coluccia R, Tassi A, Indrizzi VL, Gazzotti F (1999) The infraclavicular brachial plexus block. Techniques in regional anesthesia and pain management. 3:217-221
25. Borene SC, Edwards JN, Boezaart AP (2004) At the cords, the pinkie towards: Interpreting infraclavicular motor responses to neurostimulation. Reg Anesth Pain Med 29:125-129
26. Rodriguez J, Taboada-Muniz M, Barcena M et al (2004) Median versus musculocutaneous nerve response with single injection infraclavicular coracoid block. Reg Anesth Pain Med 29:534-538
27. Wehling MJ, Koorn R, Leddell C et al (2004) Electrical nerve stimulation using a stimulating catheter: what is the lower limit? Reg Anesth Pain Med 29:230-233
28. Boezaart AP, De Beer JF, Nell ML (2003) Early experience with continuous cervical paravertebral block using a stimulating catheter. Reg Anesth Pain Med 28:406-413

CHAPTER 31

Elbow Brace in Physical Therapy

R. ROTINI, A. MARINELLI

Introduction

The elbow is a joint that, following trauma, very easily becomes stiff. In an attempt to limit the occurrence of such a complication, an articulated brace should be used in the rehabilitation phase to enable earlier movement that was impossible to obtain with the splints or casts commonly used years ago.

A specific characteristic of the brace is that it ensures articular excursion while protecting from varus-valgus stresses and, by restricting articular excursion, prevents the degrees of flexion-extension which are considered to be dangerous; furthermore, through special handles that can be applied to the brace, it is possible if necessary also to prevent undesired degrees of prono-supination. Finally, some braces can exert distractive tension on the retracted soft tissues, thus helping to increase the articular excursion in patients affected by elbow stiffness.

The use of the brace is therefore indicated both in traumatology as well as for the treatment of stiffness; in both situations, according to the case, the brace can be used both as conservative treatment, and as postoperative rehabilitation treatment.

The brace is indicated therefore for the rehabilitation of the elbow in:

1. Acute trauma: simple elbow dislocation, collateral ligaments lesion, or nonsurgical elbow fracture to allow an early and safe mobilization.
2. Post-operative care after bone fixation (distal humeral fractures, radius head fractures, olecranon fractures, coronoid process fractures), after ligament reconstruction or surgery that might jeopardize joint stability.
3. Elbow stiffness that can be treated with brace alone without soft tissue release, with the aim of exerting a progressive distraction force on the retracted soft tissues of the elbow, thus lengthening them and subsequently increasing the range of movement.
4. Post-operative course after soft tissue release. The brace in this group of patients has the purpose to limit solicitations and dangerous movements for joint stability (that can be compromised sometimes after soft tissue release), allowing early active and passive movement within the allowed range and, contemporarily, the application of a distraction force on the soft tissues to maintain the range of movement achieved in the operating room.

It is useful to remember that the aim of elbow stiffness treatment, conservative or surgical, is to re-establish at least a range of motion between 30°-130° in flexion-extension, and 50° in pronation and 50° in supination. Such a range of motion constitutes the functional arc movement that allows the most common daily activities [1].

Classification of Elbow Braces

Because clinical conditions and indications for elbow braces are very different, it is easy to understand why they come in a wide range of shapes and types.

Table 1. Elbow brace classification

Immobilization brace
   Nonarticulated
   Articulated-locked
Restriction brace
   Flexion-Extension control
   Flexion-Extension and Prono-Supination control
Mobilization brace
   Dynamic
   Progressive Static:
      Turnbuckle type (usually custom-made)
      Knob type (usually prefabricated)

As far as we know there is no brace classification to facilitate communication among health professionals involved in elbow rehabilitation: orthopedic surgeons, physiatrists, technicians, and physical therapists.

Following the splint classification system proposed by Garner in 1992 (American Society of Hand Therapist, cited by Jacobs ML) [2] we can classify the elbow brace (Table 1).

Immobilization brace: this type can be a nonarticulated or articulated locked brace; the purpose of this brace is purely to protect the limb by completely restricting its movement, and is indicated in the initial phase after trauma or surgery, when early movement cannot be allowed (Fig. 1).

Restriction brace: this braces allows a controlled range of movement. With this brace active and passive movement within the desired range of flexion and extension is allowed, whereas pronation and supination can be controlled by a special handle that can be attached if required. After trauma this brace enables early movement that can be adjusted according to the type of lesion, or surgery performed (Fig. 2).

Mobilization brace: by special mechanisms it can exert distraction forces on the retracted soft tissues and is used to maintain or increase the elbow range of movement after trauma or surgery (Fig. 3).

There are braces that can perform all three functions according to need: they can protect when the locking mechanism is fully locked; they can be adjusted to enable controlled movement when the system is partially locked; or they can act as mobilization brace if the locking mechanism is locked in tension.

Whereas immobilization and restriction braces are indicated in the initial phase of fracture/dislocation treatment or immediately after surgery, the mobilization brace is specifically indicated as treatment for elbow stiffness.

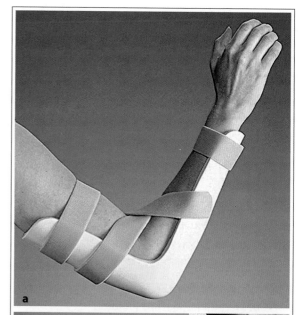

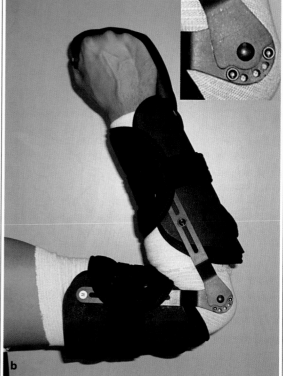

Fig. 1. Immobilization brace. (**a**) Nonarticulated brace; (**b**) Articulated locked brace

As described in detail below, mobilization braces can have an elastic or spring mechanism (dynamic braces) or an angular unlocking and locking mechanism, adjusted by bars or knobs (progressive static braces).

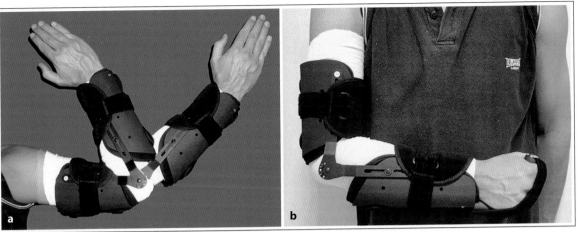

Fig. 2. Restriction brace. (**a**) Flexio-extension restriction brace; (**b**) Flexio-extension and prono-supination restriction brace

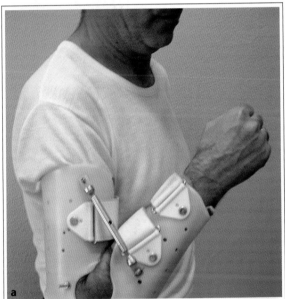

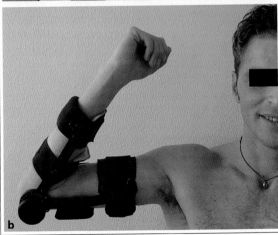

Fig. 3. Mobilization brace. (**a**) Custom made progressive static brace (Turnbuckle type); (**b**) Prefabricated progressive static brace (Knob type)

Elbow Brace Indications and Protocols

Acute Trauma

The elbow brace, after fracture or dislocation, has both a protective and rehabilitation purpose, allowing on one hand to limit the stress forces and the dangerous movements for a correct healing of the bone and the soft tissues, and on the other allowing an early movement within an allowed range.

In particular, the articulated brace is effective in the treatment of simple elbow dislocations, with only soft tissue involvement.

In these cases the aim of the brace is to prevent dangerous degrees of movement, to avoid varus-valgus stresses and to concur in an early passive and active motion in the allowed range of motion.

After elbow reduction, the joint stability is examined by performing gentle complete flexion-extension and prono-supination.

Treatment will depend on the degree of instability [3, 4].

After reduction, if the elbow is clinically and radiographically stable, a 90° flexion and intermediate prono-supination immobilization splint (non-articulated or an articulated locked brace) is applied for 3-5 days.

At the next follow-up exam, if the elbow stability is maintained throughout the entire range of movement, a brace with unlocked flexion-extension and prono-supination is indicated, and the patient is followed-up every 7-10 days for 4 weeks.

If instability persists, a brace with pronation forearm and unlocked flexion-extension is applied instead, and the brace has to be maintained for 5 weeks. If the elbow is still unstable, although the pronation position, the last 30° of extension is not allowed. In that case the brace has to be maintained for 6-8 weeks.

If the elbow is unstable also with forearm pronation and beyond 30°-40° of extension, surgical treatment must be taken into consideration.

The restriction brace is also indicated for the effective treatment of fractures; using a brace to protect the elbow from stress an early movement can be allowed, as in the treatment of Mason type 1 radial head fracture or isolated Regan-Morrey type I coronoid fracture.

Post-operative Course After Fixation or Ligament Reconstruction Surgery

In the first phase after distal humeral or olecranon or radial head fracture fixation, or radial head replacement or ligament reconstruction/repair, an immobilization brace is useful; in the second phase a restriction brace with a controlled ROM is used.

The brace protocol has to be personalized according to fixation strength and ligament stability, considering the harmful varus forces (acting on the elbow with the shoulder in abduction position and the elbow flexed) and the usefulness of early joint movement.

Conservative Treatment of Elbow Stiffness By Brace

The idea of treating elbow stiffness with devices that allow progressive distraction of soft tissues goes back centuries, as testified by a woodcut dated 1517 [5] (Fig. 4).

To indicate the brace alone as treatment for elbow stiffness, we have to assess the type of stiffness (intrinsic or extrinsic), type of end point of motion (rigid or springy), degree of stiffness (mild, moder-

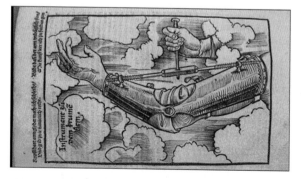

Fig. 4. von Gersdorf H: Feldbuch der Wundarznei, Strassburg 1517. Putti Donation, Rizzoli Orthopedic Institute, Bologna-Italy

ate, severe, or very severe) [6], duration of stiffness, and some of the patient's characteristics, such as age, expectations, and motivations.

Treatment of elbow stiffness by brace is indicated when defined by the following characteristics:
- extrinsic stiffness;
- moderate grade (ROM between 60° and 90°) [6];
- springy end-points of motion;
- onset not longer than 6-12 months before treatment;
- patient highly motivated.

The brace is contraindicated when one of the following characteristics is present:
- intrinsic stiffness;
- presence of heterotopic bridge ossifications;
- severe stiffness (ROM between 30° and 60°) or very severe (ROM <30°) [6];
- ulnar nerve neuropathy;
- poor patient compliance.

Mobilization braces

There are two types of mobilization braces [7]:
- dynamic brace, with elastic or spring mechanism;
- static progressive brace, that acts with flexion-extension distractive forces with turnbuckle or knob hinge.

Both types of brace (dynamic or static progressive) can be "custom made" or prefabricated (Fig. 5).

The main difference between dynamic and static progressive braces is the type of force applied. In fact, the elastic or spring mechanism produces a continuous type of stress that, according to some authors, can cause periarticular inflammation [7]. The static progressive brace determines instead an alternate stress at rest, or rather, between two successive phases of progressive stretching the tissue, although remaining in tension, has the time to relax. Therefore, over time, a biological adaptation of the tissue can be obtained.

The rational of mobilization with a brace is that, by exerting a controlled stretching force on the soft tissues for a suitable time period, such tension is able to induce gradual and progressive tissue extension (muscles, tendons, and capsules) and, in the meantime, to stimulate the growth of cells more functional for the new situation.

After all, the viscous-elastic characteristics of the soft tissues and the possibility therefore to be also modelled substantially, have been known since ancient times and are still exploited in some populations. Such populations show us how stretching a notable lengthening can be achieved through slow, gradual, and progressive phases of relaxation alter-

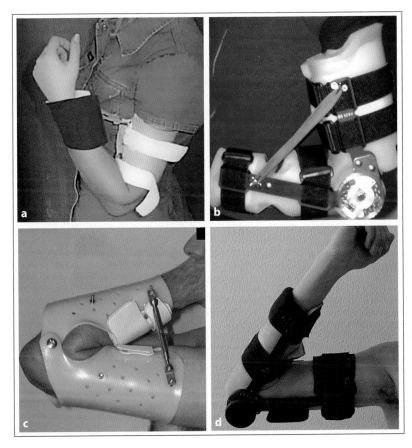

Fig. 5 a-d. Mobilization braces. (**a, b**) Dynamic braces. (**c, d**) Static braces. (**a**) Custom-made dynamic brace. (**b**) Prefabricated dynamic custom-made brace. (**c**) Custom-made static progressive brace (Turnbuckle type). (**d**) Prefabricated static progressive brace (Knob type)

nated with phases in which the tissues, despite remaining under stress, have the time to adapt (Fig. 6).

The rational principle of this method therefore is to obtain a small amount of gradual stretching to be maintained for long periods of time.

The progressive static turnbuckle type brace mostly at the last degree of flexion produces compression forces and at the last degree of ex-

tension distraction forces on the ulno-humeral joint [7, 8]. A fixed hinge attached to the splint close to the axis of rotation is necessary to absorb the dangerous stress and to transfer only to the forearm the rotational component of the force (Figs. 3a, 5c) [8].

The braces in which the force is directly applied to the axis of rotation (Figs. 3b, 5d) produce no compression or distraction forces [7] and are usually better managed by the patients.

Protocol for Using the Brace

If the tension applied is insufficient, the stretching action will be ineffective; if, however, it is excessive, or the stretching action is performed too quickly the tissues will be damaged, resulting in antalgic contracture, bleeding, increase in scarring, heterotopic ossifications, and deterioration of the stiffness (Fig. 7).

It is therefore fundamental to inform the patient that when the brace is worn a tolerable feeling of tension should be felt. Following the protocol proposed by Morrey [7], the patient should be taught how to wear the brace throughout the day

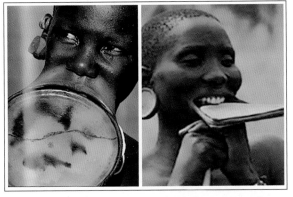

Fig. 6. Some populations hand down from generation to generation the ancient art to lengthen the soft tissue, using a slow, gradual, and progressive stretching technique

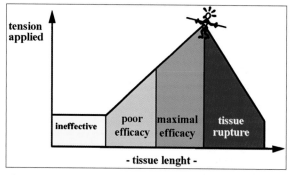

Fig. 7. Schematization of the length-tension curve of the soft tissue showing its viscoelastic properties [9]. Applying a progressive stretching to the tissue, it is progressively lengthened showing elastic behavior; beyond a certain tension degree the tissue has a plastic behavior with tear and rupture. It is therefore difficult to find the equilibrium between maximal stretching that we want to obtain (maximal elastic behavior of the tissues) and the tissue tearing (plastic behavior) we absolutely have to avoid

and that at night the brace should be held in the position that needs more correction. When the patient wakes up, active movement is performed. Three times a day, once in the morning, in the afternoon, and again at night, the position of the brace is inverted and one hour of active movement without the brace is performed (Fig. 8).

For the first 3-4 weeks the treatment is a 20-h program every day. After 3 weeks the patient is reassessed and the program modified as needed. Between the 4 to 6 weeks a 12-14-h program is usually applied until the end of the treatment.

Treating inveterate stiffness takes a long time, at least 3-4 months, and the brace is removed by suspending it gradually and checking that the range of

movement achieved has not decreased. Sometimes, treatment may take up to 1 year.

In many cases the orthopaedic elbow brace is an effective method for treating elbow stiffness. However, it is fundamental to select patients correctly, to treat the stiffness with a static progressive brace, and to use a good protocol.

Mobilization Brace for Stiffness After Soft Tissue Release

A shared opinion is that often the greatest difficulty in the treatment of a stiff elbow is not the surgical elimination of the contracture, but how to maintain the range of movement in the following post-operative phase.

Despite this, much has been written on the surgical techniques of soft tissue release, but little about the following rehabilitation methods.

Pathogenesis of the Contracture

After soft tissue release elbow stiffness has the tendency to recur in four phases: bleeding, edema, granulation tissue, and fibrosis. Such phases develop within hours, days, weeks, and months, respectively. An immobilization elbow brace is indicated in the early post-operative period, while in the following phases a mobilization brace is indicated. In these cases we prefer to use a brace that can perform both these functions.

To decrease the bleeding and edema phases it is possible to set the limb extended and unloaded, to use a compressive bandage, apply ice, and pre-

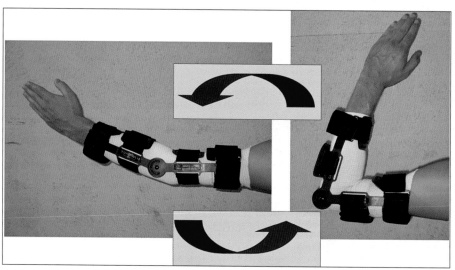

Fig. 8. During the day, three times a day the brace position is inverted; during the night sleeping in the position that needs more correction

scribe NSAIDs and continuous passive mobilization (Fig. 9) [10].

Continuous passive movement (CPM), together with the brace, is also used during the following granulation tissue phase, with the aim of reducing swelling and preventing the formation of scar tissue (Fig. 10).

It is useful to underline that CPM is useful to prevent and reduce swelling, and maintains an already present movement but by itself does not induce its increase [11]; to increase the movement through stretching of the retracted soft tissues, the only tool is the brace that, in fact, is specifically indicated in the last phase, where the fibrosis formation occurs with the following natural tendency of the soft tissues to shorten and retract.

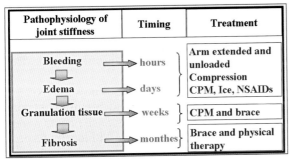

Fig. 9. Pathophysiology of soft tissue contraction and its treatment

After surgical soft tissue release, the brace can be utilized with a program different from the Morrey brace protocol [7] (that is specifically indicated for the conservative treatment of elbow contracture), alternating extension and flexion position every 40 minutes and utilizing CPM for the following 20 minutes of each hour [13].

In the fibrosis phase it is useful to combine brace treatment with exercises of:
– Active and passive movement helped by a physiotherapist, useful above all for patients who are psychologically helped by a specialist who follows them, by helping and encouraging them in this difficult rehabilitation phase; it is essential to have an experienced elbow rehabilitation physiotherapist who should be informed of the program and the obtainable objectives of the patient.
  • It is necessary to make a detailed rehabilitation report specifying the range of motion gained in the operating room; this range of motion constitutes, in fact, the highest achievable range.
  • It is important that excessive force is not applied to the joint that may lead to tissue lesions, antalgic muscular contracture, bleeding, followed by the formation of scar tissue, with a great likelihood of the development of heterotopic ossifications and worsening of the stiffness.
– Self-assisted mobilization with exercises directly performed by the patient that block the ho-

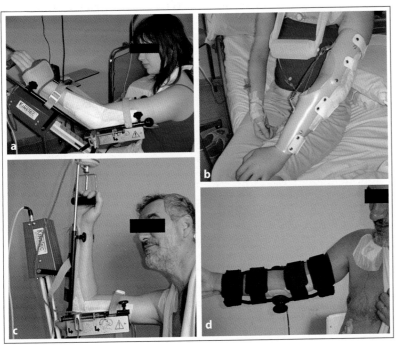

Fig. 10 a-d. Combined therapy with continuous passive movement and brace is used in the granulation tissue phase

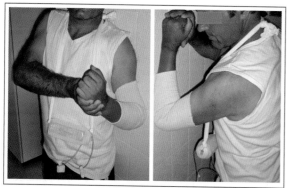

Fig. 11. Self-assisted mobilization, in a patient with continuous post-operative analgesia

molateral shoulder by leaning against a wall; with the contralateral limb the patient performs flexion and extension movements exerting progressive and increasing forces (Fig. 11).

All these exercises of mobilization performed in the first days/week after surgery draw enormous benefit by the use of methods for continuous postoperative analgesia. Through an infraclavicular or axillary block with continuous infusion of local anesthetic and also the possibility to plan boluses, it is possible to achieve appropriate analgesia of the elbow region in the postoperative period to allow an effective rehabilitation therapy.

According to personal experience, regional analgesia managed by the patient can also be continued at home, usually for some days, but in some cases continued up to 3 weeks; this is useful for the rehabilitation of the elbow.

Protocol After Arthroscopic or Open Soft Tissue Release

Before surgery Explanation of the surgical procedure and the post-operative rehabilitation program; heterotopic ossifications prophylaxis for 3 weeks after surgery: Indomethacin 25 mg, 3 times a day. In arthroscopic surgery a 2-week prophylaxis after surgery is recommended only for extensive release [12].

During surgery Loco-regional anesthesia maintained usually for 5 days after the operation (3-7 days); one or two drains; at the end of the operation we apply an immobilization elbow brace in extension and we set the limb unloaded.

First postoperative day Elbow brace in extension and limb unloaded.

Second day Removal of the drain; CPM (continuous passive movement) or passive FKT with phys-

iotherapist (after anesthetic bolus) 3 times/day for 30 minutes.

Third day Application of brace that is maintained night and day alternating the position of maximum flexion and maximum extension. In the breaks without the brace CPM is performed; if there are difficulties with the continuous motion machine passive and assisted active physical therapy is performed.

Discharge for arthroscopic soft tissue release patients.

Fourth day or Fifth day Discharge for open soft tissue release patients, with detailed information about:
- protocol for using the brace;
- analgesic and prophylaxis medical therapy;
- rehabilitation exercises and, if necessary, management of the catheter for anesthesia at home.

Fifteen to twenty-one days Continued use of the brace; beginning of active mobilization and hydrokinesitherapy.

Tree weeks Suspension of the indomethacin therapy.

Four-six weeks Suspension of CPM machine.

Four-six months: Stop using the brace. At times treatment up to one year is necessary.

If it is arthroscopically possible to obtain a full range of motion (0°-140° of flexion-extension) the CPM machine, utilized continuously night and day since the first few post-operative hours, is very effective; in fact, squeezing the soft tissue at the end of the flexion and extension movement reduces the soft tissue elbow swelling and helps to maintain the full range of motion [10, 13].

Naturally, these protocols have to be adapted to the type of surgery, patients' pain tolerance and compliance, elbow stability, skin condition, and progress made.

Conclusions

In physical therapy of the elbow, the brace constitutes an additional device to contrast the risk of stiffness. In the treatment of acute traumas or after fixation surgery, the brace has the certain advantages of being well tolerated by the patient, reducing the risks of venous stasis and reflex sympathetic dystrophy, preventing dangerous movements, while allowing those permitted (for example blocking extension and supination in severe postero-lateral rotatory instabilities). In elbow stiffness, the brace is a therapeutic device that makes it possible, in selected cases, to treat elbow contractures conservatively. Also, after soft tissue release, the brace is very useful to help maintain the range of motion gained in the operating room.

In elbow stiffness treatment the patient should always be informed of the long time the treatment may take.

The limitations of braces in elbow physical therapy are that they are expensive and are time consuming for the doctors with regards to explanations and necessary frequent follow-up exams. The task of the doctor, in fact, is not only to prescribe the brace, but also to follow the patient over time, regulating and adapting the brace based on the various stages and progress of the physical therapy.

For full success of treatment it is necessary, moreover, that the doctor really is convinced of the usefulness of the brace and that the patient is informed at every follow-up of the importance that such a device has for the treatment.

Being a removable device, managed for a long time at home, complete information, a total understanding and full collaboration of the patient are mandatory.

Despite these limitations, in our experience the use of the brace in elbow physical therapy has improved results in our patients.

Acknowledgements

The author wish to thank Anna Viganò, MD – Rizzoli Orthopaedic Institute Library for her help finding the woodcut of the XVI centuries and Fulvio Tabellini – Officine Rizzoli S.p.A. for his help in making the custom-mode static progressive braces.

References

1. Morrey BF, Askew LJ, Chao EY (1981) A biomechanical study of normal functional elbow motion. J Bone Joint Surg Am 63:872-877
2. Jacobs ML (2003) Splint classification In: Jacobs ML, Austin N (eds) Splinting the hand and upper extremity, Lippincott, New York, pp 2-18
3. O'Driscoll SW, Jupiter JB, King GJ et al (2001) The unstable elbow. Instr Course Lect 50:89-102
4. Celli A, Nicoli E, Celli L (2003) The elbow dislocation and radial head fractures. GIOT 29[Suppl 2]:S169-S175
5. von Gersdorf H (1517) Feldbuch der Wundarznei. In: Joānes Schott (ed) Strassburg. Putti Donation, Rizzoli Orthopedic Institute, Bologna
6. Morrey BF (1993) Distraction arthroplasty. Clinical applications. Clin Orthop Relat Res 293:46-54
7. Morrey BF (2000) Splints and bracing at the elbow. In: Morrey BF (ed) The Elbow and its Disorders, 3rd edn. Saunders, Philadelphia, pp 50-154
8. Szekeres M (2006) A biomechanical analysis of static progressive elbow flexion splinting. J Hand Ther 19:34-38
9. Wenner S, Smithline E (2003) Tissue healing. In: Jacobs ML, Austin N (eds) Splinting the hand and upper extremity. Lippincott, New York, pp 48-58
10. O'Driscoll SW, Giori NJ (2000) Continuous passive motion (CPM). Theory and principles of clinical application. J Rehab Res Dev 37:179-188
11. Morrey BF (2005) The posttraumatic stiff elbow. Clin Orthop Relat Res 431:26-35
12. Gofton WT, King GJ (2001) Heterotopic ossification following elbow arthroscopy. Arthroscopy 17:E2-1-5
13. O'Driscoll SW (2005) Personal communication: II SICSeG Course, Bologna, Italy December 2001

SUBJECT INDEX

Printed in October 2007